The Effective Management of Colorectal Cancer

Fourth edition

Titles of related interest in the UK Key Advances in Clinical Practice Series

SOLID TUMOURS
The Effective Management of Breast Cancer, 1st and 2nd edns
The Effective Management of Colorectal Cancer, 1st, 2nd, 3rd and 4th edns
The Effective Management of Lung Cancer, 1st, 2nd and 3rd edns
The Effective Management of Malignant Melanoma
The Effective Management of Ovarian Cancer, 1st, 2nd and 3rd edns
The Effective Management of Prostatic Cancer
The Effective Management of Renal Cell Carcinoma
The Effective Management of Urological Cancer

HAEMATOLOGICAL MALIGNANCIES
The Effective Management of Non-Hodgkin's Lymphoma, 1st and 2nd edns
The Effective Prevention and Management of Systemic Fungal Infection in Haematological Malignancy, 1st and 2nd edns
The Effective Management of Common Complications of Induction Chemotherapy in Haematological Malignancy
The Effective Management of Chronic Lymphocytic Leukaemia

SYMPTOM CONTROL
The Effective Management of Cancer Pain, 1st and 2nd edns
The Effective Prevention and Control of Symptoms in Cancer
The Effective Prevention and Management of Post-Operative Nausea & Vomiting, 1st and 2nd edns

HEALTH POLICY
NICE, CHI and the NHS Reforms: Enabling excellence or imposing control?
Clinical Governance and the NHS Reforms: Enabling excellence or imposing control?
Managed Care Networks: Principles and practice

The Effective Management of Colorectal Cancer

Fourth edition

Edited by

David Cunningham MD FRCP
*Consultant Medical Oncologist & Head, GI and Lymphoma Units,
The Royal Marsden Hospital, London and Surrey, UK*

Clare Topham MB FRCR
*Consultant Clinical Oncologist,
Royal Surrey County Hospital, Surrey, UK*

Andrew Miles MSc MPhil PhD
*Professor of Public Health Sciences &
Editor-in-Chief, Journal of Evaluation in Clinical Practice,
Barts and The London,
Queen Mary's School of Medicine and Dentistry,
University of London, UK*

Assistant Editor
*Dr. Sheela Rao MRCP, Clinical Research Fellow,
The Royal Marsden Hospital, London and Surrey, UK*

Barts and The London
Queen Mary's School of Medicine and Dentistry

British Society for Gastroenterology

British Association of Surgical Oncology

Association of Coloproctology of Great Britain and Ireland

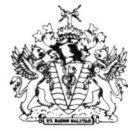

The Royal College of Radiologists

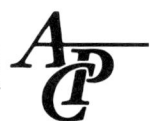

Association of Cancer Physicians

AESCULAPIUS MEDICAL PRESS
LONDON SAN FRANCISCO SYDNEY

Published by

Aesculapius Medical Press (London, San Francisco, Sydney)
PO Box LB48, London EC1A 1LB, UK

© Aesculapius Medical Press 2005

First published 2005

All rights reserved. No part of this publication may be reproduced or transmitted in any form or by any means, electronically or mechanically, including photocopying, recording or any other information storage or retrieval system, without the prior permission in writing from the publishers.

British Library Cataloguing in Publication Data
A CIP catalogue record for this book is available from the British Library

ISBN: 1 903044 43 X

While the advice and information in this book are believed to be true and accurate at the time of going to press, neither the authors nor the publishers nor the sponsoring institutions can accept any legal responsibility or liability for errors or omissions that may be made. In particular (but without limiting the generality of the preceding disclaimer) every effort has been made to check drug usages; however, it is possible that errors have been missed. Furthermore, dosage schedules are constantly being revised and new side effects recognised. For these reasons, the reader is strongly urged to consult the drug companies' printed instructions before administering any of the drugs recommended in this book.

Further copies of this volume are available from:

Claudio Melchiorri
Aesculapius Medical Press
PO Box LB48, Mount Pleasant Mail Centre, Farringdon Road, London EC1A 1LB, UK

Tel: 020 8525 8660
Email: claudio@keyadvances4.demon.co.uk

Copy edited by The Clyvedon Press Ltd, Cardiff, UK

Typeset, printed and bound in Britain
Peter Powell Origination & Print Limited

Contents

Contributors vii

Preface ix

Part 1 Genetics of colorectal cancer

1 Inherited susceptibility to colorectal cancer 3
   Sanjay Popat, Richard Hubner and Richard Houlston

2 Mismatch repair deficiency in hereditary and sporadic colorectal cancer 25
   Mark J. Arends and Ian M. Frayling

3 Genetic differences between left- and right-sided bowel cancer and their relation to prognosis and management 41
   Julian W. Adlard and Susan D. Richman

4 Clinical genetics and genetic counselling 49
   Shirley Hodgson

Part 2 Evidence and opinion for surgical intervention

5 Current thinking on the clinical significance of the two-week pathway for colorectal cancer 61
   Christopher Gandy, Valerie Morrell, Rupert Pullan and David DeFriend

6 Benefits of laparoscopic surgery in colorectal cancer 77
   Polly M. King and Robin H. Kennedy

7 Progress towards total mesorectal excision as the new 'gold standard' for rectal cancer surgery 85
   Bill Heald

8 Optimising sphincter-sparing surgery in rectal cancer 91
   Rob Glynne-Jones and Marina Wallace

9 Intensive follow-up after colorectal cancer: recent successes and future challenges 101
   Andrew G. Renehan, Matthias Egger, Mark P. Saunders, David K. Whynes and Sarah T. O'Dwyer

Part 3 Evidence and opinion for medical intervention

10 Evidence and opinion for chemotherapy in the management of early disease 121
    Robert Wade and Clare Topham

11	Evidence and opinion for combination therapy in the management of advanced disease *Ashita Waterston and Jim Cassidy*	133
12	Evidence and opinion for the use of combined modality treatment in rectal cancer *Rob Glynne-Jones and Suzy Mawdsley*	151
13	Intermittent or continuous palliative chemotherapy in metastatic colorectal cancer *Tim Maughan and Richard Stephens*	167
14	Novel approaches in the management of colorectal cancer *Anjana Kulkarni and Daniel Hochhauser*	179

Part 4 Clinical governance of colorectal cancer services

15	Recent judgements of the National Institute for Clinical Excellence: their scientific basis, clinical credibility and moral implications *Catherine A. McBain and Mark P. Saunders*	195
16	Risk adjustment in colorectal cancer surgery: the role of hierarchical models in comparative clinical audit *P. P. Tekkis, J. D. Stamatakis, M. R. Thompson and C. G. Marks*	209
17	The development of colorectal cancer services through the implementation of the National Cancer Plan and the operation of cancer networks *Roger James*	227
Index		*233*

Contributors

Julian W. Adlard MBBS MRCP FRCR MMedSci, Clinical Research Fellow/Specialist Registrar, Cookridge Hospital, Leeds, UK

Mark J. Arends MB ChB BSc PhD FRCPath, Department of Pathology, University of Cambridge, Addenbrooke's Hospital, Cambridge, UK

David DeFriend MD FRCS, Consultant Colorectal Surgeon, Department of Colorectal Surgery, Torbay Hospital, Torquay, UK

Matthias Egger MD MFPHM, Department of Social and Preventive Medicine, University of Bern, Switzerland

Ian M. Frayling MA MB BChir PhD MRCPath, Department of Medical Genetics, University of Cambridge, Addenbrooke's Hospital, Cambridge, UK

Christopher Gandy FRCS MB ChB, Specialist Registrar in General Surgery, Department of Colorectal Surgery, Torbay Hospital, Torquay, UK

Rob Glynne-Jones FRCP FRCR, Consultant Clinical Oncologist and Macmillan Lead Clinician in Gastrointestinal Cancer, Mount Vernon Cancer Centre, Mount Vernon Hospital, Northwood, Middlesex, UK

Bill Heald OBE MChir FRCS, Professor of Surgery, University of Southampton & Director of Surgery, North Hampshire Hospital, Basingstoke

Shirley Hodgson BM BCh DM FRCP, Professor of Cancer Genetics and Consultant Clinical Geneticist, St George's Hospital Medical School, London, UK

Richard S Houlston MD PhD FRCP FRCPath, Reader in Molecular and Population Genetics, Section of Cancer Genetics, Institute of Cancer Research, Surrey, UK

Richard Hubner BA MRCP, Specialist Registrar, Department of Medicine, Royal Marsden Hospital, Surrey, UK

Roger James FRCR, Clinical Director of the Kent Cancer Network, UK

Robin H. Kennedy MS FRCS, Consultant Surgeon, Yeovil District Hospital, UK

Polly M. King BSc MBBS MRCS, Research Fellow, Yeovil District Hospital, UK

C. G. Marks, MChir FRCS, Consultant Colorectal Surgeon, and Professor of Surgical Oncology, Department of Surgery, Royal Surrey County Hospital, Guildford, UK

Tim Maughan MB BS MRCP FRCR, Professor of Clinical Oncology, Velindre Hospital, Cardiff, UK

Catherine A. McBain MB ChB MRCR FRCR, Clinical Research Fellow, Department of Clinical Oncology, Christie Hospital NHS Trust, Manchester, UK

Suzy Mawdsley FRCR, Clinical Research Fellow, The Gray Cancer Institute, UK

Valerie Morrell SRN, Colorectal Cancer Audit Assistant, Department of Colorectal Surgery, Torbay Hospital, Torquay, UK

Sarah T. O'Dwyer MD FRCS FRCS(Edin), Consultant Colorectal Surgeon, Department of Surgery, Christie Hospital NHS Trust, Manchester, UK

Sanjay Popat BSc MRCP PhD, Clinician Scientist Fellow and Honorary Specialist Registrar, Section of Cancer Genetics, Institute of Cancer Research, Surrey, UK

Rupert Pullan, MA DM FRCS, Consultant Colorectal Surgeon, Department of Colorectal Surgery, Torbay Hospital, Torquay, UK

Andrew G. Renehan PhD FRCS FDS, Senior Research Fellow, Department of Surgery, Christie Hospital NHS Trust, Manchester, UK

Susan D. Richman BSc MSc PhD, Senior Scientific Officer, Cancer Research UK, University of Leeds, UK

Mark P. Saunders MB BS PhD MRCP FRCR, Consultant Clinical Oncologist, Department of Clinical Oncology, Christie Hospital NHS Trust, Manchester, UK

J. D. Stamatakis MS FRCS, Consultant General and Colorectal Surgeon, Princess of Wales Hospital, Bridgend, UK

Richard Stephens PhD, Cancer Division, MRC Clinical Trials Unit, London, UK

P. P. Tekkis FCRS, RSO in Colorectal Surgery, Department of Surgery, St Mark's Hospital, Harrow, UK

Clare Topham MB FRCR, Consultant Clinical Oncologist, St. Luke's Cancer Centre, Royal Surrey County Hospital, Guildford, Surrey, UK

M. R. Thompson MD FRCS, Consultant Colorectal Surgeon, Queen Alexandra Hospital, Portsmouth, UK

Robert Wade MRCP, Specialist Registrar in Clinical Oncology, Royal Surgery County Hospital, Guildford, UK

M. H. Wallace MS FRCS, Consultant Colorectal Surgeon, West Herts Health Trust, UK

David K. Whynes PhD, School of Economics, University of Nottingham, Nottingham, UK

Preface

After lung and breast cancer, colorectal cancer is the most common cause of death from malignant disease in Western countries. In England and Wales, there are approximately 30,000 new cases annually resulting in approximately 17,000 deaths and worldwide it has been estimated there are at least half a million new cases of colorectal cancer each year. About 10% of colorectal cancer cases have some family history of the disease and epidemiological studies have consistently shown that first-degree relatives of colorectal cancer cases have a 2 to 3-fold increase in risk compared with the general population, providing strong evidence for the role of genetic factors. It is to a detailed description of our current knowledge in the field of colorectal cancer genetics that Popat and colleagues and Arends and Frayling turn in the opening two chapters of the book and their contributions set the scene well for the detailed account of the molecular and environmental factors governing the predisposition to and pathogenesis of colorectal cancer which forms the subject of Part One of this Fourth Edition volume. The differences in presenting symptoms and surgical management of right-sided colon cancer and distal colon or rectal cancer are well known. There is now also increasing evidence of differences in the molecular pathology of sporadic large bowel cancers arising proximal to the splenic flexure and those arising more distally. This may be due, as Adlard and Richman point out in Chapter 3, to differences in function, embryological development or exposure to intra-luminal carcinogens. Right-sided cancers, as these authors discuss, are more likely to show high-level microsatellite instability due to inactivation of mismatch repair genes. Other genes are also epigenetically silenced by gene promoter hypermethylation, more often in right-sided cancers. For example, MGMT inactivation is associated with guanine to adenine mutations in the *K-ras* oncogene and low level microsatellite instability. Left-sided large bowel cancers are more likely to show p53 mutations and over-expression of vascular endothelial growth factor and thymidylate synthase. These factors may worsen the prognosis of distal cancers, and reduce responsiveness to fluorouracil chemotherapy. In contrast, cancers showing microsatellite instability have been associated with an improved prognosis in the absence of chemotherapy but an increased resistance to 5-fluorouracil-based chemotherapy. The responses of colorectal cancers to irinotecan and oxaliplatin, farnesyl transferase and tyrosine kinase inhibitors and anti-VEGF antibodies, may also vary according to the site and genetics of individual tumours, leading to the future possibility of targeted therapy based on molecular pathology.

Two major patterns of genomic instability are seen in sporadic colorectal cancers: chromosomal instability in the majority and microsatellite instability in around 15%. Microsatellite instability (MSI) is due to defective DNA mismatch repair (MMR), usually caused by *MLH1* silencing by promoter methylation. Hereditary non-polyposis colorectal cancer (HNPCC) accounts, as Hodgson describes in Chapter 4, for 1–2% of colorectal cancers, caused by inheritance of a mutated MMR gene, usually *MSH2 I* or MLH1, but occasionally others (e.g. *MSH6* or IPMS2). HNPCC gene carriers are also liable to develop extra-colonic tumours, especially cancers of endometrium, ureter, renal pelvis, ovary, stomach, small intestine, and skin (sebaceous tumours). Distinguishing HNPCC from sporadic MMR-deficient cancers requires, as Hodgson discusses, consideration of the family history and examination of the tumours for MSI and abnormal MMR protein expression. Extracted tumour DNA, examined at multiple microsatellite loci, shows MSI at high frequency (MSI-H) in HNPCC tumours and immunohistochemical analysis of ML, MSH2, MSH6 and PMS2 protein expression in HNPCC tumours shows three different expression patterns: a) homogeneously positive for the four proteins (normal): b) homogeneously negative for one or two of the proteins (abnormal); and c) patchy/weakly positive for one or two of the proteins (abnormal). Abnormal expression of MSH6 is significantly associated with abnormal MSH2 expression (MSH6 forms dimers with MSH2), and abnormal expression of PMS2 is significantly associated with abnormal MLH1 expression (PMS forms dimers with MLH1). Hodgson is clear that, unlike sporadic MMR-deficient colon cancers, almost all of which show abnormal MLH1 expression, HNPCC tumours do not always exhibit abnormal MMR protein expression. Thus, tumour analysis by MMR immunohistochemistry and MSI testing are necessary to provide a comprehensive picture of molecular abnormality, for use with family history data to diagnose HNPCC cancers. This greatly helps in interpreting sequence changes found on mutation screening, and may save resources by limiting MMR gene mutation screening to one HNPCC gene.

We turn in Part Two, through Chapters 6–9, to a detailed review of the evidence base for surgical intervention in colorectal cancer. The NHS cancer plan states that survival of common cancers within the UK falls short of American and European standards, with delays in presentation, referral and treatment all contributing to this observation and which are proving increasingly unacceptable to patients. However, there is little evidence that they affect outcome. The 2-week rule for colorectal cancer was introduced in July 2000 and states that patients with suspected cancer should be seen by a specialist within 2 weeks. This was the first in a series of rules culminating in a one-month rule from referral to definitive treatment. Evidence-based research guidelines have been produced with the aim of maximising pick up rates but avoiding excessive referrals. The Colorectal Unit of South Devon NHS trust has produced an audit comparing short-term outcome measures in patients referred under the 2-week rule and traditional referrals and Gandy and his co-workers, writing in Chapter 5, describe the results of their study of the effects of the rule. The authors outline how 194 elective patients were studied as part of their investigation and how the yields for colorectal cancer were higher for the two-week rule clinic (16%) compared to the standard colorectal clinic (3.7%). Of the patients with colorectal cancer presenting via normal clinics, 47% are described by the authors as having been eligible for a two-week referral. The ratio of rectal to colonic tumours was higher for the two-week rule referrals and those identified as potentially curative resections were comparable for both referral routes. Times from referral to appointment and referral to surgery were significantly lower for two-week rule referrals as were times from diagnosis to surgery. This was independent of tumour site. The data discussed by Gandy and colleagues are consistent with those of other studies, with higher detection rates, shorter times during each step of the cancer journey, but with no effect on numbers or curative resections or pathological stage. The majority of colorectal cancer cases continue to present via conventional referral pathways and this finding will need to be addressed if these "clinics" are to meet their full potential.

In 1998, initial data became available demonstrating a reduction in post-operative pain and hospital stay, along with quality of life improvement, following laparoscopic surgery for colorectal cancer. Since that time, various studies have shown benefits in short term recovery following laparoscopic surgery and a seminal study published in *The Lancet* in 2002 showed clear improvement in survival for Stage III cancer following laparoscopic colonic resection. In Chapter 6, King and Kennedy describe the long-term outcomes from this particular surgical approach within their practice. Interestingly, the authors have recently reported that, through use of an Enhanced Recovery Programme, post-operative hospital stay after laparoscopic surgery is now a median of three days for colonic procedures and six days for rectal procedures. It seems increasingly clear from data such as these that laparoscopic surgery for colorectal cancer does not therefore confer a higher mortality or local recurrence rate and that there are significant reductions in hospital stay, with attendant improvement sin the quality of life of the patient.

The summer of 2002 saw the introduction of two key words in the literature on rectal carcinoma: 'TME Workshop'. And it is to the procedure of total mesorectal excision (TME) that Heald turns in Chapter 7. Papers attesting to a major impact on rectal cancer outcomes in Norway, Sweden and Holland are the background to two major papers in the *British Journal of Surgery*, one from Ireland and one from Sweden plus a leading article from Singapore entitled 'Adjuvant therapy for rectal cancer cannot be based on the results of other surgeons'. Indeed, it is now essentially accepted that each surgeon must audit his or her own results and that medical and radiation oncologists must know these results before they can advise their patients appropriately. Within the context of TME, Heald agrees that local recurrence is largely a failure of surgical technique. The key realities that must now dominate our future thoughts on rectal cancer management, Heald feels, are now focused on the embryological plane between the mesorectal viceral envelope (a hindgut structure embryologically) and the surrounding parities. The fundamental importance of the TME workshops he describes, which have had such a major impact in so many countries, is that surgeons can learn to follow this plane faithfully and to deliver a specific tissue block which is the caudal component of the hindgut with its visceral mesentery around it. This same 'holy plane' can now be visualized, as he describes, before surgery by high quality fine slice MRI examinations. It is becoming increasingly clear that we need a pre-operative staging system and that we need to plan adjuvant therapy in a selective manner based upon this staging system so that adjuvant therapies may be given before and not after surgery. Surgery should become the final episode in a planned management schedule and must reach the very high standard of 'specimen orientated surgery' in which the surgeon puts as his first priority the perfect excision of an intact mesorectal envelope. Furthermore, such an approach can avoid sphincter sacrifice in around 80–90% (compared with the current 50–60%) of cases and it should also seek to preserve the autonomic nerves of sexual function which have so often been damaged by conventional abdominoperineal and anterior resection.

There is increasing enthusiasm for the use of preoperative synchronous chemoradiation (SCRT) in rectal cancer and it is to the clinical value of this intervention that Glynne-Jones and Wallace turn in Chapter 8. The rationale for this approach, as these authors describe, has been fuelled in parts by the hopes of facilitating a sphincter sparing procedure if the tumour regresses sufficiently. Despite relatively recent data from Germany on the quality of life when an abdominoperitoneal excision of the rectum is compared to an anterior resection, the vast majority of patients in Europe have an almost pathological terror of the prospect of a colostomy. Hence, specialist rectal cancer surgeons are under increasing pressure to preserve organ and function wherever possible. Significant shrinkage of a tumour can allow an easier resection, particularly within the confines of a narrow pelvis in males and also may justify the surgeon in accepting a narrower distal margin without increasing risks of local recurrence. Indeed, many surgeons now consider 1 cm as an adequate distal margin and this is even more acceptable following SCRT. However, there is considerable variation in the sphincter preserving rates for rectal cancer from published trials. It is not clear why, in some series, very distal tumours close to the anorectal ring can be resected with sphincter preservation where in other series this is not the case. Hopefully, forthcoming trials will come to answer this question definitively, as the authors anticipate. Should all resectable tumours, which appear borderline for sphincter-sparing procedures receive preoperative chemoradiation to facilitate sphincter sparing? When performing SPS, should surgeons perform a frozen section analysis of the distal margin and donut to ensure there is no microscopic evidence of residual disease at or close to this resection margin? What is the late function if a surgeon performs an ultra-low anterior resection after preoperative

SCRT? Is the quality of life really better than that experienced by a patient who undergoes APER? Glynne-Jones and Wallace pose and discuss these critical questions and we move from their detailed analysis to the question of follow-up and the monitoring of long term outcomes.

Given that colorectal cancer is the second commonest cause of cancer-related mortality in Europe, the issue of follow-up is, axiomatically, very important indeed. Until recently, the merits of follow-up have remained unproven. In 2002, Renehan and his colleagues published in the *British Medical Journal* a systematic review and meta-analysis of all randomised controlled trials (RCTs), identified five RCTs ($n = 1342$) and demonstrated that intensive follow-up was associated with a reduction in all-cause mortality (combined risk ratio 0.81, 95% confidence interval 0.70 to 0.94, $p = 0.007$). They discuss the significance of their results in extended detail within Chapter 9. The beneficial effect was most pronounced, as the authors show, in trials that employed computed tomography and frequent measurements of serum carcinoembryonic antigen (risk ratio 0.73, 0.60 to 0.89, $p = 0.002$). Simultaneously, the Cochrane Colorectal Cancer Group independently reported their review on intensive follow-up and arrived at similar conclusions. A number of international investigations wrote responses to this study and Renehan and associates usefully summarise that debate. Given that a number of questions remained outstanding as part of their study, not least the issue of cost, the authors describe how they performed an economic evaluation (cost-effectiveness analysis) of intensive follow-up using the effectiveness data from the meta-analysis and costings based on NGS mean reference costs. Benefits of intensive versus conventional follow-up were calculated as life years (LY) gained per subject and cost differences expressed as the incremental cost-effectiveness ratio (ICER). Sensitivity analyses were also performed. For all five RCTs combined, the ICER was between £3500 and £4000. This ratio compares favourable to other cancer mortality prevention health strategies such as breast and cervical screening. The two recently published meta-analyses represent important advances in this controversial aspect of colorectal cancer management but fall short of a prescriptive regimen for surveillance and large trials are now required to identify which components of follow-up are most beneficial.

We have dedicated Part Three of the book, through Chapters 10–14, to detailed reviews of the evidence base for medical intervention in colorectal cancer. As Wade and Topham discuss in the opening chapter of this Part, standard chemotherapy in the UK is bolus 5-FU and LV either weekly for 24 weeks or for five days per month for 6 months. The X-ACT data reported at the American Society for Clinical Oncology meeting last year (2004) showed a statistically significant superior relapse-free survival for capecitabine with a trend to superior disease free survival and overall survival. Toxicity for capecitabine in this study was less than for 5-FU with the exception of hand-foot syndrome and the trial was able to demonstrate that oral capecitabine was at least as good as bolus FU. The authors proceed to discuss the results of the MOSAIC study which, as they describe, compared infusional 5-FU and LV with oxaliplatin, 5-FU and LV, showing a 3-year disease-free survival in Stage III patients of 72% for the oxaliplatin arm compared with 65% with 5-FU and LV. In Stage II patients there was a 3% benefit for the oxaliplatin arm and the incidence of Grade 3 neuropathy was 12% overall, falling to 0.5% at 18 months. They go on to review the study comparing bolus 5-FU and irinotecan with bolus 5-FU alone reported by Salz (which showed no benefit for the addition of irinotecan) and discuss the large study of infusional 5-FU plus or minus irinotecan that has recently been completed. The role of the biological agents cetuximab and bevacizumab are also discussed by the authors, providing a broad and detailed introduction to the benefits of chemo- and biological therapy in the management of early disease.

The development and introduction into clinical practice of at least 6 new drugs for the management of colorectal cancer (raltitrexed, capecitabine, irintotecan, oxaliplatin, cetuximab, bevacizumab) over the last decade or so has undoubtedly improved the options for patients with advanced disease. Of course, not all drugs are freely available and for all these drugs the definitive evidence needed to define optimal therapy is simply not available at the present time. The clinical data which are currently available support the notion that combination cytotoxic therapy in advanced colorectal cancer is more active and more toxic than single agent 5-FU. Some sources believe there are insufficient comparative data to conclude whether oxaliplatin or irinotecan should be the first line combination partner with a fluoropyrimidine. Cassidy, for example, favours oxaliplatin on the basis that there are more data on salvage (potentially curative) surgery in such patients and he feels, writing with Waterston in Chapter 11, that it makes perfect sense to give patients and clinicians the option. The EGFR and VEGF targeted agents are very promising but it is premature, as Waterston and Cassidy discuss, to conclude how and in which setting these agents will be best employed. There is, as these authors remind us, an almost infinite number of potential strategies for patients now. Nevertheless, the evolving field of molecular diagnostics, prognostication and prediction of response is an exciting and encouraging area of development in the management of colorectal cancer and will hopefully allow us more intelligently to select appropriate therapy in the coming years.

The optimal management of *rectal* cancer continues to represent an increasing challenge for oncologists. Although surgery remains the mainstay of treatment, a high risk of local recurrence and poor survival has historically been reported for these patients. The main prognostic factors remain the extent of the primary tumour (T stage), regional lymph node status (N stage) and whether there is sufficient circumferential resection margin, and it is to the management of this disease that Glynne-Jones and Mawdsley turn in Chapter 12. The authors, in their particularly detailed and informative contribution, remain clear that we desperately need the results of the current trials, mostly planned more than a decade ago, to refine and to design the next generation of studies incorporating the new drugs and all the achievements in surgery and pathology. Future improvements in overall survival will almost certainly depend on the integration of all modalities, especially the new chemotherapy drugs irinotecan, oxaliplatin and capecitabine, and possibly the newer molecular targets.

A recurring question in the management of colorectal cancer has often been, then; 'what precisely are the optimal regimens?'. Much evidence has been established in a range of other cancers which demonstrates that shorter courses of chemotherapy can be equally as effective as those of longer duration in terms of survival. Maughan and Stephens, writing in Chapter 13, are concerned with this observation and their chapter presents and discusses the studies which have compared intermittent and continuous palliative chemotherapy for patients with metastatic colorectal cancer. They discuss many provocative results which challenge the orthodoxy that for optimal outcomes patients should be treated with cytotoxic chemotherapy until disease progression. That shortened exposures to chemotherapy may have beneficial economic as well as clinical benefits is not lost on the authors and their view is that the studies they discuss point towards the potential for an altered paradigm for treatment of patients with metastatic colorectal cancer in the more modern era of effective combination chemotherapy and novel cytostatic agents.

Over the past decade there have been major advances in our understanding of the molecular factors involved in the development and progression of colorectal cancer. Kulkarni and Hochhauser explain in Chapter 14, the closing chapter of Part Three of this volume, how this knowledge is already being translated into novel strategies using agents directed against various intracellular targets. Beginning with a description of the importance of microarray technology, these authors continue by reviewing our current understanding of the biological and clinical significance of the epidermal growth factor receptor, the use of the new monoclonal antibodies such as cetuximab, tyrosine kinase inhibitors such as gefitinib, the role of integrins, fibroblast growth factor and vascular endothelial growth factor, COX-2 inhibitors, proteosome inhibitors and histone deacetylase inhibitors. While these discoveries certainly herald a new era in the understanding of the processes of angiogenesis, invasion and metastasis in colorectal cancer and provide fascinating insights into the potential shape of future therapeutics, there are nevertheless significant cost-benefit issues which have as yet remained only partially considered and health economic research into the use of these new agents is now required.

We have dedicated Part Four, the concluding Part, through Chapters 15–17, to a detailed consideration of the clinical governance of colorectal cancer services. Cassidy, writing with Waterston in Chapter 11, and several other authors, refers to the constraints on clinical practice and therefore patient choice, exerted by NICE and in the opening chapter of this final Part, McBain and Saunders contribute a thoughtful account of the scientific basis, clinical credibility and moral implications of the judgements of NICE as they relate to the management of colorectal cancer. The guidance on the use of irinotecan, oxaliplatin and raltitrexed in the management of advanced colorectal cancer was published in March 2002 following prolonged consideration by the Institute of the reports submitted to it by a range of interested bodies. A final advisory document (FAD) was published in April 2001 and, after a successful appeal against NICE's decision-making process, a revised FAD was released in December 2001. Following a second appeal, the final guidance was published on 7 March 2002 and has remained controversial among practising clinicians, academics and patients alike. NICE is due to review its guidance on the management of advanced CRC again later this year (2005) with reference to the substantial body of evidence that has accumulated since the initial judgement was made, but McBain and Saunders are sceptical that these data will properly be taken into account by NICE and feel it likely that the UK will become even more out of step with the treatments being offered in North America and much of Europe. Surgery, as Tekkis and colleagues remind us in Chapter 16, is now in the era of objective assessment and professional accountability, with increasing emphasis being placed on the clinical effectiveness and quality of healthcare provision to the individual patient. Meaningful comparisons of outcomes between or within hospitals are, as they point out, possible if care is taken adequately to adjust for patient risk factors. In this stimulating chapter, these authors review the uses of mortality prediction models, data quality and standardization, the definition of clinical outcomes and the dimensions of risk as well as hierarchical models in colorectal surgery and the MBO colorectal cancer model, before concluding with a set of useful, associated recommendations. The final contribution, Chapter 17, which closes the volume, is contributed by James and is concerned with the operational organisation and funding of colorectal cancer services.

In this 4th Edition volume we have aimed to be as succinct as possible but as detailed as necessary. Consultants in gastroenterology, gastrointestinal surgery and medical and clinical oncology and their trainees are likely to find the book of invaluable use to their continuing professional development and specialist training, respectively, and we recommend this volume heartily for these purposes. We anticipate, also, that the book will prove of substantial use to clinical nurse specialists in these fields, to oncology pharmacists and to the planners, commissioners and managers of cancer services when in dialogue with their practising colleagues. Finally, we thank Sanofi-Aventis Ltd for the grant of unrestricted educational sponsorship that contributed to the costs of organizing the 7th national UK Key Advances update symposium on colorectal cancer held in collaboration with the British Society for

Gastroenterology, the Association of Coloproctology of Great Britain and Ireland, the British Association of Surgical Oncology, the Association of Cancer Physicians and The Royal College of Radiologists at The Royal College of Physicians of London at which synopses of many of the constituent chapters of this volume were presented.

David Cunningham MD FRCP
Clare Topham MB FRCR
Andrew Miles MSc MPhil PhD

London, July 2005

PART 1

Genetics of colorectal cancer

Chapter 1

Inherited susceptibility to colorectal cancer

Sanjay Popat, Richard Hubner and Richard S. Houlston

Introduction

Colorectal adenocarcinoma (CRC) is the commonest cause of death from malignancy in UK men, after lung and prostate cancer (http://www.statistics.gov.uk/). Despite surgical and medical advances in patient management, the overall mortality rate from CRC remains poor, with surgery still the most effective form of curative treatment.

Identifying genes predisposing to CRC is becoming increasingly important, not only to further the understanding of CRC pathobiology but also to allow identification of individuals at increased risk. Such individuals can then be offered targeted screening and entry into chemoprevention trials. In the future, specific tailored treatments may become available.

Although most cases of CRC occur sporadically, around 10% of all cases have a family history of the disease. The risk to first-degree relatives of patients with CRC has consistently been shown in epidemiological studies to be increased by about 3-fold (Peto & Houlston 2001). Here, we review the role and the mechanisms of action of CRC predisposition genes.

The adenoma carcinoma sequence

The concept that most colorectal cancers develop from normal epithelium through sequentially worsening degrees of adenomatous dysplasia was initially derived from histological observations (Muto *et al*. 1975). Based upon this concept of an adenoma carcinoma sequence, Fearon & Vogelstein (1990) proposed a genetic pathway model for the pathogenesis of sporadic CRC (Figure 1.1). Although the total accumulation of mutations is the principal factor, the model proposed that the causative mutations in tumour suppressor and oncogenes occur in a specific order in most (but not all) colorectal cancers (specifically, *APC* gene mutations, followed by global hypomethylation, *KRAS* mutations, and *DCC* gene mutations, and finally mutations in *TP*53). This model of colorectal carcinogenesis was proposed over 10 years ago, and has been termed the chromosomal unstable pathway, reflecting the high prevalence of aneuploidy observed. Since then, considerable data have allowed further elaboration to take into account alternative mechanisms for CRC development.

```
                    ┌─────────────────────┐
                    │  Normal epithelium  │
                    └──────────┬──────────┘
       APC/β Catenin  │         APC/β Catenin
                      ▼
                ┌──────────────┐         DAN mismatch
                │ Early adenoma│         repair genes
                └──────┬───────┘
                    K-Ras
                      ▼
                ┌──────────────┐
                │ Late adenoma │
                └──────┬───────┘
                     p53
              18q loss of
              heterozygosity
                      ▼                    TGFβRII, BAX,
                ┌──────────────┐           E2F4, TCF-4
                │  Carcinoma   │
                └──────────────┘
```

(Left arrow: CHROMOSOMAL INSTABILITY PATHWAY; Right arrow: MICROSATELLITE INSTABILITY PATHWAY)

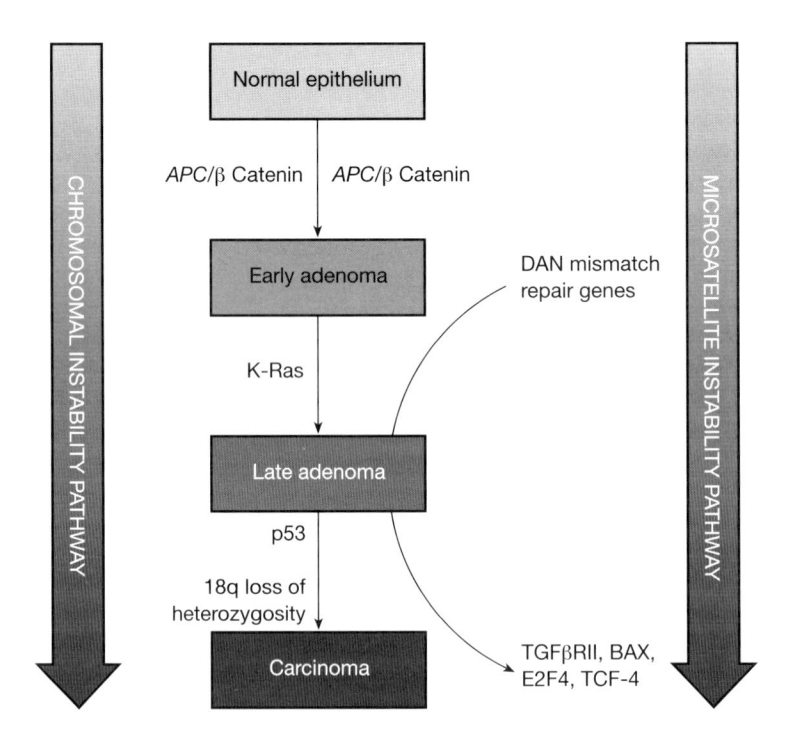

Figure 1.1 The adenoma carcinoma sequence of colorectal carcinogenesis (after Fearon & Vogelstien 1990). Genetic events in the formation of tumours without microsatellite instability are indicated on the left-hand side of the adenoma-carcinoma sequence, whereas genetic events in the formation of tumours with microsatellite instability are indicated on the right-hand side.

Mechanisms of CRC susceptibility: caretakers, gatekeepers and landscapers

Based on observations of retinoblastoma, Knudson (1971) proposed that individuals with an autosomal dominant predisposition to cancer inherited one genetic alteration (hit) at a predisposition locus, rate limiting for tumour formation. A second subsequent hit at the same locus then inactivates the remaining normal allele, allowing the cancer phenotype to develop (Knudson 1971). This 'two hit' hypothesis has been the underlying concept behind much of the initial data on CRC pathogenesis.

Following on from this concept, Kinzler and Vogelstein (1998) subsequently proposed a generalised mechanistic process for colorectal carcinogenesis. In this model, classic tumour suppressor genes, e.g. *APC,* function as 'gatekeepers', preventing carcinogenesis through direct control of cell growth. Thus, inactivation of gatekeepers directly contributes to malignancy development, and restoration of the missing gatekeeper function leads to neoplasia suppression. Second, DNA repair proteins (e.g. the mismatch repair genes, *MSH2* and *MLH1*) indirectly suppress neoplasia, and inactivation of caretakers increases the somatic mutation rate, but is never prerequisite to initiate neoplasia. Restoration of function of these genes does not, however, affect cell growth. Finally, changes in the stromal component of lesions (eg the clonal stromal component of the hamartomas of juvenile polyps and the inflammatory infiltrate in ulcerative colitis) were hypothesised to result in an altered terrain for epithelial cell growth, thereby increasing CRC likelihood. This 'landscaper' effect is exemplified by germline mutations in *SMAD4*, which predispose to hamartomatous polyps in patients with juvenile polyposis (JPS).

These concepts of 'gatekeeper' and 'caretaker' genes are, however, not entirely mutually exclusive, since 'caretaker' functions of *APC* have been identified (Fodde *et al.* 2001), as have 'gatekeeper' functions of the mismatch repair genes (Fishel 1998).

Familial adenomatous polyposis

The first gene mutated in sporadic CRC is *APC*. *APC* maps to chromosome 5q21 (Bodmer *et al.* 1987) and somatic mutations are detected in around 70% of sporadic CRCs (Solomon *et al.* 1987; Cottrell *et al.* 1992; Powell *et al.* 1992). Germline mutations in *APC* are, however, much rarer, and cause familial adenomatous polyposis (FAP) (Groden *et al.* 1991).

FAP is an autosomal dominantly inherited adenomatous polyposis syndrome characterised by the development of hundreds or thousands of adenomas throughout the colon and rectum during the second decade of life. The population frequency is about 1 in 10,000 and it accounts for less than 1% of all cases of CRC. Without prophylactic proctocolectomy, most affected individuals develop CRC by the age of 40, since one or more polyps will have inevitably progressed to carcinoma.

Several extracolonic features of FAP are recognised. Polyps may develop in the upper gastrointestinal tract and malignancies may occur at extracolonic sites, including the ampulla of Vater and brain. There is also a small increased risk of papillary thyroid carcinoma in young women and hepatoblastoma in children (Giardiello *et al.* 1991a, 1993). Other features of FAP include: congenital hypertrophy of the retinal pigment epithelium (CHRPE), observed in about 80% of FAP patients (Burn *et al.* 1991; Giardiello *et al.* 1991b); epidermoid cysts, most notably on the scalp (approximately 70% of patients); osteomas of the mandible (more than 90% of patients); and dental anomalies, e.g. supernumary and unerupted teeth (about 30% of patients). Desmoid tumours occur in 5–10% of FAP patients (more often in women, than men). The leading cause of death in patients that have undergone proctocolectomy is duodenal carcinoma (about 6% of patients), followed by local infiltration by desmoids (Powell *et al.* 1993).

These clinical features are evidence for the role of *APC* in the regulation of both colonic and extracolonic tissues. The *APC* gene comprises 15 exons, encoding a 2843 amino acid protein in its commonest isoform (Thliveris *et al.* 1996). Exon 10a is located downstream of exon 10, and is the subject of alternative splicing, adding an additional 18 amino acids to the APC protein when transcribed (Xia *et al.* 1995). The gene is unusual in that one exon (exon 15) comprises most (more than 75%) of the coding sequence of *APC*. Exon 15 is also the commonest target for both germline and somatic mutations. The protein is multifunctional and contains several domains that allow it to interact with several molecules in the wnt signalling pathway (Figure 1.2) (Bienz & Clevers 2000).

Although germline inactivating mutations (observed in FAP) are distributed throughout the entire gene, somatic mutations (observed in sporadic CRC) tend to be clustered at the 5' end of exon 15 between amino acid residues 1280–1500, termed the mutation cluster region (MCR) (Miyake *et al.* 1994). This overlaps with the 15 and 20 amino acid repeat domains that have been implicated in β-catenin interactions (Su *et al.* 1993) and the SAMP domains that interact with axin (Behrens *et al.* 1998).

As predicted by the Knudson model, APC acts as a tumour suppressor and mutations in one copy are typically coupled with chromosomal deletions in the remaining wild-type allele. However, bi-allelic activation may occur through other routes. In some cases, deletions of the wild-type *APC* allele are not observed. Rather, deletions occur in the inherited mutated allele, accompanied by new somatic mutations in the remaining allele (Spirio *et al.* 1998).

Regardless of their mechanism, more than 90% of all *APC* mutations result in the formation of a premature stop codon, and thus a truncated gene product (Miyoshi *et al.* 1992). This observation provides a rationale for using the protein truncation test (PTT) as a primary screening tool to detect mutations in clinical practice. In the PTT assay, amplified cDNA or genomic DNA is translated into protein in the presence of a labelled amino acid. The sample is then electrophoresed through polyacrylamide and the resulting protein products, either full-length or truncated, detected by autoradiography. Truncated proteins are indicative of the presence of a mutation causing a premature stop codon.

APC genotype and FAP phenotype

Studies of patients with FAP have shown interesting genotype-phenotype correlates with regard to the site of germline *APC* mutations, thereby allowing targeted follow-up. Mutations in the central region of the molecule are associated with a profuse polyposis phenotype, and hence a high risk of early-onset CRC. By contrast, mutations at the 5' end, proximal to codon 157, or at the 3' end distal to codon 1900, give an attenuated phenotype. Attenuated FAP (AFAP) is characterised by relatively few adenomas and an onset of CRC delayed to after the fifth decade of life (Spirio *et al.* 1993; Gardner *et al.* 1997) and may present as sporadic CRC in the setting of a new *APC* mutation. Mutations between codons 463 and 1387 are associated with CHRPE (Olschwang *et al.* 1993), and mutations between codons 1445 and 1578 are

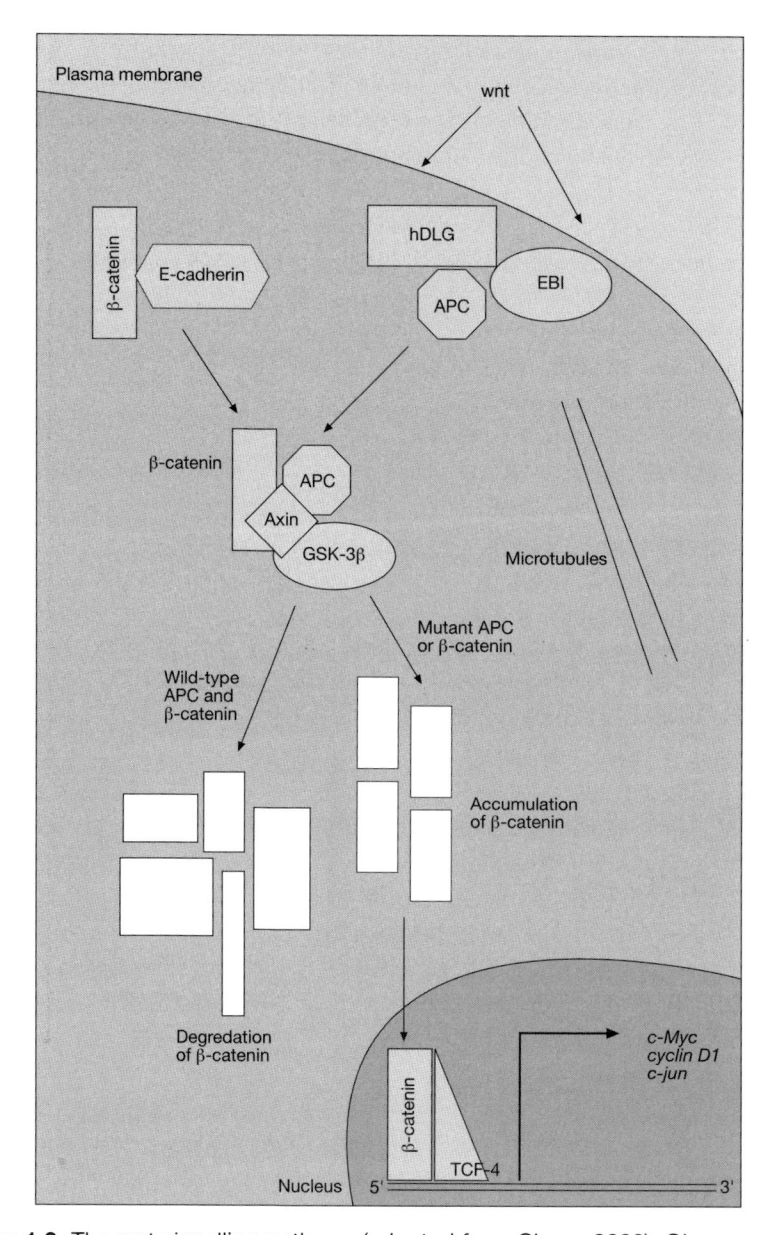

Inherited susceptibility to colorectal cancer 7

Figure 1.2 The wnt signalling pathway (adapted from Chung 2000). Glycogen sythase kinase-3β complexes and phosphorylates APC, b-catenin, and axin. Phosphorylation of β-catenin targets it for degradation via a ubiquitin-mediated proteasomal pathway. Truncated APC results in a disrupted complex and accumulated β-catenin. Free cytoplasmic β-catenin is translocated to the nucleus, where after interaction with transcription factors such as T-cell factor and lymphoid enhancer factor, up-regulation of wnt target genes (including *c-Myc, cyclin D1, c-jun, fra-1*) occurs. β-catenin binds with E-cadherin in a mutually exclusive manner at the plasma membrane. The nature of the wnt signal is unknown.

associated with an increased risk of desmoid tumour formation (Caspari *et al.* 1995). However, these correlates are not uniform and families with identical mutations may display variable phenotypes, giving evidence for the existence of modifier genes that may influence the severity of FAP.

Hamartomatous polyp syndromes

Hamartomas consist of normal looking elements of tissue, arranged so that the normal architecture is lost and replaced by another pattern of tissue organisation. They may occur either sporadically or as part of an inherited polyposis syndrome. These syndromes are associated with an increased risk of CRC and are described below.

Peutz-Jeghers syndrome

Peutz-Jeghers syndrome (PJS) is an autosomal dominantly inherited disorder affecting around 1 in 200,000. Approximately 50% of affected individuals are isolated cases (Bartholomew *et al.* 1962). PJS is characterised by the association of melanin pigmentation on the lips, perioral region, buccal mucosa, and hands, arms and feet, with gastrointestinal polyposis, and these are pathognomonic (Tomlinson & Houlston 1997). These macules may also be found around the eyes, genitalia, anus, and hands and feet of patients. Rarely, hyperpigmented macules may present without polyposis. Pigmentation is usually present in early childhood but tends to fade by the middle of the third decade.

Polyps may be distributed almost anywhere along the gastrointestinal tract, and have been observed at the following frequencies: small bowel (78%), stomach (38%), colon (42%), and rectum (28%) (Hemminki 1999). In addition, polyps may also be found in extraintestinal sites. Most patients present with recurrent episodes of colicky abdominal pain in early childhood. Presentation can be variable and is related to the site of polyposis. Intussusception is well recognised and rectal bleeding is not uncommon (Tomlinson & Houlston 1997).

While the polyps in PJS are hamartomas, they may become malignant (Gruber *et al.* 1998). Jejunal and other small bowel tumours have been reported in some patients (Lin *et al.* 1977; Matuchansky *et al.* 1979; Lehur *et al.* 1984). However, the absolute risk of malignancy is probably lower than has been reported, as many reports are undoubtedly subject to ascertainment bias.

The risk of intestinal and extraintestinal malignancy is increased about 15-fold in PJS patients, compared to normal controls, with around one half of patients dying from malignancy by the age of 57 (Boardman *et al.* 1998; Giardiello *et al.* 1987; Spigelman *et al.* 1989). The commonest malignancies are adenocarcinomas of the colon, small intestine, stomach and pancreas. Extraintestinal malignancies reported include ovarian sex-cord tumours (10–14% of females) and Sertoli cell tumours. Both breast and cervical cancers have been reported with an increased frequency.

Germline mutations in *LKB1* have been shown to cause PJS. *LKB1* maps to chromosome 19p13.3 and functions as a classical tumour suppressor, with PJS tumours showing loss of the wild-type allele (Hemminki *et al.* 1998). However, mutations in *LKB1* account for only about half of all familial and sporadic cases (Kikorkala *et al.* 1999). Although some mutations may go undetected, such as those due to large deletions or mutations in regulatory elements, families unlinked to 19p13.3 have been reported indicating that PJS is heterogeneous (Hemmiki *et al.* 1998; Jenne *et al.* 1998; Jiang *et al.* 1999; Westerman *et al.* 1999; Yoon *et al.* 2000). Furthermore, a second PJS susceptibility locus on chromosome 19q13.4 has been proposed (Mehenni *et al.* 1997). However, the gene responsible at this locus has yet to be identified, and is the focus of current research.

Juvenile polyposis syndrome and other hamartomatous polyposis syndromes

Juvenile polyposis (JPS) is a rare autosomal dominantly inherited condition characterised by hamartomatous polyps, usually within the colon but occasionally arising in the stomach and small bowel (Jass *et al.* 1988). These polyps are typified by a predominant stroma, cystic spaces and an abundant lamina propria lacking smooth muscle, so distinguishing them from PJS polyps. Although the JPS polyps themselves have a low malignant potential, the epithelial cells within and surrounding the polyp are at increased risk of neoplastic transformation as a result of their abnormal microenvironment ('landscaper' theory). Unlike solitary juvenile polyps, which may affect up to 2% of children and adolescents and have little or no malignant potential, JPS patients have an approximate 10–70% lifetime risk of CRC (Jass *et al.* 1988; Murday & Slack 1989). Extracolonic features are well recognised in JPS, observed in about 10–20% of patients. Such features include cleft lip or palate, and malrotations (Desai *et al.* 1998). JPS has also been observed in association with arteriovenous malformations, but it is unclear whether this represents a distinct syndrome.

Juvenile polyps may also occur as a manifestation of a number of dominantly transmitted rare familial cancer syndromes: Cowden syndrome (CS (MIM 158350); characterised by multiple hamartomas, macrocephaly, trichilemmomas, and a high risk of benign and malignant neoplasms of the thyroid, breast, uterus and skin); Bannayan-Riley-Ruvalcaba syndrome (Bannayan-Zonana syndrome: BRRS, BZS; characterised by mental retardation, macrocephaly, lipomatosis, haemangiomas and genital pigmentation); and Gorlin syndrome (GS; characterised by multiple naevoid basal carcinomas, skeletal abnormalities and odontogenic keratinocytes, macrocephaly, intracranial calcification and cranifacial abnormalities). The juvenile polyps in CS, BRRS and GS seem to have a low malignant potential (Murday & Slack 1989).

Germline mutations in *SMAD4* have been shown to cause JPS in a proportion of families (Howe *et al.* 1998; Houlston *et al.* 1998). *SMAD4* maps to chromosome

18q21.1, and encodes a protein involved in the TGFb signalling pathway. Most germline mutations produce a truncated *SMAD4* protein, which results in inactivated function. No mutations in the other members of the SMAD family of proteins have been detected in JPS patients (Bevan *et al*. 1999). The frequency of *SMAD4* mutations among American JPS patients is approximately 35–60%, compared with 3–28% of JPS families originating from mainly Europe. Germline truncating mutations in *BMPR1A* have also been described in families segregating JPS (Howe *et al*. 2001). *BMPR1A* maps to chromosome 10q21–q22, and encodes a bone morphogenic protein receptor serine-threonine kinase, which belongs to the TGFb receptor–SMAD superfamily. Further work on defining other sequence variants conferring an increased risk of juvenile polyps is ongoing.

Hereditary non-polyposis colon cancer syndrome

Hereditary non-polyposis colon cancer syndrome (HNPCC), formerly known as Lynch syndromes types I and II, is one of the commonest forms of inherited predisposition to CRC, accounting for 2–5% of all CRC. HNPCC differs from sporadic CRC by an earlier age of onset (mean age approximately 44 years), a predominance to the proximal colon (60–70%) and an increased probability to synchronous or metachronous CRCs (25%) (Lynch *et al*. 1988, 1993). HNPCC tumours also tend to have a mucinous histology, poor differentiation, and a peri- or intratumoural lymphocytic infiltrate. Many studies have demonstrated a better prognosis in HNPCC CRC compared with sporadic CRC, and the precise cause for this remains unclear. Compared with the risk to the general population, individuals with HNPCC have an 80% probability of developing CRC by the age of 65. They are also at an increased risk of developing a second primary CRC. In addition, affected individuals are at increased risk of a number of extracolonic malignancies, with women at an increased risk of endometrial cancer. In fact, women have a higher lifetime risk of developing endometrial cancer (60%) than CRC (54%). Affected individuals are also at increased risk of developing cancers of the stomach (13%) and ovaries (12%). Although the risks of developing malignancies of the small bowel, biliary tract, uroepithelium, kidney and central nervous system are increased, they do not exceed 4%. Despite this, there is marked interfamilial phenotypic variation.

HNPCC kindreds are defined by specific clinical criteria. The initial criteria used (Amsterdam I criteria) (Vasen *et al*. 1991) were found to be too strict by most clinicians for use in the identification of possible HNPCC kindreds for mutational analysis. Furthermore, the criteria did not take into account extracolonic malignancies. To resolve these issues, new clinical criteria were proposed (Amsterdam II criteria, Vasen *et al*. 1999) (see Table 1.1). In addition, the National Cancer Institute workshop on HNPCC has published criteria to target kindreds for mutational analyses (Bethesda guidelines; Rodriguez-Bigas *et al*. 1997) (see Table 1.2). These are more sensitive but less specific than either the Amsterdam I or

Amsterdam II criteria in identifying kindreds segregating pathogenic mutations (Syngal et al. 2000).

Table 1.1 Revised Amsterdam criteria (Amsterdam II criteria; Vasen et al. 1999)

There should be at least three relatives with a HNPCC-associated cancer (cancer of the colorectum, endometrium, small bowel, ureter, or renal pelvis) *and*:

1. One should be a first-degree relative of the other two
2. At least two successive generations should be affected
3. At least one should be diagnosed before age 50
4. Familial adenomatous polyposis (FAP) should be excluded
5. Tumours should be verified by pathological examination

Table 1.2 Bethesda guidelines (Rodriguez-Bigas et al. 1997)

1. Individuals with cancer in families that meet the Amsterdam criteria
2. Individuals with two HNPCC-related cancers, including synchronous and metachronous CRC or associated extracolonic cancers*
3. Individuals with CRC and a first-degree relative with CRC and/or HNPCC-related extracolonic cancer and/or a colorectal adenoma: one of the cancers diagnosed at age <45 years, and the adenoma diagnosed at age <40 years
4. Individuals with CRC or endometrial cancer diagnosed at age <45 years
5. Individuals with right-sided CRC with an undifferentiated pattern (solid/cribriform) on histopathology diagnosed at age <45 years
6. Individuals with signet-ring-cell-type CRC diagnosed at age <45 years
7. Individuals with adenomas diagnosed at age <40 years

*Endometrial, ovarian, gastric, hepatobiliary, or small bowel or transitional cell carcinoma of the renal pelvis or ureter

HNPCC arises as a result of germline mutation in one of the several DNA mismatch repair (MMR) genes to date: *MSH2, MLH1, PMS1, PMS2, MSH3, MSH6* (Fishel et al. 1993; Leach et al. 1993; Peltomaki et al. 1993; Bronner et al. 1994; Nicolaides et al. 1994; Yin et al. 1997). Although a germline mutation in any of the six MMR genes above may cause HNPCC, most mutations detected occur in *MHS2* or *MLH1*, with germline mutations widely distributed throughout the 16 exons of *MHS2* or the 19 exons of *MLH1* (Peltomaki et al. 1997). Most are point mutations. In *MHS2*, this results in primarily frameshifts (60%) or premature truncations (23%), whereas frameshifts (40%) or missense mutations of unknown significance (31%) are typically observed in families with a mutant *MLH1* gene. The molecular basis for clinical phenotypes remains to be defined for the majority of genotypes. However, carriers of germline *hMHS2* mutations have been shown to have an increased risk of extraintestinal tumours of the uroepithelium, stomach and ovary (Vasen et al. 1996).

The MMR genes control the repair of DNA base-pair mismatches and are responsible for ensuring correct DNA synthesis during replication. DNA polymerases are error-prone enzymes, especially at areas containing highly repetitive nucleotide sequences, such as microsatellite DNA. Microsatellites are repeating sequences of DNA composed of mono-, di-, tri- or tetranucleotide repeats, scattered throughout the genome. Even in normal cells, these sites are inherently unstable, and inappropriate base insertion or DNA replication slippage at these sites results in insertion or deletion loops consisting of multiples of the nucleotide repeat sequence. These loops are normally repaired, but in the absence of efficient mismatch repair enzymes, they become 'permanent' and result in alleles of differing sizes at the next round of replication. Over several generations, multiple different sized alleles at that microsatellite locus may accumulate within a tumour with defective mismatch repair genes, and this is termed 'microsatellite instability' (MSI). Microsatellite instability therefore acts as a surrogate marker of aberrant MMR (Figure 1.3).

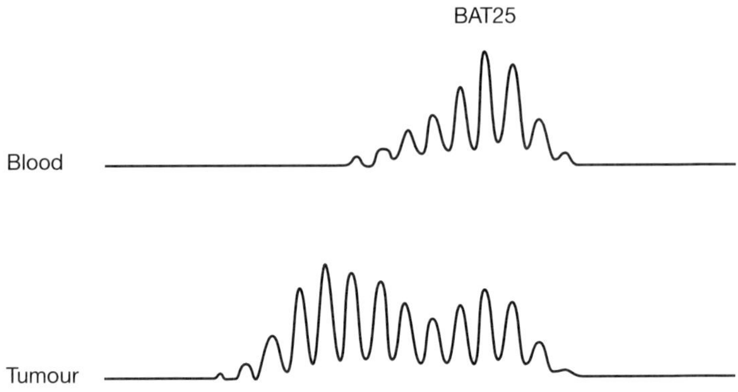

Figure 1.3 Genotyping of germline DNA (from blood) and somatic DNA (from tumour) at the microsatellite locus BAT-25. Microsatellite instability is shown in the somatic (tumour) DNA.

Although a tumour from an HNPCC kindred with MSI is most likely to represent an underlying mutation in an MMR gene, about 5% of these tumours do not demonstrate MSI. Hence, a negative result for MSI will not preclude HNPCC as a diagnosis. Furthermore, approximately 13% of sporadic CRCs display MSI (Aaltonen et al. 1998) due to somatic rather than germline MMR gene inactivation. Hence, tumours displaying MSI do not necessarily imply a diagnosis of HNPCC.

There has been some debate as the exact definition of the MSI phenotype. Criteria have range from instability at any microsatellite locus, to at least 30% of the loci studied. A consensus has been brought nearer by the identification of BAT26, a microsatellite marker that is highly sensitive and specific in identifying MMR deficient tumours. A recent National Cancer Institute workshop has proposed a consensus panel of mononucleotide and dinucleotide microsatellite markers for MSI testing. On this basis, tumours could be classified as demonstrating high-frequency MSI (MSI-H, two or more markers unstable), low-frequency MSI (MSI-L, one marker unstable), or microsatellite stability (MSS, no markers unstable) (Boland *et al*. 1998).

Inactivation of both alleles of *MHS2* or *MLH1* is necessary to generate the MSI-H phenotype, and this occurs through several routes. Loss of heterozygosity (LOH) is often coupled with point mutations of *MHS2* or *MLH1*, consistent with the Knudson two-hit model: these tumour suppressors are examples of 'caretakers'. Epigenetic mechanisms may also play a role. Transcription of *MLH1* can be silenced by hypermethylation of CpG islands in its promoter, and this is likely to be the primary mechanism underlying the MMR deficient phenotype in sporadic CRCs (Herman *et al*. 1998).

MMR defects are thought to lead to tumorigenesis through accumulation of widespread mutations within short repetitive sequences. Most MSI is likely to be functionally insignificant since most microsatellites are distributed in non-coding regions of the genome. However, once loss of mismatch repair has occurred, not only microsatellite but all nucleotide repeat sequences become targets for insertion/deletion-type mutations. A number of genes have been identified which have mono- or dinucleotide repeat sequences in exonic DNA. Mutations in MMR deficient tumours have been found in many of these genes: the type II TGFb receptor (*TGFBR2*), the IGF II receptor (*IGFIIR*), the apoptosis regulator Bax, the cell cycle transcription factor E2F-4, TCF-4, caspase 5, the intestinal homeobox factor CDX2, and *MHS3* and *MSH6*. The latter provides a unique positive feedback loop in which tumours with MSI can enhance their own phenotype.

Current evidence indicates that tumours with MSI probably develop along a genetic pathway different to sporadic MSS tumours. The early part of the pathways may be the same, and observations have established the overriding importance of *APC* in the initiation of tumorigenesis. However, once loss of mismatch repair occurs, tumours displaying MSI probably develop along a different pathway, in which the process of tumour initiation is accelerated.

Evidence for additional colorectal adenoma/carcinoma susceptibility genes

Cohort analysis of twins has suggested that about 35% of all colorectal cancer can be ascribed to an inherited genetic susceptibility (Lichtenstein *et al*. 2000). However, less than 5% can be ascribed to dominant syndromes for which mutations have been shown to be causative (Burt *et al*. 1990; Bonaiti-Pellie 1999): *APC*, DNA mismatch repair genes, *SMAD4* and *LKB1*. Of the known mutations, the DNA mismatch repair genes undoubtedly make the largest contribution. Segregation analyses provide compelling evidence that about 15% of all colorectal cancer might be attributable to the action of dominantly acting predisposition genes (Cannon-Albright *et al.* 1988; Houlston *et al.* 1992). Partitioning the familial risks in pedigrees segregating adenomata provides strong *a priori* evidence that a significant proportion of the inherited predisposition to CRC is mediated through the susceptibility to adenoma formation. These family studies indicate that the familial risks of CRC in relatives of adenoma cases (relative risk (RR) = 2.0, 95% confidence interval (CI): 1.55–2.55) parallel those seen in relatives of CRC probands (Johns & Houlston 2001). This supports the notion put forward by Cannon-Albright *et al.* (1988) who, on the basis of segregation analysis, proposed that there could be a relatively common dominant predisposition to adenomatous polyps, colorectal cancer, or both. Direct evidence for the existence of additional colorectal cancer predisposition genes with lower penetrance than *APC*, is provided by CRC families that show evidence against linkage to known loci (Lewis *et al.* 1996) or identify novel loci, not associated with mismatch repair deficiency: exemplified by *CRAC1* (Tomlinson *et al.* 1999).

The *CRAC1* locus maps to chromosome 15q14-22 and was first detected by a combination of linkage and loss of heterozygosity analysis in an Ashkenazi family segregating a susceptibility to colorectal adenomata and CRC in a dominant manner. Further evidence for a susceptibility locus in this region comes from work by Park *et al.* (2000), who found some evidence for a tumour suppressor on chromosome 15q21.1 by deletion mapping. The precise predisposition allele at this locus has yet to be identified, but is not likely to contribute significantly to sporadic CRC (Popat *et al.* 2003).

The *EXO1* gene on chromosome 1q42-43 is another recently described putative CRC susceptibility locus (Wu *et al.* 2001). Wu et al. screened *EXO1* for sequence variants in a cohort of HNPCC and HNPCC-like kindreds and detected variants specific to the affected individuals. However, the precise role of *EXO1* in CRC pathogenesis, if any, has yet to be elucidated.

Perhaps the most interesting recent development in CRC susceptibility has been the demonstration that sequence variation in *MYH* can predispose to multiple colorectal andenomas and CRC (Al-Tassan *et al.* 2002). Al-Tassan *et al.* (2002) reported on a single Welsh family with three affected members and recessive inheritance of multiple colorectal adenomas and carcinoma, and demonstrated an excess of somatic mutations consisting of the substitution of a thymidine:adenine pair for a guanine:cytosine pair (G:C→T:A) in *APC*, transversions typical of changes secondary to oxidative damage (see Figure 1.4). Oxidative repair genes were tested for germline changes and two missense variants (Y165C and G382D) were detected in *MYH*. *MYH*, alongside *MTH1* and *OGG1* is a member of the human base-excision repair pathway, and its products have a pivotal role in the repair of mutations caused by reactive oxygen species generated during aerobic metabolism. Intriguingly, by contrast to other CRC susceptibility alleles, pathogenic mutations appear to act in a recessive fashion. The phenotypes associated with *MYH* sequence variation have been assessed by Sieber *et al.* (2003), who investigated 152 patients with multiple (3–100) colorectal adenomas and 107 *APC*-negative probands with classical FAP (more than 100 adenomas). Six patients with multiple adenomas (ranging from 18–100) and eight with FAP had biallelic germline *MYH* variants. None of the FAP patients had severe disease (more than 1000 adenomas), but three had extracolonic disease. The precise role of *MYH* sequence variants in colorectal carcinogenesis remains to be defined. However, recent work has suggested that *MYH*-associated cancers may follow a distinct genetic pathway, with some features of both the chromosomal instability and MSI pathway (Lipton *et al.* 2003).

Low-penetrance genes

The penetrance of a gene is defined as the probability of developing a specific phenotype given the presence of that causal genotype. Highly penetrant mutations in *APC* and the MMR genes may cause a substantial proportion of colorectal cancers at young ages, but are unlikely to be responsible for a high proportion of all cases. However, it is possible that penetrance susceptibility loci could do so. Highly penetrant mutations confer large relative risk and generate large pedigrees (see Figure 1.5). Hence, these loci may be amenable to detection by linkage strategies. Low-penetrance susceptibility loci confer only modest risks. For example, a susceptibility locus conferring a 2-fold increase in risk of CRC, present at a population frequency of 0.2, will only generate a relative risk of 1.06. Such loci will be difficult or impossible to detect by linkage, because the number of affected relative pairs required will be prohibitively large. The commonest method used for the identification of common low-penetrance alleles is through association studies. These are based on the comparison of the frequencies of polymorphic genotypes in cases and controls. Alleles positively associated with the disease are analogous to risk factors in epidemiology and may either be causally related to disease risk, or be in linkage disequilibrium with a disease-causing variant.

Putative low-penetrance CRC susceptibility genes can be broadly delineated into those coding for: carcinogen metabolism enzymes (e.g. *CYP1A1, NAT2, GSTM1, GSTT1*), methylation enzymes (*MTHFR*), microenvironmental modifiers (*PLA2G2A, APOE*), and oncogenes and tumour suppressors (*H-ras*-VNTR, *APC* I1307K).

Interest in the I1307K missense sequence variant of *APC* was first generated when Laken *et al.* (1997) investigated the risk of CRC in Ashkenazim with this variant. They demonstrated that *APC* I1307K was present in 6% of Ashkenazi controls, compared to 10% of CRC cases and 28% of cases with a positive family history of CRC. The precise mechanism by which the sequence variant predisposes to CRC is thought to be by the creation of a poly-(A_8) tract, instead of the normal A_3TA_4 sequence, thereby increasing the rate of somatic mutation. A systematic review of this and other published polymorphisms and risk of CRC has been undertaken (Houlston

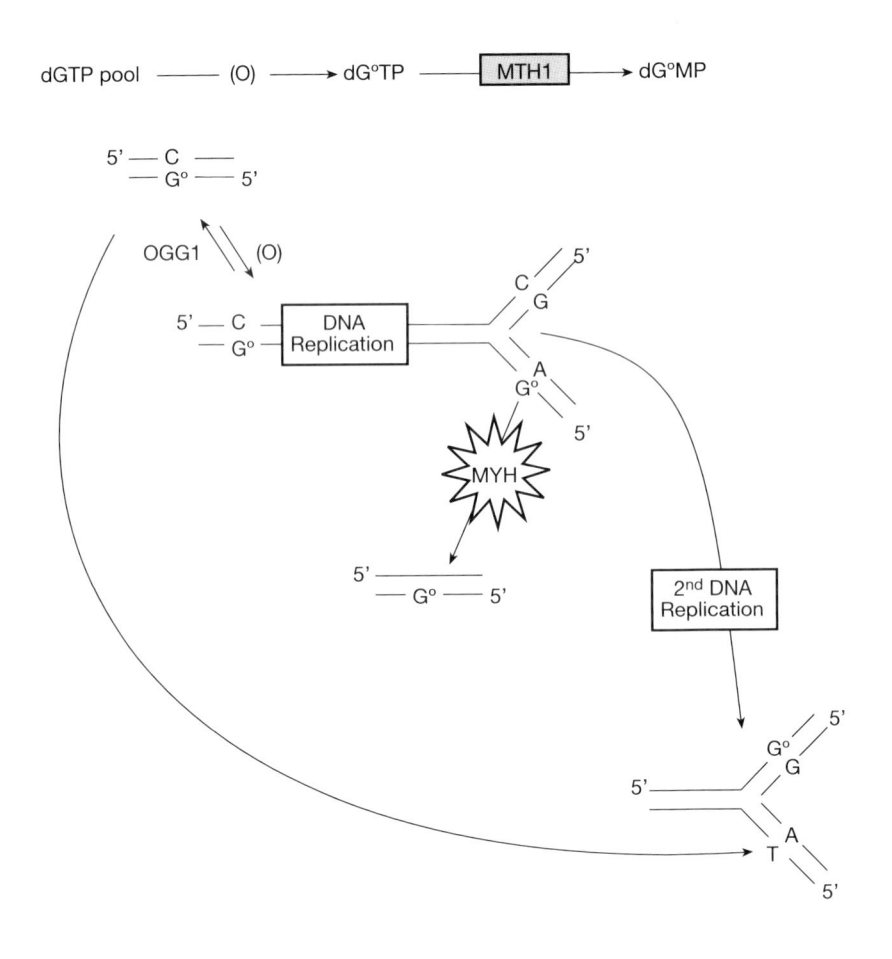

Figure 1.4 Repair of mutations involving 8-oxoguanine (G°) by the proteins: MTH1, OGG1, and MYH (adapted from Marra & Jiricny 2003). Reactive oxygen species (O) modify the nucleotide pool to produce 8-oxoguanine triphosphate (dG°TP). These are subsequently detoxified by MTH1. G° is incorporated into newly synthesized DNA from unhydrolyzed dG°TP during replication by DNA polymerase, and 8-oxoguanine–cytosine (G°:C) or (8-oxoguanine–adenine (Go:A)) mispairs are formed. Oxidation of guanines gives rise to G°:C mispairs, which revert to guanine–cytosine (G:C) pairs, due to OGG1. In the presence of uncorrected G°:C mispairs, DNA polymerase preferentially inserts adenine opposite 8-oxoguanine, forming G°:A mispairs at DNA replication. Removal of the mispaired adenine by MYH and subsequent base-excision repair converts G°:A to G°:C, which is then repaired by OGG1. Uncorrected Go:A mispairs give rise to G:C→T:A transversions in 50% of progeny DNA after replication.

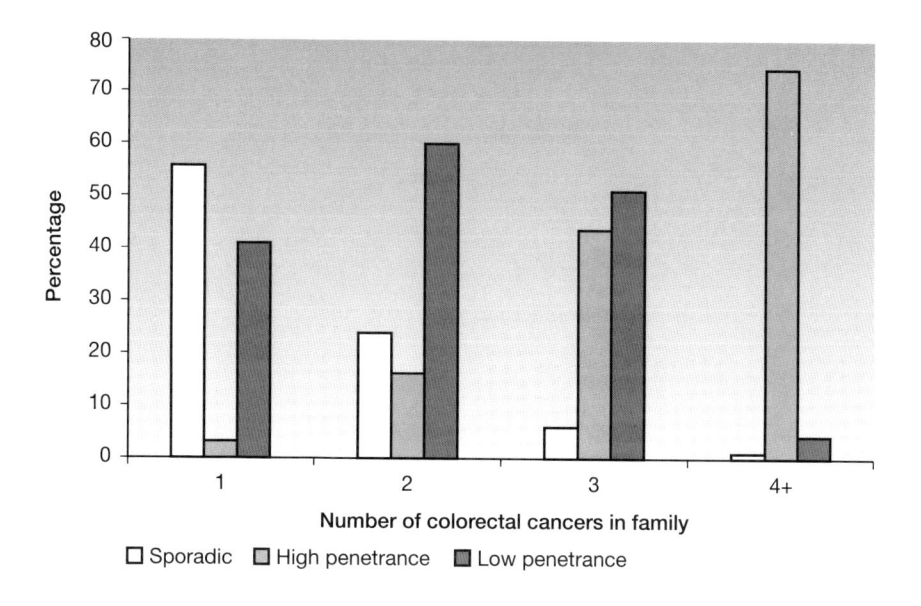

Figure 1.5 Possible role of high and low penetrance genes to familial clustering of colorectal cancer.

& Tomlinson 2001). Fifty studies of the effect of common alleles of 13 genes on the risk of CRC were identified. After pooling results from published studies, significant associations were only seen at three polymorphisms: *APC*-I1307K (odds ratio (OR) 1.58; 95% CI: 1.21–2.07), *HRAS-1* VNTR (OR 2.50; 95% CI: 1.54–4.05) and *MFTR*$^{val/val}$ (OR 0.76; 95% CI: 0.62–0.92).

A case–control study of 1244 Ashkenazim has identified a potential low-penetrance CRC susceptibility allele. Gruber *et al*. (2002) showed that patients with CRC were significantly more likely to be carriers of a specific allele at the *BLM* locus (*BLM*^{Ash}) than matched controls (OR 2.34, 95% CI 1.5–3.7). *BLM* encodes a RecQ DNA helicase, and inactivating germline mutations at this locus result in Bloom syndrome, a syndrome of small stature, immunodeficiency, male infertility, and predisposition to various cancers. The *BLM*^{Ash} allele contains a frame-shift mutation in exon 10 that results in premature translation termination. Further evidence for the role of this allele in the predisposition to CRC comes from a mouse model, in which mice heterozygous at *Blm* developed twice the number of intestinal tumours when crossed with mice carrying an *APC* mutation (Goss *et al*. 2002).

These sequence variants therefore represent the strongest candidates for low-penetrance CRC susceptibility alleles. Although their genotypic risks are modest, their high population frequency implies that they might well have considerable impact on the incidence of CRC.

Conclusion

Considerable insights into the genetic basis of CRC have been made, with the identification of high penetrance (e.g. *APC, MSH2* and *MLH1*) and low-penetrance (e.g. *APC* I1307K) predisposition alleles. These insights have been applied in clinical practice to aid diagnosis, screening, and evidence-based therapeutic intervention of individuals with increased risk of CRC. In the near future, as molecular technologies become more cost-effective and mechanised, it is likely that molecular genotyping for risk, prognostic and therapeutic indicators will become more widespread and move from the setting of the research laboratory into the clinic.

Acknowledgements

Sanjay Popat receives a Clinician Scientist Fellowship from the Department of Health.

References

Aaltonen, L. A., Salovaara, R., Kristo, P., Canzian, F., Hemminki, A., Peltomaki, P., Chadwick, R. B., Kaariainen, H., Eskelinen, M., Jarvinen, H. *et al.* (1998). Incidence of hereditary nonpolyposis colorectal concer and the feasibility of molecular screening for the disease. *New England Journal of Medicine* **338**, 1481–1487.

Al-Tassan, N., Chmiel, N. H., Maynard, J., Fleming, N., Livingston, A. L., Williams, G. T., Hodges, A. K., Davies, D. R., David, S. S., Sampson, J, R. & Cheadle, J. P. (2002). Inherited variants of MYH associated with somatic G:C→T:A mutations in colorectal tumors. *Nature Genetics* **30**, 227–232.

Bartholomew, L. G., Morre, C. E., Dahlin, D. C. & Waugh, J. M. (1962). Intestinal polyposis associated with mucocutaneous pigmentation. *Surgery, Gynecology and Obstetrics* **115**, 1–11.

Bevan, S., Woodford-Richens, K., Rozen, P., Young, J., Dunlop, M., Neale, K., Houlston, R. & Tomlinson, I. (1999). Screening SMAD1, SMAD2, SMAD3 and SMAD5 for germline mutations in juvenile polyposis syndrome. *Gut* **45**, 406–408.

Behrens, J., Jerchow, B. A., Wurtele, M., Grimm, J., Asbrand, C., Wirtz, R., Kuhl, M., Wedlich, D. & Birchmeier W. (1998). Functional interaction of an axin homolog, conductin, with beta-catenin, APC, and GSK3 beta. *Science* **280**, 596–599.

Bienz, M. & Clevers, H. (2000). Linking colorectal cancer to wnt signalling. *Cell* **103**, 311–320.

Boardman, L. A., Thibodeau, S. N., Schaid, D. J., Lindor, N. M., McDonnell, S. K., Burgart, L. J., Ahlquist, D. A., Podratz, K. C., Pittelkow, M. & Hartmann, L. C. (1998). Increased risk for cancer in patients with the Peutz-Jeghers syndrome. *Annals of Internal Medicine* **128**, 896–899.

Bodmer, W. F., Bailey, C. J., Bodmer, J., Bussey, H. J., Ellis, A., Gorman, P., Lucibello, F. C., Murday, V. A., Rider, S. H. & Scambler, P. *et al.* (1987). Localization of the gene for familial adenomatous polyposis on chromosome 5. *Nature* **328**, 614–616.

Boland, C. R., Thibodeau, S. N., Hamilton, S. R., Sidransky, D., Eshleman, J. R., Burt, R. W., Meltzer, S. J., Rodriguez-Bigas, M. A., Fodde, R., Ranzani, G. N. *et al.* (1998). A National Cancer Institute workshop in microsatellite instability for cancer detection and familial predisposition: development of international criteria for the determination of microsatellite instability in colorectal cancer. *Cancer Research* **58**, 5248–5257.

Bonaiti-Pellie, C. (1999). Genetic risk factors in colorectal cancer. *European Journal of Cancer Prevention* **8**, S27–S32.

Bronner, C. E., Baker, S. M., Morrison, P. T., Warren, G., Smith, L. G., Lescoe, M. K., Kane, M., Earabino, C., Lipford, J. & Lindblom, A. *et al.* (1994). Mutation in the DNA mismatch repair gene homolog MLH1 is associated with hereditary nonpolyposis colon cancer. *Nature* **368**, 258–261.

Burn, J., Chapman, P., Delhanty, J., Wood, C., Lalloo, F., Cachon-Gonzalez, M. B., Tsioupra, K., Church, W., Rhodes, M. & Gunn, A. (1991). The UK Northern Region genetic register for familial adenomatous polyposis coli: use of age of onset, congenital hypertrophy of the retinal pigment epithelium, and DNA markers in risk calculations. *Journal of Medical Genetics* **28**, 289–296.

Burt, R. W., Bishop, D. T., Lynch, H. T., Rozen, P. & Winawer, S. J. (1990). Risk and surveillance of individuals with heritable factors for colorectal cancer. WHO Collaborating Centre for the Prevention of Colorectal Cancer. *Bulletin of the World Health Organization* **68**, 655–665.

Cannon-Albright, L. A., Skolnick, M. H., Bishop, D. T., Lee, R. G. & Burt, R. W. (1998). Common inheritance of susceptibility to colonic adenomatous polyps and associated colorectal cancers. *New England Journal of Medicine* **319**, 533–537.

Caspari, R., Olschwang, S., Friedl, W., Mandl, M., Boisson, C., Boker, T., Augustin, A., Kadmon, M., Moslein, G., Thomas, G. *et al.* (1995). Familial adenomatous polyposis: desmoid tumours and lack of ophthalmic lesions (CHRPE) associated with APC mutations beyond codon 1444. *Human Molecular Genetics* **4**, 337–340.

Chung, D. C. (2000). The genetic basis of colorectal cancer: insights into critical pathways of tumorigenesis. *Gastroenterology* **119**, 854–865.

Cottrell, S., Bicknell, D., Kaklamanis, L. & Bodmer, W. F. (1992). Molecular analysis of APC mutations in familial adenomatous polyposis and sporadic colon carcinomas. *The Lancet* **340**, 626–630.

Desai, D. C., Murday, V., Phillips, R. K., Neale, K. F., Milla, P. & Hodgson, S. V. (1998). A survey of phenotypic features of juvenile polyposis. *Journal of Medical Genetics* **35**, 476–481.

Fearon, E. R. & Vogelstein, B. (1990). A genetic model for colorectal tumorigenesis. *Cell* **61**, 759–767.

Fishel, R., Lescoe, M. K., Rao, M. R., Copeland, N. G., Jenkins, N. A., Garber, J., Kane, M. & Kolodner, R. (1993). The human mutator gene homolog MSH2 and its association with hereditary nonpolyposis colon cancer. *Cell* **75**, 1027–1038.

Fishel, R. (1998). Mismatch repair, molecular switches, and signal transduction. *Genes and Development* **12**, 2096–2101.

Fodde, R., Kuipers, J., Rosenberg, C., Smits, R., Kielman, M., Gaspar, C., van Es, J. H., Breukel, C., Wiegant, J., Giles, R. G. *et al.* (2001). Mutations in the APC tumor supressor gene cause chromosomal instability. *Nature Cell Biology* **3**, 433–438.

Gardner, R. J., Kool, D., Edkins, E., Walpole, I. R., Macrae, F. A., Nasioulas, S. & Scott, W. J. (1997). The clinical correlates of a 3¢ truncating mutation (codons 1982-1983) in the adenomatous polyposis coli gene. *Gastroenterology* **113**, 326–331.

Giardiello, F. M., Welsh, S. B., Hamilton, S. R., Offerhaus, G. J., Gittelsohn, A. M., Booker, S. V., Krush, A. J., Yardley, J. H. & Luk, G. D. (1987). Increased risk for cancer in the Peutz-Jeghers syndrome. *New England Journal of Medicine* **316**, 1151–1153.

Giardiello, F. M., Offerhaus, G. J., Krush, A. J., Booker, S. V., Tersmette, A. C., Mulder, J. W., Kelley, C. N. & Hamilton, S. R. (1991a). Risk of hepatoblastoma in familial adenomatous polyposis. *Journal of Pediatrics* **119**, 766–768.

Giardiello, F. M., Offerhaus, G. J., Traboulsi, E. I., Graybeal, J. C., Maumenee, I. H., Krush, A. J., Levin, L. S., Booker, S. V., Hamilton, S. R. (1991b). Value of combined phenotypic markers in identifying inheritance of familial adenomatous polyposis. *Gut* **32**, 1170–1174.

Giardiello, F. M., Offerhaus, G. J., Lee, D. H., Krush, A. J., Tersmette, A. C., Booker, S. V., Kelley, N. C. & Hamilton, S. R. (1993). Increased risk for thyroid and pancreatic carcinoma in familial adenomatous polyposis. *Gut* **34**, 1394–1396.

Goss, K. H., Risinger, M. A., Kordich, J. J., Sanz, M. M., Straughen, J. E., Slovek, L. E., Capobianco, A. J., German, J., Boivin, G. P. & Groden, J. (2002). Enhanced tumor formation in mice heterozygous for Blm mutation. *Science* **297**, 2051–2053.

Groden, J., Thliveris, A., Samowitz, W., Carlson, M., Gelbert, L., Albertsen, H., Joslyn, G., Stevens, J., Spirio, L., Robertson, M. *et al.* (1991). Identification and characterization of the familial adenomatous polyposis coli gene. *Cell* **66**, 589–600.

Gruber, S. B., Entius, M. M., Petersen, G. M., Laken, S. J., Longo, P. A., Boyer, R., Levin, A. M., Mujumdar, U. J., Trent, J. M., Kinzler, K. W. *et al.* (1998). Pathogenesis of adenocarcinoma in Peutz-Jeghers syndrome. *Cancer Research* **58**, 5267–5270.

Gruber, S. B., Ellis, N. A., Rennert, G., Offit, K, Scott, K. K., Almog, R., Kolachana, P., Bonner, J. D., Kirchhoff, T., Tomsho, L. P. *et al.* (2002). *BLM* heterozygosity and the risk of colorectal cancer. *Science* **297**, 2013.

Hemminki, A., Markie, D., Tomlinson, I., Avizienyte, E., Roth, S., Loukola, A., Bignell, G., Warren, W., Aminoff, M., Hoglund, P. *et al.* (1998). A serine/threonne kinase gene defective in Peutz-Jeghers syndrome. *Nature* **391**, 184–187.

Hemminki, A. (1999). The molecular basis and clinical aspects of Peutz-Jeghers syndrome. *Cellular and Molecular Life Sciences* **55**, 735–750.

Herman, J. G., Umar, A., Polyak, K., Graff, J. R., Ahuja, N., Issa, J. P., Markowitz, S., Willson, J. K., Hamilton, S. R., Kinzler, K. W. *et al.* (1998). Incidence and functional consequences of hMLH1 promoter hypermethylation in colorectal carcinoma. *Proceedings of the National Academy of Sciences of the United States of America* **95**, 6870–6875.

Houlston, R. S., Collins, A., Stack, J. & Morton, N. E. (1992). Dominant genes for colorectal cancer are not rare. *Annals of Human Genetics* **56**, 99–103.

Houlston, R. S., Bevan, S., Williams, A., Young, J., Dunlop, M., Rozen, P., Eng, C., Markie, D., Woodford-Richens, K., Rodriguez-Bigas, M. *et al.* (1998). Mutations in DPC4 (SMAD4) cause juvenile polyposis syndrome, but only account for a minority of cases. *Human Molecular Genetics* **7**, 1907–1912.

Houlston, R. S. & Tomlinson, I. P. M. (2001). Polymorphisms and colorectal tumor risk. *Gastroenterology* **121**, 282–301.

Howe, J. R., Roth, S., Summers, R. W., Jarvinen, H. J., Sistonen, P., Tomlinson, I. P. M., Houlston, R. S., Bevan, S., Mitros, F. A., Stone, E. M. *et al.* (1998). Mutations in the Smad4/DPC4 gene in juvenile polyposis. *Science* **280**, 1086–1088.

Howe, J. R., Bair, J. L., Sayed, M. G., Anderson, M. E., Mitros, F. A., Petersen, G. M., Velculescu, V. E., Traverso, G., Vogelstein, B. (2001). Germline mutations of the gene encoding bone morphogenetic protein receptor 1A in juvenile polyposis. *Nature Genetics* **28**, 184–187.

Jass J. R., Williams, C. B., Bussey, H. J., Morson, B. C. (1988). Juvenile polyposis: a precancerous condition. *Histopathology* **13**, 691–630.

Jenne, D. E, Reimann, H., Nezu, J., Friedel, W., Loff, S., Jeschke, R., Muller, O., Back, W. & Zimmer, M. (1998). Peutz-Jeghers syndrome is caused by mutations in a novel serine threonine kinase. *Nature Genetics* **18**, 38–43.

Jiang, C.-Y., Esufali, S., Berk, T., Gallinger, S., Cohen, Z., Tobi, M., Redston, M. & Bapat, B. (1999). STK11/*LKB1* germline mutations are not identified in most Peutz-Jeghers syndrome patients. *Clinical Genetics* **56**, 136–141.

Johns, L. E. & Houlston, R. S. (2001). A systematic review and meta-analysis of familial colorectal cancer risks. *American Journal of Gastroenterology* **96**, 2992–3003.

Kikorkala, A., Avizienyte, E., Tomlinson, I. P., Tiainen, M., Roth, S., Loukola, A., Hemminki, A., Johansson, M., Sistonen, P., Markie, D. *et al.* (1999). Mutations and impaired function of LKB1 in familial and non-familial Peutz-Jeghers syndrome and a sporadic testicular cancer. *Human Molecular Genetics* **8**, 45–51.

Kinzler, W. K. & Vogelstein, B. (1998). Landscaping the cancer terrain. *Science* **280**, 1036.

Knudson, A. G. Jr (1971). Mutation and cancer: statistical study of retinoblastoma. *Proceedings of the National Academy of Sciences of the United States of America* **68**, 820–823.

Laken, S. J., Petersen, G. M., Gruber, S. B., Oddoux, C., Ostrer, H., Giardiello, F. M., Hamilton, S. R., Hampel, H., Markowitz, A., Klimstra, D. *et al.* (1997). *Nature Genetics* **17**, 79–83.

Leach, F. S., Nicolaides, N. C., Papadopoulos, N., Liu, B., Jen, J., Parsons, R., Peltomaki, P., Sistonen, P., Aaltonen, L. A., Nystrom-Lahti, M. *et al.* (1993). Mutations of a mutS homolog in hereditary nonpolyposis colorectal cancer. *Cell* **7**, 1215–1225.

Lehur, P.-A., Madarnas, P., Devroede, G., Perey, B. J., Menard, D. B. & Hamade, N. (1984). Peutz-Jeghers syndrome: association of duodenal and bilateral breast cancers in the same patient. *Digestive Diseases and Sciences* **29**, 178–182.

Lewis, C. M., Neuhausen, S. L., Daley, D., Black, F. J., Swensen, J., Burt, R. W., Cannon-Albright, L. A. & Skolnick M. H. (1996). Genetic heterogeneity and unmapped genes for colorectal cancer. *Cancer Research* **56**, 1382–1388.

Lichtenstein, P., Holm, N. V., Verkasalo, P. K., Iliadou, A., Kaprio, J., Koskenvuo, M., Pukkala, E., Skytthe, A. & Hemminki, K. (2000). Environmental and heritable factors in the causation of cancer-analyses of cohorts of twins from Sweden, Denmark, and Finland. *New England Journal of Medicine* **343**, 78–85.

Lin, J. I., Caracta, P. F., Lidner, A. & Gutzman, L. G. (1977). Peutz-Jeghers polyposis with metastasizing duodenal carcinoma. *Southern Medical Journal* **70**, 882–884.

Lipton, L., Halford, S. E., Johnson, V., Novelli, M. R., Jones, A., Cummings, C., Barclay, E., Seiber, O., Sadat, A., Bisgaard, M. L. *et al.* (2003). Carcinogenesis in MYH-associated polyposis follows a distinct genetic pathway. *Cancer Research* **15**, 7595–7599.

Lynch, H. T., Watson, P., Lanspa, S. J., Marcus, J., Smyrk, T., Fitzgibbons, R. J. Jr, Kriegler, M. & Lynch, J. F. (1988). Natural history of colorectal cancer in hereditary nonpolyposis colorectal cancer (Lynch syndromes I and II). *Diseases of the Colon and Rectum* **31**, 439–444.

Lynch, H. T., Smyrk, T. C., Watson, P., Lanspa, S. J., Lynch, J. F., Lynch, P. M., Cavalieri, R. J. & Boland, C. R. (1993). Genetics, natural history, tumour spectrum, and pathology of hereditary non-polyposis colorectal cancer. An updated review. *Gastroenterology* **104**, 1535–1549.

Marra, G. & Jiricny, J. (2003). Multiple colorectal adenomas – is their number up? *New England Journal of Medicine* **348**, 845–847.

Matuchansky, C., Babin, P., Coutrot, S., Druart, F., Barbier, J. & Maire, P. (1979). Peutz-Jeghers syndrome with metastasizing carcinoma arising from a jejunal hamartoma. *Gastroenterology* **77**, 1311–1315.

Mehenni, H., Blouin, J.-L., Radhakrishna, U., Bhardwaj, S. S., Bhardwaj, K., Dixit, V. B., Richards, K. F., Bermejo-Fenoll, A., Leal, A. S., Raval, R. C. *et al.* (1997). Peutz-Jeghers syndrome: confirmation of linkage to chromosome 19p13.3 and identification of a potential second locus, on 19p13.4. *American Journal of Human Genetics* **61**, 1327–1334.

Miyaki, M., Konishi, M., Kikuchi-Yanoshita, R., Enomoto, M., Igari, T., Tanaka, K., Muraoka, M., Takahashi, H., Amada, Y., Fukayama, M. *et al.* (1994). Characteristics of somatic mutation of the adenomatous polyposis gene in colorectal tumors. *Cancer Research* **54**, 3011–3020.

Miyoshi, Y., Nagase, H., Ando, H., Horii, A., Ichii, S., Nakatsuru, S., Aoki, T., Miki, Y., Mori, T. & Nakamura, Y. (1992). Somatic mutations of the APC gene in colorectal tumors: mutation cluster region in the APC gene. *Human Molecular Genetics* **1**, 229–233.

Murday, V. & Slack, J. (1989). Inherited disorders with colorectal cancer. *Cancer Survey* **8**, 139–157.

Muto, T., Bussey, H. J. & Morson, B. C. (1975). The evolution of cancer of the colon and rectum. *Cancer* **36**, 2251–2275.

Nicolaides, N. C., Papadopoulos, N., Liu, B., Wei, Y. F., Carter, K. C., Ruben, S. M., Rosen, C. A., Haseltine, W. A., Fleischmann, R. D., Fraser, C. M. *et al.* (1994). Mutations of two PMS homologues in hereditary nonpolyposis colon cancer. *Nature* **371**, 75–80.

Olschwang, S., Tiret, A., Laurent-Puig, P., Muleris, M., Parc, R. & Thomas, G. (1993). Restriction of ocular fundus lesions to a specific subgroup of APC mutations in adenomatous polyposis coli patients. *Cell* **75**, 959–968.

Park, W. S., Park, J. Y., Oh, R. R., Yoo, N. J., Lee, S. H., Shin, M. S., Lee, H. K., Han, S., Yoon, S. K., Kim, S. Y. *et al.* (2000). A distinct tumor suppressor gene locus on chromosome 15q21.1 in sporadic form of colorectal cancer. *Cancer Research* **60**, 70–73.

Peltomaki, P., Aaltonen, L. A., Sistonen, P., Pylkkanen, L., Mecklin, J. P., Jarvinen, H., Green, J. S., Jass, J. R., Weber, J. L., Leach, F. S. *et al.* (1993). Genetic mapping of a locus predisposing to human colorectal cancer. *Science* **269**, 810–812.

Peltomaki, P. & Vasen, H. F. A. (1997). Mutations predisposing to hereditary nonpolyposis colorectal cancer: database and results of a collaborative study. *Gastroenterology* **113**, 1146–1158.

Peto, J. & Houlston, R. S. (2001). Genetics and the common cancers. *European Journal of Cancer* **37** (Suppl. 8), S88–S96.

Popat, S., Stone, J., Houlston, R. S. (2003). Allele imbalance in colorectal cancer at the *CRAC1* (colorectal adenoma and carcinoma) locus in early-onset colorectal cancer. *Cancer Genetics and Cytogenetics* **145**, 70–73.

Powell, S. M., Zilz, N., Beazer-Barclay, Y., Bryan, T. M., Hamilton, S. R., Thibodeau S. N., Vogelstein, B. & Kinzler, K. W. (1992). APC mutations. *Nature* **359**, 235–237.

Powell, S. M., Petersen, G. M., Krush, A. J., Booker, S, Jen, J., Giardiello, F. M., Hamilton, S. R., Vogelstein, B. & Kinzler, K. W. (1993). Molecular diagnosis of familial adenomatous polyposis. *New England Journal of Medicine* **329**, 1982–1987.

Rodriguez-Bigas, M. A., Boland, C. R., Hamilton, S. R., Henson, D. E., Jass, J. R., Khan, P. M., Lynch, H., Perucho, M., Smyrk, T., Sobin, L. *et al.* (1997). A National Cancer Institute workshop on hereditary nonpolyposis colorectal cancer syndrome: meeting highlights and Bethesda guidelines. *Journal of the National Cancer Institute* **89**, 1758–1761.

Sieber, O., Lipton, L., Carbtree, M., Heinimann, K., Fidalgo, P., Phillips, R. K. S., Bisgaard, M.-L., Orntoft, T. F., Aaltonen, L. A., Hodgson, S. V. *et al.* (2003). Multiple colorectal adenomas, classical adenomatous polyposis and germ-line mutations in *MYH*. *New England Journal of Medicine* **348**, 791–799.

Solomon, E., Voss, R., Hall, V., Bodmer, W. F., Jass, J. R., Jeffreys, A. J., Lucibello, F. C., Patel, I. & Rider, S. H. (1987) Chromosome 5 allele loss. *Nature* **328**, 616–619.

Spigelman, A. D., Murday, V. & Phillips, R. K. (1989). Cancer and the Peutz-Jeghers syndrome. *Gut* **30**, 1588–1590.

Spirio, L., Olschwang, S., Groden, J., Robertson, M., Samowitz, W., Joslyn, G., Gelbert, L., Thliveris, A., Carlson, M., Otterud, B. *et al.* (1993). Alleles of the APC gene: an attenuated form of familial polyposis. *Cell* **75**, 337–340.

Spirio, L. N., Samowitz, W., Robertson, J., Robertson, M., Burt, R. W., Leppert, M. & White, R. (1998). Alleles of APC modulate the frequency and classes of mutations that lead to colonic polyps. *Nature Genetics* **20**, 385–388.

Syngal, S., Fox, E. A. & Eng, C. (2000). Sensitivity and specificity of clinical criteria for hereditary nonpolyposis colorectal cancer-associated mutations in *MSH2* and *MLH1*. *Journal of Medical Genetics* **37**, 641–645.

Su, L.-K., Vogelstein B. & Kinzler, K. W. (1993). Association of the APC tumor suppressor protein with catenins. *Science* **262**, 1734–1737.

Thliveris, A., Albertsen, H., Tuohy, T., Carlson, M., Groden J., Joslyn G., Gelbert L., Samowitz W., Spirio L. & White R. (1996). Long-range physical map and deletion characterization of the 1100-kb NotI restriction fragment harbouring the APC gene. *Genomics* **34**, 268–270.

Tomlinson, I. P. M. & Houlston, R. S. (1997). The Peutz-Jeghers syndrome. *Journal of Medical Genetics* **34**, 1007–1011.

Tomlinson, I. P. M., Rahman, N., Frayling, I. M., Mangion, J., Barfoot, R., Hamoudi, R., Seal, S., Northover, J. M. A., Thomas, H. J. W. & Neale, K. *et al.* (1999). Evidence for a gene predisposing to colorectal adenoma and carcinoma (CRCA1) on chromosome 15q14-22. *Gastroenterology* **116**, 789–795.

Vasen, H. F., Mecklin J. P., Khan, P. M. & Lynch, H. T. (1991). The International Collaborative Group on Hereditary Non-Polyposis Colorectal Cancer (ICG-HNPCC). *Diseases of the Colon and Rectum* **36**, 424–425.

Vasen, H. F. A. & Wijnen J. T. (1996). Cancer risk in families with hereditary nonpolyposis colorectal cancer diagnosed by mutational analysis. *Gastroenterology* **110**, 1020–1027.

Vasen, H. F., Watson, P., Mecklin, J. P. & Lynch, H. T. (1999). New clinical criteria for hereditary nonpolyposis colorectal cancer (HNPCC, Lynch syndrome) proposed by the International Collaborative Group on HNPCC. *Gastroenterology* **116**, 1453–1456.

Westerman, A. M., Entius, M. M., Boor, P. P. C., Koole, R., de Baar, E., Offerhaus, G. J. A., Lubinski, J., Lindhout, D., Halley, D. J. J., de Rooij, F. W. M. *et al.* (1999). Novel mutations in the *LKB1*/STK11 gene in Dutch Peutz-Jeghers families. *Human Mutation* **13**, 476–481.

Wu, Y., Berends, M. J., Post, J. G., Mensink, R. G., Verlind, E., Van Der Sluis, T., Kempinga, C., Sijmons, R. H., van der Zee, A. G., Hollema, H. *et al.* (2001). Germline mutations of EXO1 gene in patients with hereditary nonpolyposis colorectal cancer (HNPCC) and atypical HNPCC forms. *Gastroenterology* **120**, 1580–1587.

Xia, L., St Dennis, K. A. & Bapat, B. (1995). Evidence for a novel exon in the coding region of the adenomatous polyposis coli (APC) gene. *Genomics* **28**, 359–591.

Yin, J., Kong, D., Wang, S., Zou, T. T., Souza, R. F., Smolinski, K. N., Lynch, P. M., Hamilton, S. R., Sugimura, H., Powell, S. M. *et al.* (1997). Mutation of hMSH3 and hMSH6 mismatch repair genes in genetically unstable colorectal and gastric carcinomas. *Human Mutation* **10**, 474–478.

Yoon, K. A., Ku, J. L., Choi, H. S., Heo, S. C., Jeong, S. Y., Park, Y. J., Kim, N. K., Kim, J. C., Jung, P. M. & Park, J. G. (2000). Germline mutations of the STK11 gene in Korean Peutz-Jeghers syndrome patients. *British Journal of Cancer* **82**, 1403–1406.

Chapter 2

Mismatch repair deficiency in hereditary and sporadic colorectal cancer

Mark J. Arends and Ian M. Frayling

Introduction

Carcinogenesis within the colorectum is a multi-step process, which involves the transition from normal epithelium through adenomatous changes with increasing dysplasia and tumour size, to carcinoma. Originally described as a pathological stepwise set of changes, this adenoma–carcinoma sequence is associated with progressive accumulation of genetic changes (Fearon & Vogelstein 1990) (see Figure 2.1).

There are two major pathways of accumulation of genetic alterations and these are associated with different patterns of genomic instability. Chromosomal instability can be detected in the majority and microsatellite instability (MSI) in around 15% of colorectal cancers (Lothe *et al*. 1993; Abdel-Rahman *et al*. 2001). Subsequently, it has been shown that MSI occurs in 20% of colon cancers, but only 1–2% of rectal cancers. In both pathways, the transition from normal epithelium to adenoma is very strongly associated with inactivation of adenomatous polyposis coli (*APC*) gene product function, either through mutation and/or loss of the *APC* gene itself, which is seen in up to 85% of colorectal adenomas and carcinomas, or via activating mutations of the beta-catenin (*CTNNB1*) gene, the product of which is normally down-regulated by wild-type APC protein, and is involved in transcriptional regulation of other genes such as *c-myc*. Also in both pathways, mutational activation of the *K-ras* oncogene at specific codons (12, 13 or 61) is seen in 40–50% adenomas and carcinomas. In the chromosomal instability pathway, there is mutation and/or allele loss of a number of tumour suppressor genes, including *SMAD4* (also known as *DPC4*) and *p53*, during progression to malignancy (Kinzler & Vogelstein 1996). In the second pathway, MSI occurs due to defective DNA mismatch repair (MMR), usually caused by *MLH1* gene silencing by promoter hypermethylation in sporadic tumours (Cunningham *et al*. 1998; Esteller *et al*. 2001). Deficient MMR allows accumulation of unrepaired mismatches as mutations, especially in repetitive sequences known as microsatellites. The microsatellites usually affected are either dinucleotide repeats (e.g. …CACACACA…) or mononucleotide repeats (e.g. …AAAAAAAA…). Such genetic changes have been commonly identified in coding microsatellites in the *TGF-betaRII* gene (functions in the same pathway as SMAD4, mediating growth inhibition by TGF-beta) and the *Bax* gene (Bax functions in the same apoptosis-inducing pathway as p53) (Abdel-Rahman *et al*. 1999). As well as occurring in 20% of sporadic colon cancers, deficient MMR is characteristic of tumours in hereditary non-polyposis colorectal cancer (HNPCC) (Jass 1998; Toft & Arends 1998).

Historical background

An early description of affected families was by Lynch in 1966, who reported a family with colorectal, gastric and endometrial cancers, a family later found to have been described by Warthin in 1913. Lynch compared the family with others similarly afflicted, and made the distinction between those only affected by colorectal cancer (Lynch syndrome Type 1) and those affected by a variety of cancers, but mainly colorectal and endometrial (Lynch syndrome Type 2; also known as family cancer syndrome). The families had a similar predisposition to young-onset bowel cancer as those with familial adenomatous polyposis (FAP), but without the polyposis. Hence, the term used to describe Lynch syndrome became hereditary non-polyposis colorectal cancer (HNPCC) (Lynch *et al*. 1993, 1997, 1998). Unlike FAP, there is no obvious macroscopic feature to distinguish HNPCC from the large numbers of families with familial colorectal cancer due to other genes, most of which have not yet been identified.

Hereditary non-polyposis colorectal cancer

HNPCC accounts for 1–2% of colorectal cancers (Mecklin *et al*. 1995; Lynch *et al*. 1997; Lynch & de la Chapelle 1999). HNPCC colorectal tumours often develop at an earlier age, show an apparent predilection for the proximal colon compared with sporadic tumours that are more commonly distal, and are less aggressive than sporadic colorectal cancers (Lynch *et al*. 1993; Thibodeau *et al*. 1993; Gryfe *et al*. 2000). HNPCC patients are more likely to develop multiple colorectal cancers and extracolonic tumours (Watson & Lynch 1993, 1994), especially cancers of the endometrium (Mecklin & Jarvinen 1991) (the most prevalent extracolonic tumour), and also tumours of ureter, renal pelvis, ovary, stomach, small intestine, hepatobiliary tract, CNS (glioblastomas) and skin (Thibodeau *et al*. 1993; Watson & Lynch 1994; Mecklin *et al*. 1995; Toft & Arends 1998). The cutaneous neoplasms are usually keratoacanthonas or complex sebaceous gland tumours of skin, initially described as the key feature of Muir-Torre syndrome, when associated with internal malignancies (Cohen et al. 1991; Kolodner et al. 1994), although this is now recognised as part of HNPCC (see Table 2.1).

HNPCC is caused by autosomal dominant inheritance of a mutated MMR gene. Although the odds of HNPCC gene carriers developing HNPCC-associated tumours generally increase with age, HNPCC exhibits incomplete penetrance, i.e. gene carriers do not inevitably develop HNPCC-associated tumours. Moreover, given the numerous different types of HNPCC-associated tumours, expression of HNPCC can

Table 2.1 Tumour types and frequencies associated with HNPCC

Tumour type	Approximate lifetime risk (both sexes, unless specified)	Comment
Colorectal cancer	Males, 70–80% Females, 40–50%	Tumours equally common throughout colon and rectum
Endometrial cancer	Females, 40–60%	Mostly endometrioid
Ovarian cancer	Females, 5%	
Gastric cancer	5%	Varies widely
Brain cancer	2–5%	Mostly glioblastoma
Urothelial	2–5%	Renal pelvis and ureter transitional cell carcinomas
Small bowel	1%	Primary adenocarcinomas
Hepato-biliary tract	Uncertain	Risk uncertain
Pancreas	Uncertain	Risk uncertain
Non-melanoma skin	Undefined	Sebaceous adenomas/carcinomas and keratoacanthomas (in combination with an internal cancer = Muir-Torre syndrome)

be highly variable (Table 2.1). For reasons that remain obscure, some individuals with HNPCC may develop multiple tumours, while others develop none.

Germline *MSH2* and *MLH1* gene mutations together account for the majority (over 90%) of HNPCC families (Leach *et al.* 1993; Fishel *et al.* 1993; Aaltonen *et al.* 1993; Peltomaki *et al.* 1993a,b, 2001a,b; Bronner *et al.* 1994; Wheeler *et al.* 2000a; Terdiman *et al.* 2001). These may be non-sense mutations predicting the production of a truncated protein, mis-sense mutations, splice site mutations or large deletions/rearrangements (Gryfe *et al.* 2000). Germline mutations in other known DNA MMR genes such as *MSH6/GTBP, PMS2* and *MSH3* account for rather less than 10% of HNPCC families (Nicolaides *et al.* 1994; Yin *et al.* 1997; Wu *et al.* 1999; Wijnen *et al.* 1999; Loukola *et al.* 2000; Parc *et al.* 2000; Wagner *et al.* 2001). Although *PMS1* was putatively identified as an HNPCC gene, it is now considered to be a non-functional pseudogene.

DNA mismatch repair function

The primary function of the MMR system is to eliminate base-to-base mismatches and insertion–deletion loops that arise due to polymerase slippage errors during DNA replication (see Figure 2.1). In MMR defective cells, base-to-base mismatches result in the inappropriate substitution of one base for another and typically occur within sections of non-repetitive DNA, whereas insertion–deletion loops usually involve the loss or gain of repeat units in mono- and dinucleotide microsatellites, such as $(A)_n$ and

(CA)$_n$, though longer repeat units can also be affected. For repair of single base mismatches, MSH2 heterodimerizes with MSH6 to form the hMutSalpha complex, which recruits MLH1 and PMS2. In the case of insertion–deletion loops, MSH2 heterodimerizes with MSH3, to form the hMutSbeta complex that recruits MLH1 and MLH3 (Papadopolos *et al*. 1994; Kolodner & Marsischky 1999). These multi-protein complexes then function to coordinate the excision of the more recently synthesised DNA strand containing the mismatch or insertion/deletion error, which is followed by synthesis of the correct complementary DNA strand and ligation.

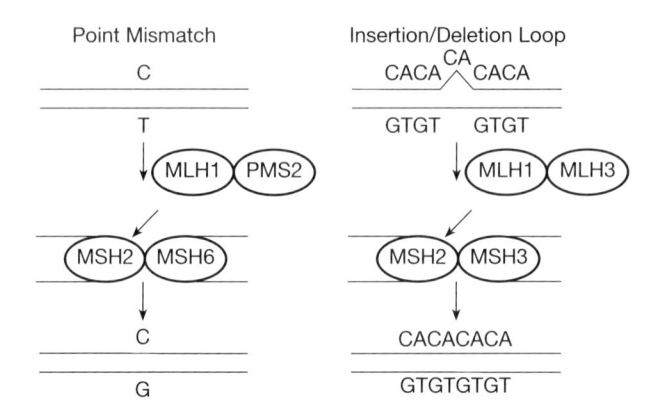

Figure 2.1 DNA mismatch repair function in humans. A complex of MSH2-MSH6 binds to point mismatches, whereas a complex of MSH2 and MSH3 binds to insertion–deletion loops. These complexes bound to mismatched DNA then bind complexes of MLH1 with either PMS2 or MLH3. The mismatches are then resolved, and repair is achieved.

In HNPCC, individuals inherit one mutant MMR gene and during tumour formation the remaining wild-type MMR allele is inactivated or lost, with consequent failure to express any normal MMR protein, and so loss of mismatch repair function occurs. This in turn leads to an accumulation of unrepaired mismatches, particularly in repetitive sequences, which result in mutations during DNA replication, manifest as microsatellite instability (MSI). Tumours in which MSI is found in >29% of microsatellites tested are described as having MSI-H (for high frequency). MSI-H is found in over 95% of HNPCC colorectal cancers (Wheeler *et al*. 2000a).

Defective MMR: selectable advantage and promoter of tumour progression

The selectable advantage conferred on tumour cells by the acquisition of MMR deficiency is contentious (Tomlinson *et al*. 1996; Tomlinson & Bodmer 1999; Fishel 2001). It does not seem to be a simple rise in mutation rate, although loss of MMR undoubtedly biases mutations to occur in mononucleotide tracts in the coding regions of genes. It may be that loss of MMR interferes with some forms of DNA damage-induced apoptosis and thus enhances cell survival after such DNA damage that is usually recognised by the MMR system (Toft *et al*. 1999, 2002). It appears that loss of MMR only occurs in colorectal tumours after *APC* mutation, ie loss of MMR acts to promote rather than initiate tumours (Homfray *et al*. 1998). That some prior mutation has to take place in another gene (presumably *APC* in the case of colorectal tumours), before a loss of MMR function becomes a selectable advantage may also explain why HNPCC patients are only predisposed to tumours at a limited range of sites. That HNPCC is a disorder that leads to tumour promotion rather than initiation is also supported by a number of very rare families in which individuals have inherited a mutant MMR allele from each parent. These individuals who have inherited two mutant alleles in a recessive pattern of inheritance are constitutionally MMR deficient from conception, in a manner analogous to other inborn errors of metabolism (Trimbath *et al*. 2001). Their phenotype is to develop multiple cutaneous neurofibromata and café-au-lait spots, multiple colorectal adenomas, primary brain tumours and leukaemia, with death usually before the age of 10 years—quite unlike that of HNPCC, but similar to the other recessively inherited DNA repair disorders, such as xeroderma pigmentosum, Fanconi's anaemia and Bloom's syndrome, etc. HNPCC is unusual as a DNA repair disorder in that it predisposes to the eventual somatic loss of a DNA repair function in tumours.

In HNPCC, the evidence suggests that the rate of progression through the adenoma–carcinoma sequence is more rapid, consistent with the concept that HNPCC predisposes to tumour promotion, rather than initiation. HNPCC cases can develop several adenomas, but not polyposis (defined as more than 100 adenomatous polyps in the large bowel), often under the age of 50 years, whereas sporadic adenomas in this age group are uncommon. HNPCC adenomas also have a greater tendency to show aggressive features, including villous or serrated architecture, large size, and high-grade dysplasia (Jass 1998). There is an increased occurrence of interval cancers in HNPCC, overall suggesting the need for frequent surveillance in known HNPCC cases.

HNPCC: pathological features and diagnosis

Colorectal cancers in HNPCC display certain pathological features. They occur equally throughout the colon and rectum, in contrast to the general population, in which colorectal cancers occur mostly in the rectum and sigmoid colon. Thus, the bowel cancers in HNPCC are said to be more often 'right-sided', but this is an artefact of the bias towards 'left-sided' tumours outside of HNPCC. They are more likely to have mucinous or poorly differentiated histology, an expansile growth pattern, and lymphocytic infiltration, both surrounding the tumour in 'Crohn's-like' lymphoid aggregates and individual lymphocytes infiltrating through tumour epithelium (Ward *et al*. 2001). On examination of the molecular attributes, over 95% of HNPCC-associated tumours exhibit MSI, but so do about 15% of the same type of cancers occurring sporadically (Peltomaki *et al.* 1993b). Thus, MSI did not prove to be a specific test for HNPCC. Subsequent attempts have been made to develop better techniques to ascertain HNPCC cases. In order to select families for the original linkage studies, criteria were established by the International Collaborative Group (ICG) on HNPCC meeting in Amsterdam, the so-called 'Amsterdam criteria': three or more relatives with histologically proven colorectal cancer, one of whom is a first-degree relative of the other two; colorectal cancer involving at least two generations; and at least one family member affected before the age of 50 years. These were necessarily stringent, ie specific but not sensitive. Although they have come to be used in clinical practice to diagnose HNPCC, this was not their original purpose. One successful alternative approach has been to analyse those features of family history that predict finding a germline mutation (Wijnen *et al.* 1998, 1999). This model shows that a family only just fulfilling the Amsterdam criteria have odds of an *MSH2* or *MLH1* mutation of only about 20%. The ICG-HNPCC subsequently produced a more useful and comprehensive definition (see Table 2.2).

Table 2.2 International collaborative group definition of HNPCC

1. Familial clustering of colorectal and/or endometrial cancer.
2. Associated cancers: gastric, ovary, ureter/renal pelvis, brain, small bowel, hepatobiliary tract and skin (sebaceous tumours).
3. Development of cancer at an early age.
4. Development of multiple cancers.
5. Features of colorectal cancer: (a) predilection for proximal (right-sided) colon; (b) improved survival; (c) multiple colorectal cancer; (d) increased proportion of mucinous tumours, and tumours with marked host-lymphocytic infiltration and lymphoid aggregation at the tumour margin.
6. Features of colorectal adenoma: (a) the numbers vary from one to a few; (b) increased proportion of adenomas with villous histology and (c) high-grade dysplasia, (d) probably rapid progression from adenoma to carcinoma.
7. High frequency of microsatellite instability (MSI-H).
8. Immunohistochemistry: loss of MLH1, MSH2, MSH6 or PMS2 protein expression in tumours.
9. Germline mutation in MMR gene: *MSH2, MLH1, (MSH6, PMS2,* or others).

Note: Any combination of 1–9 may be present, but 9 alone defines HNPCC.
Source: Vasen H. F. A. *et al.* (1999).

Diagnosis of HNPCC can be problematic. HNPCC is not the only form of familial colorectal cancer: familial adenomatous polyposis (FAP) must be excluded, as well as other familial causes. Germline mutation detection is possible, but cannot detect 100% of HNPCC cases, as HNPCC is genetically heterogeneous (genes affected include *MSH2, MLH1, MSH6, PMS2* and others), is allelically heterogeneous (due largely to many private mutations), is frequently associated with mis-sense mutations (that can be difficult to intepret in isolation), and is phenocopied (Jass *et al.* 2002). Mutation detection is a finite resource, is not 100% efficient, and therefore cannot, in itself, be used to exclude HNPCC.

HNPCC tumour analysis: combined MMR immunohistochemistry and MSI testing

A recently developed approach has been to analyse tumours from suspected HNPCC families with a combination of MSI testing of tumour DNA and investigation for abnormalities of MMR protein expression in the tumours using immunohistochemistry (IHC). Immunohistochemistry, using antibodies to the MMR proteins, MLH1 and MSH2, can demonstrate abnormal MMR protein expression in HNPCC tumours (Wilson *et al.* 1995; Leach *et al.* 1996; Thibodeau *et al.* 1996; Dietmaier *et al.* 1997; Fink *et al.* 1997; Marcus *et al.* 1999; Cawkwell *et al.* 1999; Chaves *et al.* 2000). Experience in Cambridge of immunohistochemical analysis of MLH1, MSH2, MSH6 and PMS2 protein expression in HNPCC tumours has shown that there are three different expression patterns: (a) homogeneously positive for the four proteins (the normal appearance in unaffected non-HNPCC tumours and in normal tissues); (b) homogeneously negative for one or two of the proteins (abnormal pattern); and (c) patchy/weakly positive for one or two of the proteins (abnormal pattern) (Jimenez-Linan *et al.* 2004). Abnormal expression of MSH6 is significantly associated with abnormal MSH2 expression, a function of MSH6 stabilisation when bound with MSH2 to form heterodimers. Similarly, abnormal expression of PMS2 is significantly associated with abnormal MLH1 expression, as PMS2 also forms dimers with MLH1. Loss of expression or abnormal staining (eg patchy/weak or cytoplasmic) indicates the affected protein and hence mutant gene in the tumour (Figure 2.2).

This is best interpreted in terms of the clinical setting, family history and pathological features of the tumour(s). If consistent loss or abnormality of the same MMR protein is observed across a family, or in more than one tumour from the same individual, it is very strong evidence of HNPCC. Abnormality of MSH2, with or without abnormality of MSH6, will generally indicate a mutation in *MSH2* (and similarly MLH1, with or without abnormality of PMS2, will generally indicate a mutation in *MLH1*). However, in those rare families with mutations in *MSH6* their tumours usually show abnormality of MSH6 alone (and similarly PMS2 abnormality alone would imply a mutation in *PMS2*). One limitation of IHC is that about 30% of HNPCC-associated tumours with MMR deficiency, and thus MSI, do not have abnormal MMR protein immunostaining, whereas the vast majority of, if not all, tumours with abnormal IHC have MSI. The presence or absence of MSI indicates normal or abnormal MMR, whereas abnormal IHC, when present, will indicate the gene at fault as well as MSI. Thus, the two techniques are complementary.

Testing for MSI involves analysis of a range of microsatellites. It is now evident that there are subtle differences in the information obtained from different

MLH1

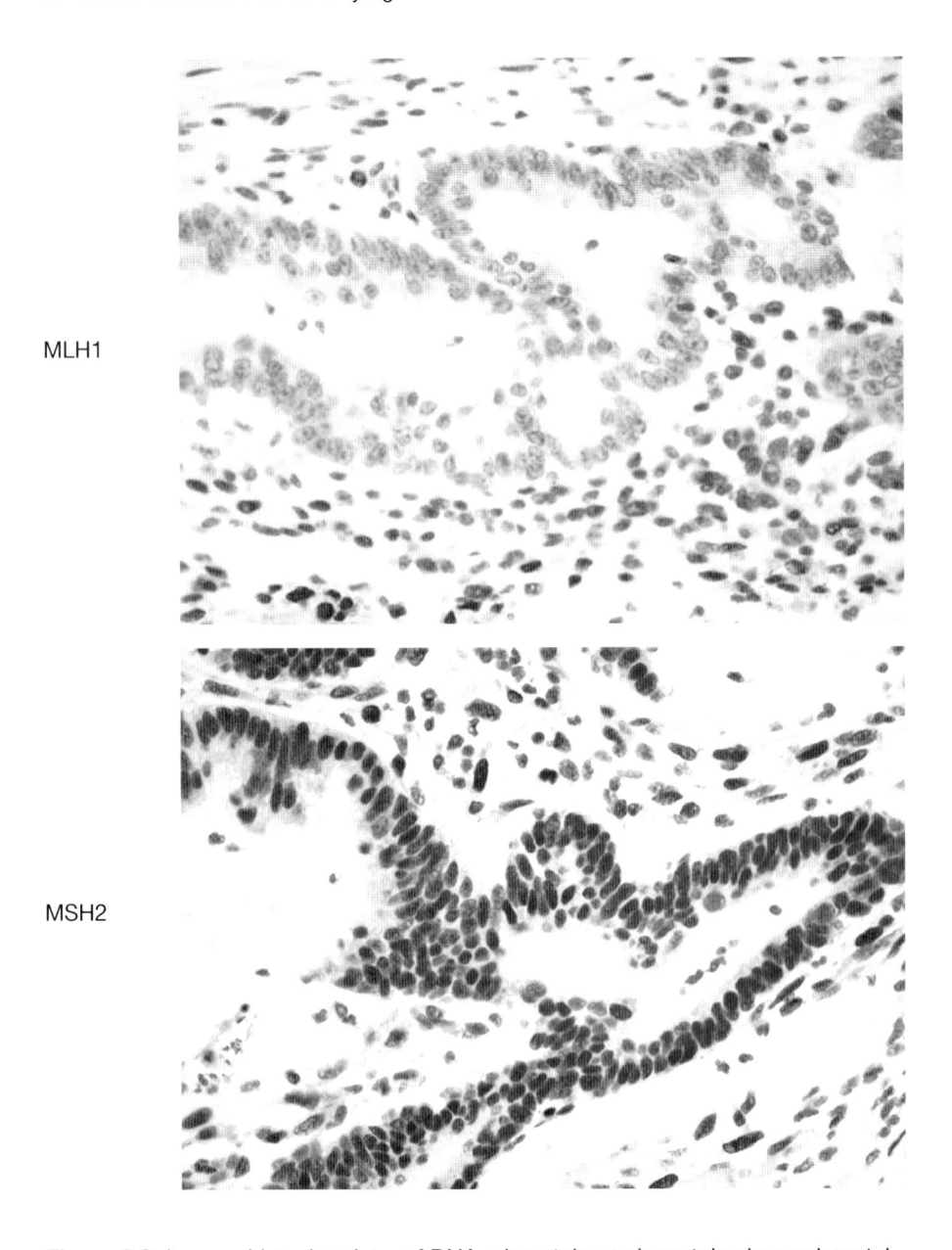

MSH2

Figure 2.2 Immunohistochemistry of DNA mismatch repair proteins in a colorectal cancer from an HNPCC patient with a germline mutation in *MLH1*. The antibodies specific to either MLH1 (top panel) or MSH2 (bottom panel) are bound to the cells within the tissues and stained red-brown; non-specific blue counterstaining is used to show nuclei not expressing MSH2 or MLH1. Note that normal tissues (lymphoid and stromal cells) express both proteins. The cancer cells stain strongly for MSH2, but they lack MLH1 staining.

microsatellites (Lamberti *et al.* 1999; Frayling 2002). Overall, a diagnosis of MSI in a tumour is based on testing several loci, at least five (defined by the ICG-HNPCC), and finding instability in at least two of the markers tested (Boland *et al.* 1998). In practice, tumours are classified as MSI-H (for high frequency), if more than 29% of markers tested show MSI, or as microsatellite stable (MSS) if no markers show MSI, and MSI-L (for low frequency), if >0% but <29% of markers show MSI. Tumours with MSI-H are likely to show loss of MMR on IHC, and exhibit other pathological features, such as mucinous histology and lymphocytic infiltration, whereas MSS and MSI-L tumours often do not to show these properties. Some have found that MSI-L tumours are more likely to have lost expression of another DNA repair protein (MGMT), but recent work has shown that if enough microsatellites are tested instability will sooner or later be observed in all tumours (Halford *et al.* 2002). Thus, MSS and MSI-L tumours would appear to represent one group of tumours, distinct from MSI-H tumours. Microsatellites which are mononucleotide repeats, e.g. $(A)_n$ or $(C)_n$, appear to be more specific for MSI-H, compared with dinucleotide (or greater) repeats, e.g. $(CA)_n$.

Experience in Cambridge suggests that a pragmatic approach to MSI testing is appropriate. Tumour DNA can be reliably extracted from three or four 10 μm paraffin sections, or from a single 50 μm section, of histopathologically confirmed tumour (Frayling 2002). A panel of 10 microsatellite markers is used, including 5 markers combined in a single PCR multiplex reaction (Sutter *et al.* 1999), and the panel is designed to cover both MSI-H and MSI-L/MSS detection, with 3 mono-nucleotide markers (*BAT-25, BAT-26, BAT-40*) and 7 dinucleotide markers (*D5S346, ACTC, D17S250, D13S153, D5S406, D5S107, D2S123*). The PCR primers are fluorescently tagged with differently coloured dyes to allow exploitation of fluorescent technology by use of DNA analysers that can detect multiple colours. Thus, all the PCR products can be run together in one lane. Microsatellite instability is defined as 'the presence of extra alleles', and this is sensitively detected using standard fluorescent DNA fragment analysis software (see Figure 2.3) (Frayling 2002).

Although about 20% of sporadic colon cancers exhibit MSI, only a small proportion of these, perhaps 1 or 2 in 20, will be due to HNPCC. However, most of the 1–2% of rectal cancers with MSI are due to HNPCC (Nilbert *et al.* 1999). Likewise, MSI is only very rarely found in sporadic adenomas, but the adenomas found in HNPCC commonly, but by no means always, have MSI (Loukola *et al.* 1999; Frayling 1999). Thus, finding MSI in an adenoma or rectal cancer is good evidence of HNPCC.

Of the 20% of sporadic colon cancers with MSI, approximately three-quarter (15%) are due to *MLH1* promoter hypermethylation causing epigenetic silencing of *MLH1* (Kuismanen *et al.* 2000). Of the remaining quarter (5%), about half are found to be due to HNPCC on further examination (Thibodeau *et al.* 1998). *MLH1* promoter hypermethylation can also be found in a few HNPCC tumours, as the mechanism of

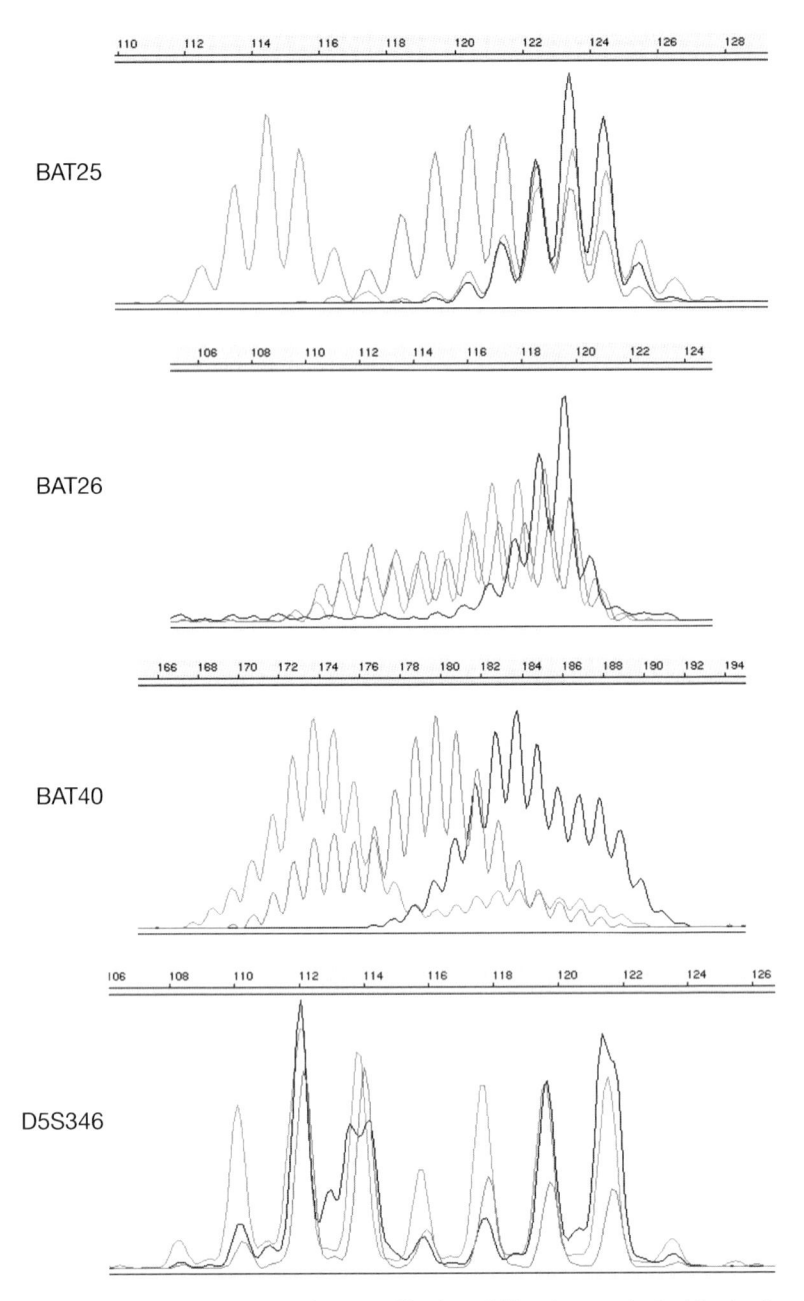

Figure 2.3 High-frequency microsatellite instability demonstrated by testing DNA extracted from two adenomas (one as a red trace, the other in blue) resected from the same HNPCC case, compared to normal blood DNA (black trace) of the same individual. The microsatellites BAT25, BAT26 and BAT40 (all mononucleotide markers) and D5S346 (dinucleotide marker) are shown. Extra alleles are clearly present in the blue and red traces compared to the normal black trace for all markers tested.*

* The Editors regret that it has not been possible to reproduce this illustration in colour and readers are invited to contact the authors directly for a colour e-mail.

inactivation of the wild-type gene, so it is not entirely specific for sporadic cancers (Wheeler et al. 2000a, 2000b). Colorectal cancers with MSI, whether sporadic or due to HNPCC, have generally been found to have a better prognosis in terms of survival, at least in part due to a better response to 5-fluorouracil (5-FU)-based chemotherapy (Elsaleh et al. 2000; Houlston et al. 2001).

Conclusions

Tumour analysis by both mismatch repair protein immunohistochemistry and microsatellite instability testing is necessary to provide a comprehensive picture of molecular abnormality, for use in conjunction with family history data and other pathological features, in order to diagnose HNPCC cancers. Even without germline mutation detection, this combination allows diagnosis or exclusion of HNPCC. With germline mutation detection, the tumour analysis data permit appropriate interpretation of mutations, especially those predicting amino acid mis-senses and mRNA splicing abnormalities. This combined approach based on tumour analysis becomes increasingly powerful when (a) there are several tumours available for examination from the same individual, and/or (b) there are several tumours available from different affected individuals in the family, and/or (c) either adenomas and/or rectal cancers are available for study. Given the utility of tumour analysis in the investigation of HNPCC and in the provision of information highly relevant to prognosis and treatment responsiveness of sporadic colorectal cancers, there is now an increasingly strong argument that such tumour analysis should become part of routine practice for sporadic and suspected HNPCC colorectal tumours.

Acknowledgements

We thank Lisa Happerfield and Nikki Wood (Molecular Histopathology, Addenbrooke's Hospital, Cambridge), Jeremy Jass (Brisbane), Gabriela Moslein (Dusseldorf), Melissa Southey (Melbourne) and Ian Tomlinson (Cancer Research UK, London) for contributions to development of this analytical approach.

References

Aaltonen, L. A., Peltomaki, P., Leach, F. S., Sistonen, P., Pylkkanen, L., Mecklin, J. P., Jarvinen, H., Powell, S. M., Jen, J. & Hamilton, S. R. (1993). Clues to the pathogenesis of familial colorectal cancer. *Science* **260**, 812–816.

Abdel-Rahman, W. M, Georgiades, I. B., Curtis, L. J., Arends, M. J. & Wyllie, A. H. (1999). Role of BAX mutations in mismatch repair-deficient colorectal carcinogenesis. *Oncogene* **18**, 2139–2142.

Abdel-Rahman, W. M., Katsura, K., Rens, W., Gorman, P. A., Sheer, D., Bicknell, D., Bodmer, W. F., Arends, M. J., Wyllie, A. H. & Edwards, P. A. (2001). Spectral karyotyping suggests additional subsets of colorectal cancers characterized by pattern of chromosome rearrangement. *Proceedings of the National Academy of Sciences of the United States of America* **98**, 2538–2543.

Boland, C. R., Thibodeau, S. N., Hamilton, S. R., Sidransky, D., Eshleman, J. R., Burt, R. W., Meltzer, S. J., Rodriguez-Bigas, M. A., Fodde, R., Ranzani, G. N. et al. (1998). A National Cancer Institute workshop on microsatellite instability for cancer detection and familial predisposition: development of international criteria for the determination of microsatellite instability in colorectal cancer. *Cancer Research* **58**, 5248–5257.

Bronner, C. E., Baker, S M., Morrison, P. T., Warren, G., Smith, L. G., Lescoe, M. K., Kane, M., Earabino, C., Lipford, J. & Lindblom, A. (1994). Mutation in the DNA mismatch repair gene homologue hMLH1 is associated with hereditary non-polyposis colon cancer. *Nature* **368**, 258–261.

Cawkwell, L., Gray, S., Murgatroyd, H., Sutherland, F., Haine, L., Longfellow, M., O'Loughlin, S., Cross, D., Kronborg, O. & Fenger, C. et al. (1999). Choice of management strategy for colorectal cancer based on a diagnostic immunohistochemical test for defective mismatch repair. *Gut* **45**, 409–415.

Chaves, P., Cruz, C., Lage, P., Claro, I., Cravo, M., Leitao, C. N. & Soares, J. (2000). Immunohistochemical detection of mismatch repair gene proteins as a useful tool for the identification of colorectal carcinoma with the mutator phenotype. *Journal of Pathology* **191**, 355–360.

Cohen, P. R., Kohn, S. R. & Kurzrock, R. (1991). Association of sebaceous gland tumours and internal malignancy: the Muir-Torre syndrome. *American Journal of Medicine* **90**, 606–613.

Cunningham, J. M., Christensen, E. R., Tester, D. J., Kim, C. Y., Roche, P. C., Burgart, L. J. & Thibodeau, S. N. (1998). Hypermethylation of the hMLH1 promoter in colon cancer with microsatellite instability. *Cancer Research* **58**, 3455–3460.

Dietmaier, W., Wallinger, S., Bocker, T., Kullmann, F., Fishel, R. & Ruschoff, J. (1997). Diagnostic microsatellite instability: definition and correlation with mismatch repair protein expression. *Cancer Research* **57**, 4749–4756.

Elsaleh, H., Powell, B., Soontrapornchai, P., Joseph, D., Goria, F., Spry, N., Iacopetta, B. (2000). p53 gene mutation, microsatellite instability and adjuvant chemotherapy: impact on survival of 388 patients with Dukes' C colon carcinoma. *Oncology* **58**, 52–59.

Esteller, M., Fraga, M. F., Guo, M., Garcia-Foncillas, J., Hedenfalk, I., Godwin, A. K., Trojan, J., Vaurs-Barriere, C., Bignon, Y. J., Ramus, S. et al. (2001). DNA methylation patterns in hereditary human cancers mimic sporadic tumorigenesis. *Human Molecular Genetics* **10**, 3001–3007.

Fearon, E. R. & Vogelstein, B. (1990). A genetic model for colorectal tumorigenesis. *Cell* **61**, 759–767.

Fink, D., Nebel, S., Aebi, S., Zheng, H., Kim, H. K., Christen, R. D. & Howell, S. B. (1997). Expression of the DNA mismatch repair proteins hMLH1 and hPMS2 in normal human tissues. *British Journal of Cancer* **76**, 890–893.

Fishel, R. , Lescoe, M. K., Rao, M. R., Copeland, N. G., Jenkins, N. A., Garber, J., Kane, M. & Kolodner, R. (1993). The human mutator gene homolog MSH2 and its association with hereditary nonpolyposis colon cancer. *Cell* **75**, 1027–1038. [Erratum in: *Cell* 1994 **77**, 167.]

Fishel, R. (2001). The selection for mismatch repair defects in hereditary nonpolyposis colorectal cancer: revising the mutator hypothesis. *Cancer Research* **61**, 7369–7374.

Frayling, I. M. (1999). Microsatellite instability. *Gut* **45**, 1–4.

Frayling, I. M. (2002). Methods of molecular analysis: mutation detection in solid tumours. *Molecular Pathology* **55**, 73–79.

Gryfe, R., Kim, H., Hsieh, E. T., Aronson, M. D., Holowaty, E. J., Bull, S. B., Redston, M. & Gallinger, S. (2000). Tumor microsatellite instability and clinical outcome in young patients with colorectal cancer. *New England Journal of Medicine* **342**, 69–77.

Halford, S., Sasieni, P., Rowan, A., Wasan, H., Bodmer, W., Talbot, I., Hawkins, N., Ward, R. & Tomlinson, I. (2002). Low-level microsatellite instability occurs in most colorectal cancers and is a nonrandomly distributed quantitative trait. *Cancer Research* **62**, 53–57.

Homfray, T. F., Cottrell, S. E., Ilyas, M., Rowan, A., Talbot, I. C., Bodmer, W. F. & Tomlinson, I. P. (1998). Defects in mismatch repair occur after APC mutations in the pathogenesis of sporadic colorectal tumours. *Human Mutation* **11**, 114–120.

Houlston R. S. (2001). What we could do now: molecular pathology of colorectal cancer. *Journal of Clinical Pathology: Molecular Pathology* **54**, 206–214.

Jass, J. R. (1998). Diagnosis of hereditary non-polyposis colorectal cancer. *Histopathology* **32**, 491–497.

Jass, J. R., Walsh, M. D., Barker, M., Simms, L. A., Young, J. & Leggett, B. A. (2002). Distinction between familial and sporadic forms of colorectal cancer showing DNA microsatellite instability. *European Journal of Cancer* **38**, 858–866.

Jiménez-Liñán, M., Frayling, I. M., Happerfield, L., Wood, N. & Arends, M. J. (2004). Microsatellite instability, mutation probability and different immunohistochemical expression patterns of hMSH2, hMLH1 and hMSH6 in normal tissues and tumours from hereditary non-polyposis colorectal cancer families. (Submitted.)

Kinzler, K. & Vogelstein, B. (1996). Lessons from hereditary colorectal cancer. *Cell* **87**, 159–170.

Kolodner, R. D., Hall, N. R., Lipford, J., Kane, M. F., Rao, M. R., Morrison, P., Wirth, L., Finan, P. J., Burn, J. & Chapman, P. (1994). Structure of the human MSH2 locus and analysis of two Muir-Torre kindreds for MSH2 mutations. *Genomics* **24**, 516–526.

Kolodner, R. D. & Marsischky, G. T. (1999). Eukaryotic DNA mismatch repair. *Current Opinion in Genetics & Development* **9**, 89–96.

Kuismanen, S. A, Holmberg, M T., Salovaara, R, de la Chapelle, A., Peltomaki, P. (2000). Genetic and epigenetic modification of MLH1 accounts for a major share of microsatellite-unstable colorectal cancers. *American Journal of Pathology* **156**, 1773–1779.

Lamberti, C., Kruse, R., Ruelfs, C., Caspari, R., Wang, Y., Jungck, M., Mathiak, M., Malayeri, H. R., Friedl, W., Sauerbruch, T. *et al.* (1999). Microsatellite instability – a useful diagnostic tool to select patients at high risk for hereditary non-polyposis colorectal cancer: a study in different groups of patients with colorectal cancer. *Gut* **44**, 839–843.

Leach, F. S., Nicolaides, N. C., Papadopoulos, N., Liu, B., Jen, J., Parsons, R., Peltomaki, P., Sistonen, P., Aaltonen, L. A. & Nystrom-Lahti, M. (1993). Mutations of a mutS homolog in hereditary nonpolyposis colorectal cancer. *Cell* **75**, 1215–1225.

Leach, F. S., Polyak, K., Burrell, M., Johnson, K. A., Hill, D., Dunlop, M. G., Wyllie, A. H., Peltomaki, P., de la Chapelle, A., Hamilton, S. R. *et al.* (1996). Expression of the human mismatch repair gene hMSH2 in normal and neoplastic tissues. *Cancer Research* **56**, 235–240.

Lothe, R. A., Peltomaki, P., Meling, G. I., Aaltonen, L. A., Nystrom-Lahti, M., Pylkkanen, L., Heimdal, K., Andersen, T. I., Moller, P. & Rognum, T. O. (1993). Genomic instability in colorectal cancer: relationship to clinicopathological variables and family history. *Cancer Research* **53**, 5849–5852.

Loukola, A., Salovaara, R., Kristo, P., Moisio, A. L., Kaariainen, H., Ahtola, H., Eskelinen, M., Harkonen, N., Julkunen, R., Kangas, E. *et al.* (1999). Microsatellite instability in adenomas as a marker for hereditary nonpolyposis colorectal cancer. *American Journal of Pathology* **155**, 1849–1853.

Loukola, A., Vilkki, S., Singh, J., Launonen, V. & Aaltonen, L. A. (2000). Germline and somatic mutation analysis of MLH3 in MSI-positive colorectal cancer. *American Journal of Pathology* **157**, 347–352.

Lynch, H. T., Smyrk, T. C., Watson, P., Lanspa, S J., Lynch, J. F., Lynch, P. M., Cavalieri, R. J. & Boland, C. R. (1993). Genetics, natural history, tumour spectrum, and pathology of hereditary non-polyposis colorectal cancer: an updated review. *Gastroenterology* **104**, 1535–1549.

Lynch, H. T., Smyrk, T. & Lynch, J. (1997). An update of HNPCC (Lynch syndrome). *Cancer Genetics and Cytogenetics* **93**, 84–89.

Lynch, H. T., Smyrk, T. & Lynch, J. F. (1998). Molecular genetics and clinical-pathology features of HNPCC (Lynch syndrome): historical journey from pedigree anecdote to molecular genetic confirmation. *Oncology* **55**, 103–108.

Lynch, H. T. & de la Chapelle, A. (1999). Genetic susceptibility to non-polyposis colorectal cancer. *Journal of Medical Genetics* **36**, 801–818.

Marcus, V. A., Madlensky, L., Gryfe, R., Kim, H., So, K., Millar, A., Temple, L. K., Hsieh, E., Hiruki, T. & Narod, S. *et al.* (1999). Immunohistochemistry for MLH1 and MSH2: a practical test for DNA mismatch repair-deficient tumors. *American Journal of Surgical Pathology* **23**, 1248–1255.

Mecklin, J. P. & Jarvinen, H. (1991). Tumour spectrum in cancer family syndrome (hereditary nonpolyposis colorectal cancer). *Cancer* **68**, 1109–1112.

Mecklin, J. P., Jarvinen, H. J., Hakkiluoto, A., Hallikas, H., Hiltunen, K. M., Harkonen, N., Kellokumpu, I., Laitinen, S., Ovaska, J. & Tulikoura, J. (1995). Frequency of hereditary nonpolyposis colorectal cancer. A prospective multicenter study in Finland. *Diseases of the Colon and Rectum* **38**, 588–593.

Nicolaides, N. C., Papadopoulos, N., Liu, B., Wei, Y. F., Carter, K. C., Ruben, S. M., Rosen, C. A., Haseltine, W. A., Fleischmann, R. D. & Fraser, C. M. (1994). Mutations of two PMS homologues in hereditary nonpolyposis colon cancer. *Nature* **371**, 75–80.

Nilbert, M., Planck, M., Fernebro, E., Borg, A. & Johnson, A. (1999). Microsatellite instability is rare in rectal carcinomas and signifies hereditary cancer. *European Journal of Cancer* **35**, 942–945.

Papadopoulos, N., Nicolaides, N. C., Wei, Y. F., Ruben, S. M., Carter, K. C., Rosen, C. A., Haseltine, W. A., Fleischmann, R. D., Fraser, C. M. & Adams, M. D. (1994). Mutation of a mutL homolog in hereditary colon cancer. *Science* **263**, 1559–1560.

Parc, Y. R., Halling, K. C., Wang, L., Christensen, E. R., Cunningham, J. M., French, A. J., Burgart, L. J., Price-Troska, T. L., Roche, P. C. & Thibodeau, S. N. (2000). hMSH6 alterations in patients with microsatellite instability-low colorectal cancer. *Cancer Research* **60**, 2225–2231.

Peltomaki, P., Aaltonen, L. A., Sistonen, P., Pylkkanen, L., Mecklin, J. P., Jarvinen, H., Green, J. S., Jass, J. R., Weber, J. L. & Leach F. S. (1993a). Genetic mapping of a locus predisposing to human colorectal cancer. *Science* **260**, 810–812.

Peltomaki, P., Lothe, R. A., Aaltonen, L A., Pylkkanen, L., Nystrom-Lahti, M., Seruca, R., David, L., Holm, R., Ryberg, D. & Haugen A. (1993b). Microsatellite instability is associated with tumors that characterize the hereditary non-polyposis colorectal carcinoma syndrome. *Cancer Research* **53**, 5853–5855.

Peltomaki, P. (2001a). Deficient DNA mismatch repair: a common etiologic factor for colon cancer. *Human Molecular Genetics* **10**, 735–740.

Peltomaki, P. (2001b). DNA mismatch repair and cancer. *Mutatation Research* **488**, 77–85.

Sutter, C., Gebert, J., Bischoff, P., Herfarth, C. & von Knebel Doeberitz, M. (1999). Molecular screening of potential HNPCC patients using a multiplex microsatellite PCR system. *Molecular and Cellular Probes* **13**, 157–165.

Terdiman, J. P., Gum, J. R. Jr, Conrad, P. G., Miller, G. A., Weinberg, V., Crawley, S. C., Levin, T. R., Reeves, C., Schmitt, A., Hepburn, M. *et al.* (2001). Efficient detection of hereditary nonpolyposis colorectal cancer gene carriers by screening for tumor microsatellite instability before germline genetic testing. *Gastroenterology* **120**, 21–30.

Thibodeau, S. N., Bren, G. & Schaid, D. (1993). Microsatellite instability in cancer of the proximal colon. *Science* **260**, 816–819.

Thibodeau, S. N., French, A. J., Roche, P. C., Cunningham, J. M., Tester, D. J., Lindor, N. M., Moslein, G., Baker, S. M., Liskay, R. M., Burgart, L. J. *et al.* (1996). Altered expression of hMSH2 and hMLH1 in tumors with microsatellite instability and genetic alterations in mismatch repair genes. *Cancer Research* **56**, 4836–4840.

Thibodeau, S. N., French, A. J., Cunningham, J. M., Tester, D., Burgart, L. J., Roche, P. C., McDonnell, S. K., Schaid, D. J., Vockley, C. W., Michels, V. V. *et al.* (1998). Microsatellite instability in colorectal cancer: Different mutator phenotypes and the principal involvement of hMLH1. *Cancer Research* **58**, 1713–1718.

Toft, N. J. & Arends, M. J. (1998). DNA mismatch repair and colorectal cancer. *Journal of Pathology* **185**, 123–129.

Toft, N. J., Winton, D. J., Kelly, J., Howard, L. A., Dekker, M., te Riele, H., Arends, M. J., Wyllie, A. H., Margison, G. P. & Clarke A. R. (1999). Msh2 status modulates both apoptosis and mutation frequency in the murine small intestine. *Proceedings of the National Academy of Sciences of the United States of America* **96**, 3911–3915.

Toft, N. J., Curtis, L. J., Sansom, O. J., Leitch, A. L., Wyllie, A. H., Te Riele, H., Arends, M. J., Clarke, A. R. (2002). Heterozygosity for p53 promotes microsatellite instability and tumorigenesis on a Msh2 deficient background. *Oncogene* **21**, 6299–6306.

Tomlinson, I. P., Novelli, M. R. & Bodmer, W. F. (1996). The mutation rate and cancer. *Proceedings of the National Academy of Sciences of the United States of America* **93**, 14,800–14,803.

Tomlinson, I. & Bodmer, W. (1999). Selection, the mutation rate and cancer: ensuring that the tail does not wag the dog. *Nature Medicine* **5**, 11–12.

Trimbath, J. D., Petersen, G. M., Erdman, S. H., Ferre, M., Luce, M. C. & Giardello, F. (2001). Café-au-lait spots and early onset colorectal neoplasia: a variant of HNPCC? *Familial Cancer* **1**, 101–105.

Vasen, H. F., Watson, P., Mecklin, J. P. & Lynch, H. T. (1999). New clinical criteria for hereditary non-polyposis colorectal cancer (HNPCC, Lynch syndrome) proposed by the ICG-HNPCC. *Gastroenterology* **116**, 1453–1456.

Wagner, A., Hendriks, Y., Meijers-Heijboer, E. J., de Leeuw, W. J., Morreau, H., Hofstra, R., Tops, C., Bik, E., Brocker-Vriends, A. H., van Der Meer, C. *et al.* (2001). Atypical HNPCC owing to MSH6 germline mutations: analysis of a large Dutch pedigree. *Journal of Medical Genetics* **38**, 318–322.

Ward, R., Meagher, A., Tomlinson, I., O'Connor, T., Norrie, M., Wu, R., Hawkins, N. (2001). Microsatellite instability and the clinicopathological features of sporadic colorectal cancer. *Gut* **48**, 821–829.

Warthin, A. (1913). Heredity with reference to carcinoma. *Archives of Internal Medicine* **12**, 546–555.

Watson, P. & Lynch, H. T. (1993). Extracolonic cancer in hereditary non-polyposis colorectal cancer. *Cancer* **71**, 677–685.

Watson, P. & Lynch, H. T. (1994). The tumour spectrum in HNPCC. *Anticancer Research* **14**, 1635–1639.

Wheeler, J. M. D., Bodmer, W. F. & Mortensen, (2000a). DNA mismatch repair genes and colorectal cancer. *Gut* **47**, 148–153.

Wheeler, J. M., Loukola, A., Aaltonen, L. A., Mortensen, N. J. & Bodmer W. F. (2000b). The role of hypermethylation of the hMLH1 promoter region in HNPCC versus MSI+ sporadic colorectal cancers. *Journal of Medical Genetics* **37,** 588–592.

Wijnen, J. T., Vasen, H. F., Khan, P. M., Zwinderman, A. H., van der Klift, H., Mulder, A., Tops, C., Moller, P. & Fodde, R. (1998). Clinical findings with implications for genetic testing in families with clustering of colorectal cancer. *New England Journal of Medicine* **339**, 511–518.

Wijnen, J., de Leeuw, W., Vasen, H., van der Klift, H., Moller, P., Stormorken, A., Meijers-Heijboer, H., Lindhout, D., Menko, F., Vossen S. *et al.* (1999). Familial endometrial cancer in female carriers of MSH6 mutations. *Nature Genetics* **23**, 142–144.

Wilson, T. M., Ewel, A., Duguid, J. R., Eble, J. N., Lescoe, M. K., Fishel, R. Kelley, M. R. (1995). Differential cellular expression of the human MSH2 repair enzyme in small and large intestine. *Cancer Research* **55**, 5146–5150.

Wu, Y., Berends, M. J., Mensink, R. G., Kempinga, C., Sijmons, R. H., van Der Zee, A. G., Hollema, H., Kleibeuker, J. H., Buys, C. H. & Hofstra, R. M. (1999). Association of hereditary nonpolyposis colorectal cancer-related tumours displaying low microsatellite instability with MSH6 germline mutations. *American Journal of Human Genetics* **65**, 1291–1298.

Yin, J., Kong, D., Wang, S., Zou, T. T., Souza, R. F., Smolinski, K. N., Lynch, P. M., Hamilton, S. R., Sugimura, H., Powell, S. M. *et al.* (1997). Mutation of hMSH3 and hMSH6 mismatch repair genes in genetically unstable human colorectal and gastric carcinomas. *Human Mutation* **10**, 474–478.

Chapter 3

Genetic differences between left- and right-sided bowel cancer and their relation to prognosis and management

Julian W. Adlard and Susan D. Richman

Introduction

Carcinomas may develop in any part of the large bowel. These are most often adenocarcinomas with variable grades of differentiation. In 2000, there were 35,300 new cases of colorectal cancer in the UK (Cancer Research UK 2004), with 54% occurring in men and 46% in women: 37% were rectal cancers and 63% colon cancers. Rectal cancers are relatively more common in men (42%) than in women (33%).

Approximately 7% of carcinomas develop in the descending colon and 18% in the sigmoid colon. Therefore, taking the splenic flexure as the dividing point between the 'left' and 'right' side of the colon, about 40% of carcinomas are right-sided and 60% are left-sided (Figure 3.1). Clinical differences between proximal and distal large bowel carcinomas have been known for many years. Cancers of the right colon tend to present at a later stage, with chronic anaemia and weight loss. Cancers of the distal colon and rectum characteristically present with rectal bleeding, change in bowel habit and tenesmus. The different presentation is due predominantly to differences in diameter of bowel lumen and consistency of stools. Bowel obstruction is also likely to occur earlier with distal tumours. Bleeding is less apparent in proximal colon tumours, which may present with positive faecal occult blood tests or occasionally melaena.

The management of colorectal cancer also varies according to site. In particular, surgery differs for colon and rectal cancer due to anatomical considerations. The use of total mesorectal excision (TME) significantly reduces recurrence rates for rectal cancer. Abdomino-perineal resection may be required, particularly for low rectal cancers. Radiotherapy is useful in the treatment of rectal cancer, but is rarely used for colon cancer due to toxicity to adjacent organs such as small bowel, kidneys and liver. The use of chemotherapy for colorectal cancer has not generally varied according to site of disease. There have been suggestions that, in the adjuvant setting, 5-fluorouracil (5-FU) is less effective in rectal cancer than colon cancer. This is in part due to less evidence being available for adjuvant chemotherapy for rectal cancer. Trials are increasingly examining the role of combined chemotherapy and radiation

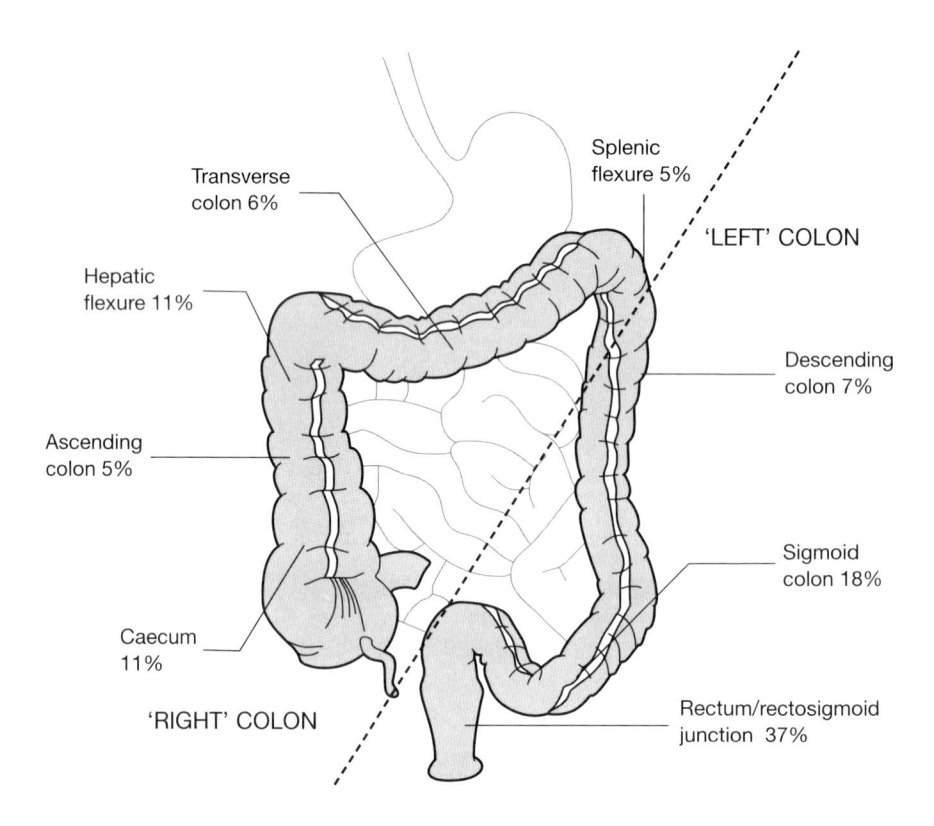

Figure 3.1 Division of the large bowel into left and right sides, and approximate distribution of cancers by site.

for rectal cancer. Some adjuvant chemotherapy trials such as MOSAIC have included only patients with colon cancer. The uncertain arm of the QUASAR trial suggests that 5-FU-based chemotherapy is also of benefit for rectal cancer (Gray et al. 2004).

Overall, the death rate from colorectal cancer is about 50%, thus representing a major cause of mortality in the UK. It is becoming clear that in addition to the differences in presentation and clinical management, there are significant genetic differences between left- and right-sided large bowel cancer. The reasons for these variations are not clear, but may be related to differences in embryological development, function or exposure to carcinogens at different sites of the large bowel. These differences may have important future implications for the assessment of prognosis and choice of therapy and are discussed in this chapter.

Microsatellite instability

Microsatellites are regions of DNA containing repetitive sequences of between one and six bases. For example, the BAT26 microsatellite is located on chromosome 7 and consists of a mononucleotide repeat of approximately 26 adenine bases. Mismatch repair proteins such as hMLH1 and hMSH2 are responsible for repair of DNA mismatches that may occur during DNA replication, either as a primary error or as the result of ionising radiation, chemical carcinogens or chemotherapy. Mismatches are most likely to occur in repetitive sequences such as microsatellites. Approximately 15% of all large bowel cancers show microsatellite instability (i.e. variations in the length of microsatellites) as the result of impaired function of mismatch repair genes. Tumours with high levels of microsatellite instability (MSI-H) are those showing MSI in 40% or more of microsatellites tested. Most often the impaired mismatch repair is as the result of inactivation of hMLH1 or hMSH2 by promoter methylation, leading to lack of protein expression when tested by immunohistochemistry.

It has been found that MSI-H is considerably more common in right-sided cancers (20–37%) than left-sided cancers (1–8%) (Gafa *et al.* 2000; Gryfe *et al.* 2000; Wright *et al.* 2000; Elsaleh *et al.* 2001). The reason for this difference is unclear. However, important differences in prognosis have also been identified. In two studies in which the majority of patients did not receive chemotherapy, MSI-H was associated with a significantly better prognosis than microsatellite stability (MSS) amounting to an absolute improvement in five-year survival of about 20% (Gryfe *et al.* 2000; Wright *et al.* 2000). MSI-H is associated with tumours showing a mucoid histological appearance and poor differentiation, but is associated with a lower stage of disease and reduced likelihood of metastases (Gryfe *et al.* 2000). A benefit in survival for MSI-H was seen in all stages of disease from I to IV. The improved survival also appears to apply to patients with MSI-H tumours occurring as a result of hereditary non-polyposis coli (HNPCC).

The question as to whether MSI-H is associated with greater response or resistance to chemotherapy has also been investigated. In cancer cell lines, MSI is associated with resistance to chemotherapeutic agents causing methylation or DNA-adducts such as temozolamide and cisplatin. It is postulated that DNA adducts caused by these agents are incompletely repaired by the mismatch repair system, leaving persistent lesions that are more lethal than the original adduct or base pair modification. A similar theory of 'futile' repair has been suggested for relative resistance to fluorouracil of mismatch repair deficient colon cancers cell lines such as HCT116 (Meyers *et al.* 2001).

In view of the cell line evidence it might therefore be expected that colorectal cancers *in vivo* with MSI-H would also be more resistant to fluorouracil. There have been conflicting reports. One Australian study has suggested that MSI (and right-sided cancers) may derive more benefit from adjuvant fluorouracil chemotherapy than MSS (or left-sided tumours) (Elsaleh *et al.* 2000). However, this was a retrospective study with only 56 MSI cases in total and was open to a number of potential biases. Also, the MSI cases who did not receive chemotherapy did not appear to have an improved prognosis which is contrary to findings in other studies mentioned above. A larger Canadian study has shown the more expected finding that MSI-H tumours are associated with an improved prognosis in the absence of chemotherapy and that adjuvant chemotherapy benefits MSS, but not MSI-H cancers (Ribic *et al.* 2003).

p53

The mutations of the p53 tumour suppressor gene occur relatively late in the Vogelstein model of colorectal carcinogenesis. Mutant p53 is usually, but not always, associated with positive staining for p53 protein on immunohistochemistry. p53 is involved in producing cell cycle arrest or apoptosis in response to DNA damage, including that resulting from chemotherapy. Several studies have shown that mutant p53 or positive immunohistochemistry is more common in left-sided bowel cancers (~55%) than in those on the right side (~34%) (Diez *et al.* 2000; Soong *et al.* 2000; Elsaleh *et al.* 2001; Gervaz *et al.* 2001; Kapiteijn *et al.* 2001; Smith *et al.* 2002). p53 mutations are also less commonly seen in MSI-H than in MSS cancers (Hawkins *et al.* 2002; Elsaleh *et al.* 2001). p53 has been associated with a worse prognosis in colorectal cancer, but there are conflicting accounts due to small sample sizes. One large study did not demonstrate a prognostic association (Soong *et al.* 2000). Mutant p53 has been linked to resistance to 5-FU in cancer cell lines (Bunz *et al.* 1999) and also in some clinical series (Anhen *et al.* 1998; Elsaleh *et al.* 2001).

Thymidylate synthase

High expression levels of thymidylate synthase have been associated with resistance to 5-FU in many studies (Adlard *et al.* 2002). TS expression may be increased in left-sided cancers and has also been noted to be increased in cancers with mutant p53 (Lenz *et al.* 1998). Therefore, mechanistically it is possible that the increased prevalence of mutant p53 and expression of thymidylate synthase in left-sided colorectal cancers could contribute to poorer prognosis and response to fluorouracil. Newer agents, such as irinotecan and oxaliplatin, may be more suitable for this group of tumours.

MGMT, *K-ras* and low-level microsatellite instability (MSI-L)

O6-methylguanine DNA methyl transferase (MGMT) removes methyl adducts from the O6 position of guanine and is responsible for cancer resistance to methylating agents such as lomustine. MGMT may protect the bowel mucosa from ingested alkylating carcinogens. One study has suggested that cancers occur more often in regions of normal bowel with low MGMT activity (Lees *et al.* 2002). MGMT is inactivated by promoter methylation in about 30% of colorectal cancers (Esteller *et al.* 2001), more commonly in right- than left-sided cancers. When O6-methyl adducts are not removed from guanine bases, DNA polymerase may misread the DNA during replication, producing an A-T base pair rather than G-C.

MGMT inactivation is associated with G to A mutations in the *K-ras* gene (Esteller *et al.* 2000), which has been associated with an adverse prognosis in colorectal cancer (Andreyev *et al.* 1998). MGMT inactivation is also associated with low-level microsatellite instability (MSI-L), possibly because of overload of the mismatch repair system (Whitehall *et al.* 2001).

Two studies have shown that K-*ras* mutations are more common in right-sided cancers (29–38%) than those on the left side (10–20%) (Bleeker *et al.* 2000; Samowitz *et al.* 2000). However, a conflicting study reported rectal cancers with more K-*ras* mutations than colonic cancers (39% versus 20%) (Smith *et al.* 2002). This study also suggested that mutations of both p53 and *K-ras* in the same cancer are rare (6%) and may suggest that *K-ras* mutations are predominantly associated with a different carcinogenesis pathway than that described by Vogelstein.

Colorectal cancers with wild-type *K-ras* may be more likely to respond to adjuvant chemotherapy than those with gene mutations (Anhen *et al. 1998*). Specific therapies may be targeted according to the tumour genotype, such as farnesyl transferase inhibitors for *K-ras* mutations and nitrosoureas for tumours with loss of function of MGMT (Adlard *et al.* 2002)

Vascular endothelial growth factor

Expression of growth factors or receptors such as vascular endothelial growth factor (VEGF) are associated with an adverse prognosis in colorectal cancer (Cascinu *et al.* 2000; White *et al.* 2002), though have not been directly linked with response or resistance to therapy. VEGF expression is reduced in cancers showing MSI-H (13%) compared with those that are MSS (38%) (Wynter *et al.* 1999). New treatments such as antibodies to VEGF or inhibitors of tyrosine kinases associated with growth factor receptors may be useful in these patients.

Conclusions

Increasing evidence is emerging of different pathways in colorectal carcinogenesis, that these differences vary with the site within the large bowel, and that they may have implications for prognosis and response to systemic therapy. The features seen predominantly in distal colonic or rectal lesions, such as aneuploidy, mutant p53, and increased VEGF expression have been associated with an adverse prognosis and possible reduced benefit from fluorouracil-based chemotherapy. In contrast, right-sided lesions are more likely to show gene hypermethylation, microsatellite instability and improved prognosis. The improved prognosis may be offset by the fact that symptoms from right-sided cancers often become evident at a later stage, and that appears to be associated with increased resistance to 5-FU-based chemotherapy.

Further large studies are required to correlate the genotype or phenotype of tumours with subsequent prognosis and response to therapy. At present, the evidence is not strong enough to allow selection of individualised systemic therapy outside clinical trials. However, the increasing number of agents becoming available for the treatment of colorectal cancer offers the future possibility of tailoring treatment to the molecular pathology of the individual tumour.

References

Adlard, J. W., Richman, S. D., Seymour, M. T., Quirke, P. (2002). Prediction of the response of colorectal cancer to systemic therapy. *Lancet Oncology* **3**, 65–82.

Andreyev, H. J., Norman, A. R., Cunningham, D. *et al.* (1998). Kirsten ras mutations in patients with colorectal cancer: the multicenter 'RASCAL' study. *Journal of the National Cancer Institute* **9**, 674–684.

Anhen, D. J., Feigl, P., Quan, G. *et al.* (1998). Ki-ras mutation and p53 overexpression predict the clinical behaviour of colorectal cancer: a Southwest Oncology Group study. *Cancer Research* **58**, 1149–1158.

Bleeker, W. A., Hayes, V. M., Karrenbeld, A. *et al.* (2000). Impact of KRAS and TP53 mutations on survival in patients with left- and right-sided Dukes' C colon cancer. *American Journal of Gastroenterology* **95**, 2953–2957.

Bunz, F., Hwang, P. M., Torrance, C. *et al.* (1999). Disruption of p53 in human cancer cells alters the responses to therapeutic agents. *Journal of Clinical Investigation* **104**, 263–269.

Cascinu, S., Staccioli, M. P., Gasparini, G. *et al.* (2000). Expression of vascular endothelial growth factor can predict event-free survival in stage II colon cancer. *Clinical Cancer Research* **6**, 1803–2807.

Diez, M., Medrano, M., Muguerza, J. M. *et al.* (2000). Influence of tumor localisation on the prognostic value of p53 protein in colorectal adenocarcinomas. *Anticancer Research* **20**, 3907–3912.

Elsaleh, H., Joseph, D., Grieu, F. *et al.* (2000). Association of tumour site and sex with survival benefit from adjuvant chemotherapy in colorectal cancer. *The Lancet* **355**, 1745–1750.

Elsaleh, H., Powell, B., McCaul, K. *et al.* (2001). P53 alteration and microsatellite instability have predictive value for survival benefit from chemotherapy in stage III colorectal carcinoma. *Clinical Cancer Research* **7**, 1343–1349.

Esteller, M., Toyota, M., Sanchez-Cespedes, M. *et al.* (2000). Inactivation of the DNA repair gene O6-methylguanine-DNA methyltransferase by promoter hypermethylation is associated with G to A mutations in K-ras in colorectal tumorigenesis. *Cancer Research* **60**, 2368–2371.

Esteller, M., Corn, P. G., Baylin, S. B. & Herman, J. G. (2001). A gene hypermethylation profile of human cancer. *Cancer Research* **61**, 3225–3229.

Gafa, R., Maestri, I., Matteuzzi, M. *et al.* (2000). Sporadic colorectal adenocarcinomas with high-frequency microsatellite instability. *Cancer* **89**, 2025–2037.

Gervaz, P., Bouzourene, H., Cerottini, J. P. *et al.* (2001). Dukes' B colorectal cancer: distinct genetic categories and clinical outcomes based on proximal or distal tumor location. *Diseases of the Colon and Rectum* **44**, 364–372.

Gray, R. G., Barnwell, J., Hills, R. *et al.* (2004). QUASAR: A randomized study of adjuvant chemotherapy (CT) versus observation including 3238 colorectal cancer patients. *Proceedings of the American Society of Clinical Oncology*, abstract 3501.

Gryfe, R., Kim, H., Hsieh, E. T. K. *et al.* (2000). Tumor microsatellite instability and clinical outcome in young patients with colorectal cancer. *New England Journal of Medicine* **342**, 69–77.

Hawkins, N., Norrie, M., Cheong, K. *et al.* (2002). CpG island methylation in sporadic colorectal cancers and its relationship to microsatellite instability. *Gastroenterology* **122**, 1376–1387.

Kapiteijn, E., Liefers, G. J., Los, L. C. *et al.* (2001). Mechanisms of oncogenesis in colon versus rectal cancer. *Journal of Pathology* **195**, 171–178.

Lees, N. P., Harrison, K. L., Hill, E. *et al.* (2002). Longitudinal variation in O6-alkylguanine DNA-alkyltransferase activity in the human colon and rectum, *British Journal of Cancer* **87**, 168–170.

Lenz, H. J., Danenberg, K. D., Leichman, C. G. *et al.* (1998). p53 and thymidylate synthase expression in untreated stage II colon cancer: associations with recurrence, survival, and site. *Clinical Cancer Research* **4**, 1227–1234.

Meyers, M., Wagner, M. W., Hwang, H.-S. *et al.* (2001). Role of the hMLH1 DNA mismatch repair protein in fluoropyrimidine-mediated cell death and cell cycle responses. *Cancer Research* **61**, 5193–5201.

Ribic, C. M., Sargent, D. J., Moore, M. J. *et al.* (2003). Tumor microsatellite-instability status as a predictor of benefit from fluorouracil-based adjuvant chemotherapy for colon cancer. *New England Journal of Medicine* **349**, 247–257.

Samowitz, W. S., Curtin, K., Schaffer, D. *et al.* (2000). Relationship of Ki-ras mutations in colon cancers to tumor location, stage, and survival: a population based study. *Cancer Epidemiology, Biomarkers and Prevention* **9**, 1193–1197.

Smith, G., Carey, F. A., Beattie, J. *et al.* (2002). Mutations in APC, Kirsten-ras, and p53 – alternative genetic pathways to colorectal cancer, *Proceedings of the National Academy of Sciences of the United States of America* **99**, 9433–9438.

Soong, R., Powell, B., Elsaleh, H. *et al.* (2000). Prognostic significance of TP53 gene mutation in 995 cases of colorectal carcinoma: influence of tumour site, stage, adjuvant chemotherapy and type of mutation. *European Journal of Cancer* **36**, 2053–2060.

White, J. D., Hewett, P. W., Kosuge, D. *et al.* (2002). Vascular endothelial growth factor-D expression is an independent prognostic marker for survival in colorectal carcinoma. *Cancer Research* **62**, 1669–1675.

Whitehall, V. L. J., Walsh, M. D., Young, J. *et al.* (2001). Methylation of O-6-methylguanine DNA methyltransferase characterises a subset of colorectal cancer with low-level DNA microsatellite instability. *Cancer Research* **61**, 827–830.

Wright, C. M., Dent, O. F., Barker M. *et al.* (2000). Prognostic significance of extensive microsatellite instability in sporadic clinicopathological stage C colorectal cancer. *British Journal of Surgery* **87**, 1197–1202.

Wynter, C. V. A., Simms, L. A., Buttenshaw, R. L. *et al.* (1999). Angiofactor VEGF is decreased in human colorectal neoplasms showing DNA microsatellite instability. *Journal of Pathology* **189**, 319–325.

Chapter 4

Clinical genetics and genetic counselling

Shirley Hodgson

Introduction

Colorectal cancer (CRC) is a common disease, occurring in approximately 1 in 35 of the UK population. Symptomatic presentation tends to be late, so endoscopic surveillance in individuals at increased risk of the condition is advocated in order to detect cancers at an earlier stage and thus improve outcomes. The problem is to define what level of familial risk is appropriate for surveillance and how frequent and in what form this should be. Long-term evaluation of screening outcome in relation to risk is required to inform future surveillance programmes (Marie *et al*. 1984; Kune *et al*. 1989; Ransohoff & Lang 1991; Stephenson *et al*. 1991; Hodgson *et al*. 1993, 1995; Burke *et al*. 1997; Markowitz & Winawer 1999; Burt 2000; Lieberman *et al*. 2000). Familial clustering of colorectal cancer may be ascribed to: rare single highly penetrant predisposing genes; commoner, lower penetrant genes; and common environmental factors; or a combination of these.

The rare conditions that are highly penetrant for cancer predisposition include the polyposes—of which familial adenomatous polyposis (FAP) is the most common. This autosomal dominant condition, occurring in 1 in 10,000 of the population, is characterised by florid adenomatous polyposis in the colon and an increased risk of gastric and duodenal polyps, hepatoblastoma, thyroid cancer, brain tumours and desmoid tumours. Black lesions known as CHRPE may be seen in the retina (congenital hypertrophy of the retinal pigment epithelium) (Tiret *et al.* 1997) and other extracolonic features include sebaceous cysts, exostoses, osteomas, supernumary teeth and fibromas. Surveillance should be initiated in the early teenage years in at-risk individuals, initially by annual sigmoidoscopy, but later by annual colonoscopy with dye-spray. Genetic testing is possible in a majority of families but not all, since the causative APC mutation cannot always be identified. In affected individuals after colectomy, surveillance of the rectal stump and duodenum should continue annually (Church *et al.* 1992; Guillem *et al.* 1992; Spirio *et al.* 1993; Campbell *et al.* 1994; Gardener *et al.* 1997; Giardiello *et al.* 1997; Wallace & Phillips 1998; Lynch 1999; King *et al.* 2000; Sieber *et al.* 2003).

Bi-allelic *MYH* mutations and 'attenuated polyposis'

Recently, it has been shown that bi-allelic germline mutations in the *MYH* gene (involved in base-excision repair of oxidative DNA damage) may account for a proportion of cases of 'attenuated polyposis', which is characterised by few to a few hundred colonic adenomas and later onset CRC. Bi-allelic germline *MYH* mutations have been detected in approximately a third of individuals with 30–100 colonic adenomas, and in approximately 10% of cases of FAP in whom no APC mutation had been detected. These individuals generally are at the milder end of the phenotypic spectrum for FAP (with fewer than 1,000 colonic adenomas) (Sieber *et al*. 2003). This is clearly of very great clinical and genetic counselling significance, since the condition is autosomal recessive, and the children of affected individuals should have a low risk of being affected (unless both parents carried germline mutations). The population frequency of *MYH* mutation carriers is about 1%, so this is a consideration. It is not known whether *MYH* heterozygotes have any increased risk of CRC although the risk is probably slight.

Other cases of 'attenuated polyposis' are caused by mutations in the 3' or 5' end of the *APC* gene, or to the E1307K *APC* mutation. The 11307K *APC* mutation confers an approximate 2-fold increase in risk of CRC, probably because it causes a poly-A tract in the gene which is hypermutable in somatic tissues (Spirio *et al*. 1993; Gardener *et al*. 1997; Giardello *et al*. 1997).

Rare autosomal dominant conditions characterised by hamartomatous gastrointestinal polyps include Peutz-Jegher syndrome, juvenile polyposis and Cowden syndrome. The genes in which inherited mutations cause these conditions are being identified. Peutz-Jegher syndrome (PJS) is an autosomal dominant condition characterised by pan-intestinal polyposis and mucocutaneous pigmentation, due to germline mutations in the *LKBI* gene. There is an increased risk of colorectal and other malignancies in this condition, including pancreatic, breast and ovarian (sex cord) tumours. Two-yearly upper and lower bowel surveillance by endoscopy is necessary for individuals with this condition; breast cancer screening and pelvic ultrasound for ovarian fibromas have also been advocated. (Tomlinson & Houlston 1997; Hemminki *et al*. 1998; Dunlop 2002a).

Juvenile polyposis (JP) is a heterogeneous condition often associated with extracolonic features. Hamartomatous polyps develop throughout the gastrointestinal tract but predominantly in the colorectum. Approximately one-third of cases are due to mutations in *BMPR1A* and one-third to mutations in *SMAD4*, but the rest remain unexplained (Zhou *et al*. 2001). Germline *PTEN* mutations cause Cowden's and Bannayan-Ruvalcaba-Smith syndromes, which may manifest juvenile polyposis, but have other phenotypic features that are diagnostic (lipomas, macrocephaly, genital pigmentation and an increased risk of breast and thyroid cancer) (Desai *et al*. 1995; Houlston *et al*. 1998; Howe *et al*. 1998; Jass *et al*. 1998; Woodford-Richens *et al*. 2000).

Hereditary non-polyposis colorectal cancer (HNPCC) is thought to be the cause of approximately 2% of all colorectal cancer. This autosomal dominant condition causes a high lifetime risk of colorectal cancer, this being more likely to be diagnosed at a young age, predominantly proximally sited and of mucinous histology, and there is a high incidence of multiple tumours, 18% presenting with synchronous cancers and 40–50% developing a second malignancy over the next 10–15 years after the first (Aarnio *et al.* 1995). There is also an increased risk of extracolonic cancers especially of the endometrium, small bowel, ureter, kidney, stomach and ovary. It is caused by inherited mutations in a group of genes involved in the repair of DNA 'mismatch' errors. About one-third of cases are caused by germline mutations in *MSH1* and a third by *MSH2* mutations. A minority are caused by *MSH6* mutations and these families are more likely to contain endometrial cancer cases, and to be microsatellite stable (MSI-S); other genes occasionally involved include *PMS1* and *PMS2* (Dunlop *et al.* 2000). The mutation cannot be identified in approximately 30% of cases.

Microsatellite instability can be detected in repetitive sequence DNA in tumour tissue as a result of failure of repair of DNA mismatches, and is characteristic in individuals with HNPCC (although it is seen in approximately 15% of sporadic cancers, probably associated with somatic methylation of *MLH1*). Lifetime risk of CRC in males with HNPCC is approximately 80%, but lower (approximately 40%) in affected females (Aarnio *et al.* 1995; Jarvinen *et al.* 1995, 2000; Syngal *et al.* 1998). Surveillance for individuals at risk of HNPCC should be by one- two-yearly colonoscopies from the age of 25 years (or earlier in families with early-onset cases) (De Vos tot Nederveen Cappel *et al.* 2002). Interval cancers have been detected in cases on two-yearly surveillance so yearly colonoscopies are preferable, but difficult to achieve in practice (Ahlquist 1995; Rodriguez-Bigas *et al.* 1997; Samowitz *et al.* 2001). Subtotal colectomy may be appropriate in cases diagnosed with a colorectal tumour. Endometrial cancer is common in HNPCC (up to 60% risk in affected women) – but screening for this has not yet been fully evaluated. Endometrial ultrasound and pipelle biopsy annually from 25 years age has been advocated.

Family testing strategy under debate

The strategy for determining which families to test for mutations is under debate. In families conforming to the Amsterdam criteria for HNPCC (three close relatives affected with CRC, one the first-degree relative of the others, two generations affected, one diagnosed below the age of 50; FAP excluded) there is a high yield of germline HNPCC mutation detection using current detection methods (up to 80%). Other family history criteria (modified Amsterdam and Bethesda criteria, which include other associated cancers as diagnostic of affected status, such as endometrial and small intestinal; see Table 4.1) have a lower yield of mutation positive cases (Rodriguez-Bigas *et al.* 1997). Individuals with a less strong family history of colon cancer have an even lower yield. Families may be classified into risk groups taking into account age at diagnosis, number of affected relatives and the presence of endometrial cancer in the family. A model proposed by Wijnen (Wijnen *et al.* 1997;

Ramsey *et al.* 2001) suggests that germline mutation testing for HNPCC should be performed in cases whose family history gives a 20% chance of identifying a mutation. (Syngal *et al.* 1998; Ramsey *et al.* 2001; Winawer *et al.* 2003a). In families with a smaller risk it is suggested that the tumour(s) be tested for microsatellite instability (MSI) and immunohistochemistry for HNPCC proteins. Only cases showing a MSI-high phenotype and/or abnormal staining for MSH2, MLH1 or MSH6 proteins would be analysed for germline mutations. (Rodriguez-Bigas *et al.* 1997; Vasen *et al.* 1999). The advantage of immunohistochemistry is that it indicates which gene is likely to harbour the causative mutation, although MSH2 and MSH6 staining may alter concurrently. At-risk individuals in families with identified HNPCC mutations can be offered predictive genetic testing. Families not found to have such mutations but with a strong family history may be at lesser risk of colorectal cancer, but recent evidence suggests that their cancer risk is still high and they should still be offered surveillance as for HNPCC (Bahmana *et al.* 2003).

Table 4.1 Clinical criteria for HNPCC

Amsterdam criteria (Vasen *et al.* 1991) (all of the criteria must be met)
1. At least three family members with colorectal cancer, two of whom are first-degree relatives
2. At least two generations affected
3. At least one individual less than 50 years old at diagnosis
4. FAP excluded

Modified Amsterdam criteria (Bellacosa *et al.* 1996)
1. Very small families, which cannot be further expanded, can be considered as HNPCC even if only two colorectal cancers are found (in the presence of the other criteria)
2. In families, with two first-degree relatives affected by colorectal cancer, the presence of a third relative with an early-onset unusual neoplasm or endometrial cancer is sufficient to consider the family as HNPCC

Bethesda criteria (Rodriguez-bigas *et al.* 1997)
1. Individuals with cancer families that meet the Amsterdam criteria
2. Individuals with two HNPCC-related cancer, including synchronous and metachronous or associated extracolonic cancers (endometrial, ovarian, hepatobiliary or small bowel cancers and transitional cell carcinoma of renal pelvis or ureter)
3. Individuals with colorectal cancer and a first-degree relative with colorectal cancer and/or HNPCC – extracolonic cancer and/or a colorectal adenoma; one of the cancers diagnosed at age <45 years, and the adenoma diagnosed at age <40 years
4. Individuals with colorectal cancer or endometrial cancer diagnosed at age <45 years
5. Individuals with right-sided colorectal cancer with an undifferentiated pattern (solid/cribriform) on histopathology diagnosed at age <45 years 6.
6. Individuals with signet-ring-cell-type colorectal cancer diagnosed at age <45 years
7. Individuals with adenomas diagnosed at age <40 years

There is an increased relative risk of colorectal cancer in the close relatives of colorectal cancer cases without features of the highly penetrant conditions described above. Risk increases as the age at diagnosis is earlier and the number of affected relatives greater. First-degree relatives of a single case have a 2- to 3-fold increased risk, rising to 4- to 5-fold in relatives of cases diagnosed below the age of 45 (Bonelli *et al.* 1988). The majority of such familial clustering is likely to be due to genes other than those causing HNPCC. Evidence to help develop the most effective screening strategy for such families is still being accumulated, but there is increasing consensus that some form of colonoscopic surveillance should be offered to individuals with a relative risk of developing CRC of four to five times the population risk. The chance of finding neoplasia below the age of 40 is small in this group, however, so some advocate that colonoscopic screening can be initiated at the age of 45, or 5 years before the earliest cancer in the family. It has also been suggested that screening should be by two colonoscopies, one at the age of 35 and one at 55 if the first was normal (Dunlop 2002b). Individuals who have a first-degree relative with CRC diagnosed below 45 years age, or with two affected first-degree relatives, are considered to qualify for such surveillance. Individuals with three close relatives affected on the same side of the family, including one first-degree relative, should also be considered for surveillance. This is based on best current evidence, but in the future it can only be evaluated in the light of further evidence from long-term audited surveillance in relation to prior risk. Screening guidelines for individuals with a family history of colorectal cancer conferring a moderately increased risk are therefore still being evaluated (Rozen *et al.* 1987; Bonelli *et al.* 1988; Ponz de Leone *et al.* 1989, 1999; St John *et al.* 1993; Dinning *et al.* 1994; Carpenter *et al.* 1995; Burke *et al.* 1997; Emery *et al.* 2000; Hampel & Peltomaki 2000; Winawer *et al.* 1993, 1997, 2003b).

Conclusion

There continues to be debate about whether to offer colonoscopic surveillance to individuals who carry germline mutations, which confer a 2-fold increase in risk of colorectal cancer. Examples are two Ashkenazi founder mutations – the *BLM ASHK* (Bloom's syndrome ancestral Ashkenazi mutation) and the *APC* 11307K mutations. It is possible that the identification of genes conferring a moderately increased risk of colorectal cancer may in the future lead to the development of multigene tests to provide a risk profile for colorectal and other cancers. However, the debate about what constitutes a sufficiently increased risk to justify colonoscopic surveillance will remain, as will the details of surveillance – when to start, and stop, and how often to perform endoscopies. New screening modalities such as computed tomographic colonography may simplify (or complicate) the issue (because of the need for colonoscopy if an abnormality is detected,) but continuing audit will undoubtedly be necessary. The development of national strategies must await the outcome of audited long-term follow-up of individuals at defined levels of risk.

References

Aarnio, M., Mecklin, J. P., Altonen, L. A. et al. (1995). Lifetime risks of different cancers in hereditary non-polyposis colorectal cancer (HNPCC) syndrome. *International Journal of Cancer* **64**, 430–433.

Ahlquist, D. A. (1995). Aggressive polyps in HNPCC: targets for screening. *Gastroenterology* **108**, 1590–1592.

Bahmana, J. et al. (2003). Prevalence of HNPCC cancers is not different between Amsterdam families with or without detectable MMR gene mutations. *Familial Cancer* **2** (Supplement 1), 25.

Bellacosa, A., Genuardi, M., Anti, M. et al. (1996). Hereditary nonpolyposis colorectal cancer: review of clinical, molecular genetics, and counselling aspects. *American Journal of Medical Genetics* **62**, 353–364.

Bonelli, L., Martines, H., Conio, M. et al. (1988). Family history of colorectal cancer as a risk factor for benign and malignant tumours of the large bowel. A case-control study. *International Journal of Cancer* **41**, 513–517.

Brewer, D., Fung, C., Chapuis, P., Bokey, E. (1994). Should relatives of patients with colorectal cancer be screened. *Diseases of the Colon and Rectum* **37**, 1328–1338.

Burke, W., Peterson, G., Lynch, P. et al. (1997). Recommendations for follow-up care of individuals with an inherited predisposition to cancer. *Journal of the American Medical Association* **277**, 915–919.

Burt, W. (2000). Colon cancer screening. *Gastroenterology* **119**, 837–853.

Campbell, W. J., Spence, R. A. & Parks T. G. (1994). Familial adenomatous polyposis. *British Journal of Surgery* **81**, 1722–1733.

Carpenter, S., Broughton, M., Marcs, C. G. (1995). A screening clinic for relatives of patients with colorectal cancer in a district general hospital. *Gut* **36**, 90–92.

Church, J. M., McGannon, E., Hull-Boiner, S. et al. (1992). Gastroduodenal polyps in patients with familial adenomatous polyposis. *Diseases of the Colon and Rectum* **35**, 1170–1173.

Desai, D. C., Neale, K. F., Talbot, I. C. et al. (1995). Juvenile polyposis. *British Journal of Surgery* **82**, 14–17.

De Vos tot Nederveen Cappel, W. H., Nagengast, F. M., Griffioen, G. et al. (2002). Surveillance for HNPCC: a long-term study on 114 families. *Diseases of the Colon and Rectum* **45**, 1588–1594.

Dinning, L., Hixson, L., Clark, L. (1994). Prevalence of distal colonic neoplasia associated with proximal colon cancers. *Archives of Internal Medicine* **154**, 853–856.

Dunlop, M. G. (2002a). Guidance on gastrointestinal surveillance for hereditary non-polyposis colorectal cancer, familial adenomatous polyposis, juvenile polyposis, and Peutx-Jeghers syndrome. *Gut* **51** (Supplement V), V21–V27.

Dunlop, M. G. (2002b). Guidance on large bowel surveillance for people with two first degree relatives with colorectal cancer or one first degree relative diagnosed with colorectal cancer under 45 years. *Gut* **51** (Supplement V), V17–V20.

Dunlop, M. G., Farrington, S. M., Nicholl, I. et al. (2000). Population carrier frequency of hMSH2 and hMLH1 mutations. *British Journal of Cancer* **83**, 1643–1645.

Emery, J., Murphy, M. & Lucassen, A. (2000). Hereditary cancer – the evidence for current recommended management. *Lancet Oncology*, **1**, 9–16.

Gardener, R. J., Kool, D., Edkins, E. et al. (1997). The clinical correlates of a 3' truncating mutation (codons 1982–1983) in the adenomatous polyposis coli gene. *Gastroenterology* **113**, 326–331.

Giardiello, F. M., Brensigner, J. D., Luce, M. C. et al. (1997). Phenotypic expression of disease in families that have mutations in the 5' region of the adenomatous polyposis coli gene. *Annals of Internal Medicine* **12,** 514–519.

Guillem, J. G., Forde, K. A., Treat, M. R. et al. (1992). Colonoscopic screening for neoplasms in asymptomatic first-degree relatives of colon cancer patients. A controlled, prospective study. *Diseases of the Colon and Rectum* **35**, 523–529.

Hampel, H. & Peltomaki, P. (2000). Hereditary colorectal cancer: risk assessment and management. *Clinical Genetics* **57**, 89–97.

Hemminki, A., Markie, D., Tomlinson, I. et al. (1998). A serine/threonine kinase gene defective in Peutz-Jeghers syndrome. *Nature* **391**, 184–187.

Hodgson, S. V., Bishop, D. T., Dunlop, M. G., Evans, D. G. & Northover, J. M. (1995). Suggested screening guidelines for familial colorectal cancer. *Journal of Medical Screening* **2**, 45–51.

Hodgson, S. V., Harocopos, C. & Gaglia, P. (1993). Screening results in a family cancer clinic: Five years experience. *Anticancer Research* **13**, 2581–2586.

Houlston, R., Bevon, R., Williams, A. et al. (1998). Mutations in DPC4/SMAD4 cause juvenile polyposis syndrome but only in a minority of cases. *Human Molecular Genetics* **7**, 1907–1912.

Howe, J. R., Roth, S., Ringold, J. C. et al. (1998). Mutations in the SMAD4/DPC4 gene in juvenile polyposis. *Science* **280**, 1086–1088.

Jass, J. R., Williams C. B., Bussey, H. J. & Morson, B. C. (1998). Juvenile polyposis – a precarious condition. *Histopathology* **1**, 619–630.

Jarvinen, H. J. et al. (1995). Screening reduces colorectal cancer rate in families with hereditary nonpolyposis colorectal cancer. *Gastroenterology* **108**(5), 1405–1411.

Jarvinen, H. J., Aarnio, M., Mustonen, H. et al. (2000). Controlled 15-year trial on screening for colorectal cancer in families with hereditary nonpolyposis colorectal cancer. *Gastroenterology* **118**, 829–834.

King, J. E., Dozois, R. R., Lindor, N. M. et al. (2000). Care of patients and their families with familial adenomatous polyposis. *Mayo Clinic Proceedings* **75**, 57–67.

Kune, G. A., Kune, S., Watson, L. F. (1989). The role of hereditary in the aetiology of large bowel cancer: data from the Melbourne Colorectal Cancer Study. *World Journal of Surgery* **13**, 124–129; discussion 129–131.

Lieberman, D. A. et al. (2000). Use of colonoscopy to screen asymptomatic adults for colorectal cancer. *New England Journal of Medicine* **343**, 162–168.

Lynch, M. L. (1999). Clinical challenges in management of familial adenomatous polyposis and hereditary nonpolyposis colorectal cancer. *Cancer Supplement* **86**, 1713–1719.

Marie, P., Morichau-Beauchant, M., Drucker, J. et al. (1984). Familial occurrence of cancer of the colon and the rectum: results of a 3-year case-control survey. *Gastroenterologie Clinical Biology* **8**, 22–27.

Markowitz, A. J. & Winawer, S. J. (1999). Screening and surveillance for colorectal cancer. *Seminars in Oncology* **26**, 485–498.

Ponz de Leone, M., Pedrone, M., Benatti, P. et al. (1999). Hereditary colorectal cancer in the general population: from cancer registration to molecular diagnosis. *Gut* **45**, 32–38.

Ponz de Leone, M., Sassatelli, R., Sacchetti, C. et al. (1989). Familial aggregation of tumours in the 3-year experience of a population-based colorectal cancer registry. *Cancer Research* **49**, 4344–4348.

Ramsey, S. D., Clarke L., Etzioni R., Higashi M., Berry K., Urban N. (2001). Cost-effectiveness of microsatellite instability screening as a method for detecting hereditary nonpolyposis colorectal cancer. *Annals of Internal Medicine* **16**, 135 (8 Part 1) 577–588.

Ransohoff, M. D. & Lang, C. A. (1991). Screening for colorectal cancer. *The New England Journal of Medicine* **325**, 37–42.

Ransohoff, D. F. & Sandler, R.S. (2002) Screening for colorectal cancer. *The New England Journal of Medicine* **346**, 40–44.

Rodriguez-Bigas, M. A. *et al*. (1997). A National Cancer Institute workshop on hereditary nonpolyposis colorectal cancer syndrome. *Journal of the National Cancer Institute* **89**, 1758–1762.

Rozen, P., Fireman, Z., Figer, A. *et al*. (1987). Family history of colorectal cancer as a marker of potential malignancy within a screening programme. *Cancer* **60**, 248–254.

St. John, D., McDermott, F., Hopper, J. *et al*. (1993). Cancer risk in the relatives of patients with common colorectal cancer. *Annals of Internal Medicine* **118**, 785–790.

Samowitz, W. S., Curtin, K., Lin, H. H. *et al*. (2001). The colon cancer burden of genetically defined hereditary nonpolyposis colon cancer. *Gastroenterology* **121**, 830–838.

Sieber, O. M., Lipton, L, Crabtree, M. *et al*. (2003). Multiple colorectal adenomas, classical adenomatous polyposis and germline mutations in MYH. *New England Journal of Medicine* **348**, 791–799.

Spirio, L., Olscharang, S., Groden, J. *et al*. (1993). Alleles of the APC gene: an attenuated form of familial polyposis. *Cell* **75**, 951–957.

Stephenson, B. M., Finan, P. J., Gascoyne, J. *et al*. (1991). Frequency of familial colorectal cancer. *British Journal of Surgery* **78**, 1162–1166.

Sweet, K. M., Bradley, T. L., Westman, J. A. (2002). Identification and referral of families at high risk for cancer susceptibility. *Journal of Clinical Oncology* **20**, 528–537.

Syngal, S., Weeks, J. C., Schrag, D., Garber, J. E. & Kuntz, K. M. (1998). Benefits of colonoscopic surveillance and prophylactic colectomy in patients with hereditary nonpolyposis colorectal cancer mutations. *Annals of Internal Medicine* **15,** 129(10), 787–796.

Tomlinson, I. P. & Houlston, R. S. (1997). Peutz-Jeghers syndrome. *Journal of Medical Genetics* **34**, 1007–1011.

Wallace, M. H. & Phillips, R. K. (1998). Upper gastrointestinal disease in patients with familial adenomatous polyposis. *British Journal of Surgery* **85**, 742–750.

Vasen, H. F., Mecklin, J. P., Khan, P. M. *et al*. (1991). The International Collaborative Group on Hereditary Non-polyposis Colorectal Cancer (ICG-HNPCC). *Diseases of the Colon and Rectum* **34**, 424–425.

Vasen, H. F., Watson, P., Mecklin, J.-P. *et al*. (1999). New clinical criteria for hereditary nonpolyposis colorectal cancer (HNPCC, Lynch syndrome) proposed by the International Collaborative Group on HNPCC. *Gastroenterology* **116**, 1453–1456.

Wijnen, J. T., Vasen, H. F. A., Meera-Khan, P. *et al*. (1998). Clinical findings with implications for genetic testing in families with clustering of colorectal cancer. *New England Journal of Medicine* **339**, 511–518.

Wijnen, J., Kahn, P. M., Vasen, H. *et al*. (1997). Hereditary non-polyposis colorectal cancer not complying with the Amsterdam criteria show extremely low frequency of mismatch repair gene mutations. *American Journal of Human Genetics* **61**, 329–335.

Winawer, S., Fletcher, R., Rex, D., Bond, J., Burt, R., Ferrucci, J., Ganiats, T., Levin, T., Woolf, S., Johnson, D. *et al*. (2003). Gastrointestinal Consortium Panel. Colorectal cancer screening and surveillance: clinical guidelines and rationale – update based on new evidence. *Gastroenterology* **124**, 544–560.

Winawer, S. J., Fletcher, R. H., Miller, L. *et al*. (1997). Colorectal cancer screening: clinical guidelines and rationale. *Gastroenterology* **112**, 594–642.

Winawer, S. J., Fletcher, R., Rex, D. *et al*. (2003a). Colorectal cancer screening and surveillance: clinical guidelines and rationale-update based on new evidence. *Gastroenterology* **124**, 544–560.

Winawer, S. J., Zauber, A. G., O'Brien, M. J. et al. (1993b). Randomized comparison of surveillance intervals after colonoscopic polypectomy. *New England Journal of Medicine* **329**, 901–906.

Woodford-Richens, K., Bevan, S., Churchman, M. et al. (2000). Analysis of genetic and phenotypic heterogeneity in juvenile polyposis. *Gut* **46**, 656–660.

Zhou, X. P., Woodford-Richens, K., Lehtonen, R. et al. (2001). Germline mutations in BMPR1A/ALK3 cause a subset of cases of juvenile polyposis syndrome and of Cowden and Bannayan-Riley-Ruvalcaba syndromes. *American Journal of Human Genetics* **69**, 704–711.

PART 2

Evidence and opinion for surgical intervention

Chapter 5

Current thinking on the clinical significance of the two-week pathway for colorectal cancer

Christopher Gandy, Valerie Morrell, Rupert Pullan and David DeFriend

Introduction

The NHS Cancer Plan 2000 states that survival of patients with common cancers in England and Wales falls short of that of the best European countries and the USA (National Cancer Institute 1998; Berrino *et al.* 1999; Coleman *et al.* 1999; NHS Executive 2000a). Delays in presentation to primary care as well as referral, diagnostic and treatment delays have been implicated (NHS Executive 2000a; Spurgeon *et al.* 2000).

The four key aims of the NHS Cancer Plan are to save lives, improve patients' experience, reduce regional and social inequalities in care and build for the future (NHS Executive 2000a; Department of Health 2001). The plan introduces several strategies intended to improve cancer survival and save lives. These include schemes to reduce the risk of developing cancer by promoting healthier lifestyles, increasing the number of patients with early stage disease through screening and public education programmes and improving access to cancer teams. This final goal will be meet by an expansion of current services and a series of rules and guidelines to speed up the assessment, investigation and treatment of patients with cancer.

Goals and targets to reduce waiting times

These new targets are being introduced in phases with the ultimate goal of no more than one-month delay from referral to starting treatment for all patients with cancer (NHS Executive 2000a; Department of Health 2002). The 'two-week rule' was the first of these targets and stated that *'Everyone with suspected cancer will be able to see a specialist within two weeks of their GP deciding they need to be seen urgently and requesting an appointment'* (NHS Executive 2000b). It was introduced for colorectal cancer in July 2000 and has had a major impact on the organisation of cancer services; it also comes with the considerable burden of data collection and reporting. The next phase of rules for colorectal cancer rolled out in April 2003 to be in place by 2005 states there should be a maximum two-month wait from referral to treatment and a one-month wait from diagnosis to treatment (NHS Executive 2000a).

This will require even more radical service reorganisation and yet greater amounts of data collection and monitoring (Cancer Services Collaborative 2001; NHS Executive 2002).

The evidence for delay in colorectal cancer

The evidence for delay in colorectal cancer has been reviewed in several national guidelines and reports. There are reports of median delays from onset of symptoms to treatment of about 10 months (Cancer Guidelines Sub-Group of the Clinical Outcomes Group 1997a). The relatively recent NHS Cancer Survey reported that half of patients with colorectal cancer were treated within two months of referral; however, unacceptable delays of over seven months were suffered by 10% of patients (Airey et al. 2002). A national audit of waiting times in 1997 reported that urgent referrals were treated on average two months quicker than non-urgent referrals (Spurgeon et al. 2000) and there is also evidence that patients referred to surgical rather than non-surgical teams receive more timely treatment (Wessex Cancer Intelligence Unit 1995; Carter & Winslet 1998). Delays occur at several points during the cancer journey. On average, patients delay reporting symptoms for three months with similar delays occurring at primary care (Cancer Guidelines Sub-Group of the Clinical Outcomes Group 1997a). Ironically, in the context of the of the two-week rule, the shortest delay occurs between referral and hospital appointment with the NHS Cancer Survey reporting more than 50% of colorectal cancer patients received a hospital appointment within one month of referral. There is no conclusive evidence that delays of this magnitude influence outcome in colorectal cancer, but over a third of patients waiting up to three months for an appointment reported a deterioration in their condition (Airey et al. 2002). Timely investigation and treatment is popular with patients (Department of Health 2001) and has been recommended to reduce psychological morbidity in colorectal cancer (Association of Coloproctology of Great Britain and Ireland 1996).

Referral guidelines

Referral guidelines for each cancer site have been developed using evidence from published literature, audit and expert opinion (NHS Executive 1999). The aim of each guideline is to avoid both overly stringent criteria which may miss a significant proportion of cancer cases, and broad criteria which would result in large numbers of 'worried well' and impose unacceptable levels of referrals on an already overburdened services (NHS Executive 2000c). The referral guidelines for colorectal cancer were developed with an intended 90% sensitivity. There is no obligation to use them and there is scope to adjust the criteria to suit local needs (NHS Executive 1999) (see Figure 5.1).

> 1. Rectal bleeding *WITH* a change in bowel habit to looser stools and/or increased frequency of defecation persistent for 6 weeks. *All ages*
>
> 2. A definite palpable right-sided abdominal mass. *All ages*
>
> 3. A definite palpable rectal (not pelvic) mass. *All ages*
>
> 4. Rectal bleeding persistently WITHOUT anal symptoms. *Over 60 yrs*
>
> 5. Change of bowel habit to looser stools and/or increased frequency of defecation, WITHOUT rectal bleeding and persistent for six weeks. *Over 60 yrs*
>
> 6. Iron deficiency anaemia WITHOUT an obvious cause (Hb < 11 g/dl in men or < 10 g/dl in postmenopausal women).

Figure 5.1 Six Department of Health criteria for two-week referral (NHS Executive 1999; Thompson 2002).

South Devon Healthcare NHS Trust Colorectal Cancer Study

There has been great interest in the impact of the two-week rule for colorectal cancer with many presentations published in abstract form but with few full publications in peer-reviewed journals. The Colorectal Unit at South Devon Healthcare NHS Trust has studied the impact of the two-week rule for colorectal cancer. As it will be some time before meaningful assessments its impact on standard outcome measures such as survival and local recurrence are known, we used short-term surrogate outcome measures of operability, pathological stage and delays within the patient's cancer journey. The study period was from July 2000 to November 2001. Two-week referrals were made by letter or on a structured pro forma using the six Department of Health high-risk criteria (NHS Executive 1999; Thompson 2002). These were faxed using a dedicated telephone line and appointments to colorectal clinics made immediately without clinical scrutiny of the referrals. With the pro forma we included guidance for the management of patients with low-risk symptoms. All two-week referrals and traditional referrals with appropriate symptoms underwent flexible sigmoidoscopy in outpatients. Subsequent investigations were based on findings at initial assessment. To date we have not introduced a specific fast-track investigation service for patients presenting via the two-week pathway so that all patients are investigated on merit.

Results

During the study period 244 patients were treated for colorectal cancer within South Devon Healthcare NHS Trust; 178 were referred electively, of whom 72 (40%) were referred to the two-week clinic and 106 (60%) presented by traditional referral routes (see Table 5.1). Age and sex ratios were comparable for the two referral routes (M:F ratio = 3:2 for both groups, $p = 0.5$, χ^2) (mean, standard deviation age = 71, 10.8 versus 74, 10.4, $p = 0.1$ Student's t-test). Of the patients referred to the non-two-week clinics, 46% (49 of 106) would have been eligible for a two-week clinic appointment. Most of these patients reported rectal bleeding and/or a change in bowel habit. Sixteen per cent were found to have an easily palpable rectal carcinoma on digital rectal examination.

Table 5.1 Referral routes

	Number of patients
Emergency referral with emergency treatment	50
Emergency referral (elective investigation & treatment)	16
Two-week clinic (colorectal unit)	72
Traditional colorectal clinic	72
Non-colorectal surgical clinic	22
Physician clinic	12
Total	**244**

For the Colorectal Unit alone, 2,503 patients were referred over the study period for investigation of suspicious colorectal symptoms: 542 (22%) referred under the two-week rule and 1,961 (78%) to the standard clinic. The cancer pick-up rates were 16% (72 patients) for the two-week referrals and 3.7% (72 patients) for the standard colorectal clinic ($p > 0.0001$, χ^2).

Operability

All 178 elective referrals and 16 emergency referrals underwent elective staging. Of these, 36 were found to have locally advanced disease or distant metastasis and received palliative treatments (see Figure 5.2). There were no significant differences in the number of patients receiving palliative treatments after staging between those referred via the two-week pathway and those referred via traditional routes ($p = 0.89$, χ^2) (See Table 5.2).

Table 5.2 Operability rates

	2-week clinic	Non-2-week clinic	Total
Potentially curative surgery	59	99	158
Palliative treatments	13	23	36
Total	**72**	**122**	**194**

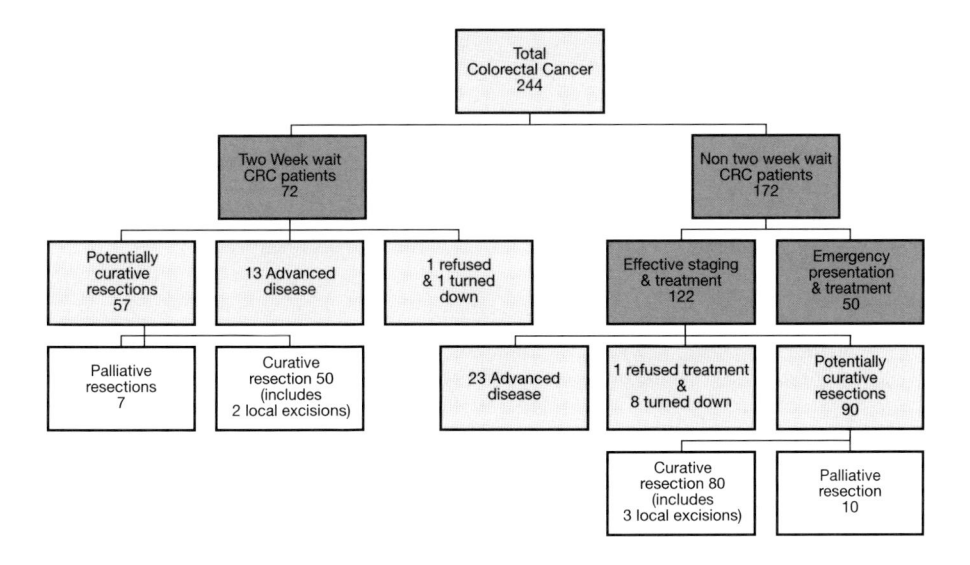

[Figure 5.2 flowchart]

Figure 5.2 Colorectal cancer referrals July 2000 to November 2001.

Potentially curative resections

Despite favourable staging, serious co-morbidity precluded potentially curative surgery in nine patients, and two patients refused treatment (see Figure 5.2). Therefore, 147 patients had potentially curative disease on staging and were candidates for resectional surgery. Of these, five had local or endoscopic treatments for early tumours or malignant polyps (see Table 5.3). The remaining 142 patients underwent laparotomy with the intention of curative resection (Figure 5.2).

Table 5.3 Surgical procedures

Procedure	Number of patients
Right hemicolectomy	33
Extended right hemicolectomy	11
Transverse colectomy	3
Left hemicolectomy	12
Sigmoid colectomy	10
Hartmanns	3
Anterior resection	51
APER	12
Subtotal colectomy	6
Local excision	5
Defunctioned only	1
Total	**147**

Palliative procedures were performed in 17 patients because of irresectable local disease (1 patient), incomplete local excision (6 patients), peritoneal deposits (2 patients) or unexpected liver metastasis (8 patients). There were no differences in numbers of potentially curative resections between the two-week group and non-two-week group ($p = 0.82$, χ^2) (see Table 5.4).).

Table 5.4 Curative resections (excludes local resections)

	2-week group	Non-2-week group	Total
Palliative procedure	7	10	17
Potentially curative resection	48	77	125
Total	**55**	**87**	**142**

Site of tumour at surgery

Eleven patients had synchronous tumours, therefore 158 tumour sites were recorded in the 147 patients who underwent laparotomy or local excision (see Figure 5.3).

The ratio of rectal to colonic tumours was significantly different between groups (two-week group 1:2 and non-two-week group 1:4 ($p = 0.04$ χ^2). However, the ratio of tumours accessible by flexible sigmoidoscopy (i.e. to splenic flexure) was not significantly different between groups (two-week group R:L = 1:2 and non-two-week group R:L 3:7 ($p = 0.7$, χ^2).

Pathological stage

Full histological assessment was available on 140 of the 142 patients who underwent laparotomy. Full histological assessment was not available on patients undergoing local or endoscopic resections or on the patient found to have locally irresectable disease. One patient undergoing right hemicolectomy was found to have a carcinoid tumour and was therefore excluded from analysis of pathological stage. Of the 11 patients with synchronous tumours the highest pathological stage was assessed.

Numbers of each stage were remarkably similar between those referred on the two-week rule and traditional referrals, with no significant differences based on Dukes' stage ($p = 0.58$, χ^2) and TNM pT ($p = 0.48$, χ^2) and pN ($p = 0.16$ χ^2) (see Figures 5.4–5.6). There was, however, a tendency for pN2 tumours in the two-week group (22% of two-week group versus 10% of non-two-week) although this did not reach statistical significance ($p = 0.058$, χ^2).

Timing of assessment and surgery

Of two-week referrals, 98% were seen within the requisite time. As expected there was a significantly shorter time from referral to assessment for the two-week group ($p < 0.0001$, t-test), which translated into a shorter time from referral to surgery ($p <$

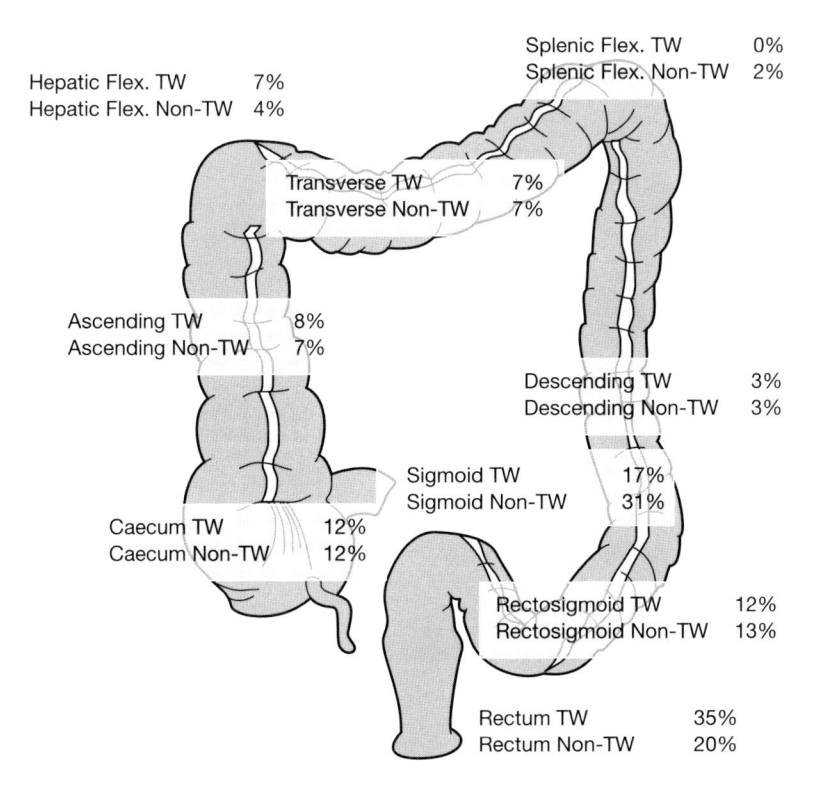

Clinical significance of the two-week pathway 67

Location	TW	Non-TW
Hepatic Flex.	7%	4%
Splenic Flex.	0%	2%
Transverse	7%	7%
Ascending	8%	7%
Descending	3%	3%
Caecum	12%	12%
Sigmoid	17%	31%
Rectosigmoid	12%	13%
Rectum	35%	20%

Figure 5.3 Percentage distribution of tumours.

0.0001, t-test) (see Figure 5.7). However, times from diagnosis to surgery were also shorter for the two-week group ($p = 0.02$, t-test) and this difference persisted on analysis of those patients referred to the colorectal team only ($p = 0.008$, t-test) (see Table 5.5).

The two-week group had a higher proportion of rectal cancers (Figure 5.3). Analysis of times to surgery by rectal and colonic tumours shows that significant differences favouring the two-week group persist for both sites (see Table 5.6).

Impact of the two-week rule on waiting times

In accordance with recommendation from the COG guidelines we have audited times from referral to diagnosis since 1997 (NHS Executive 1997). To assess the overall impact of the two-week rule on waiting times we have compared referral to diagnosis times for all patients in the study period (study group) with a similar period before the introduction of the rule in 1999–2000 (control group). Although delays were shorter for the two-week clinics there was no significant difference for the study group and control group ($p = 0.89$, unpaired t-test) (Table 5.7).

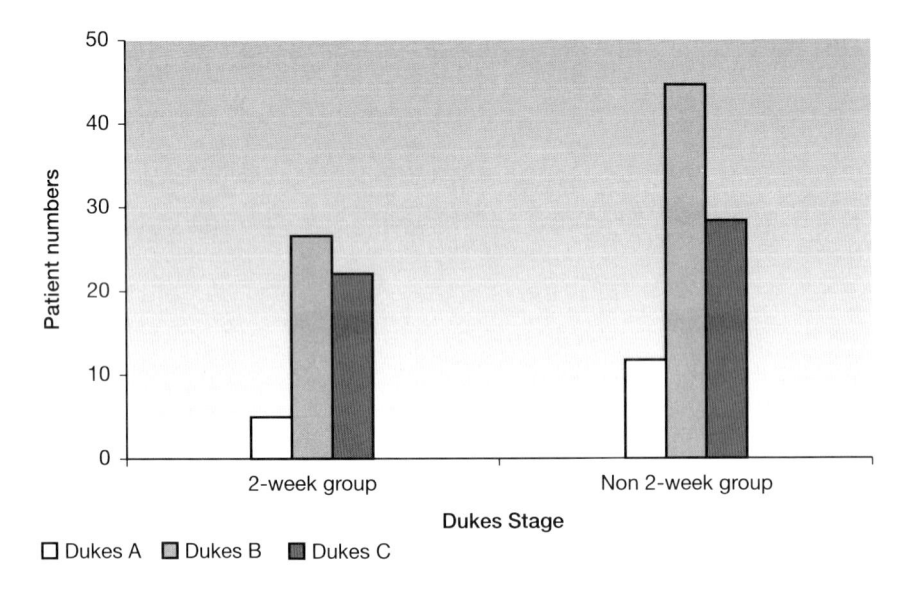

Figure 5.4 Dukes stage two-week group and non-two-week group.

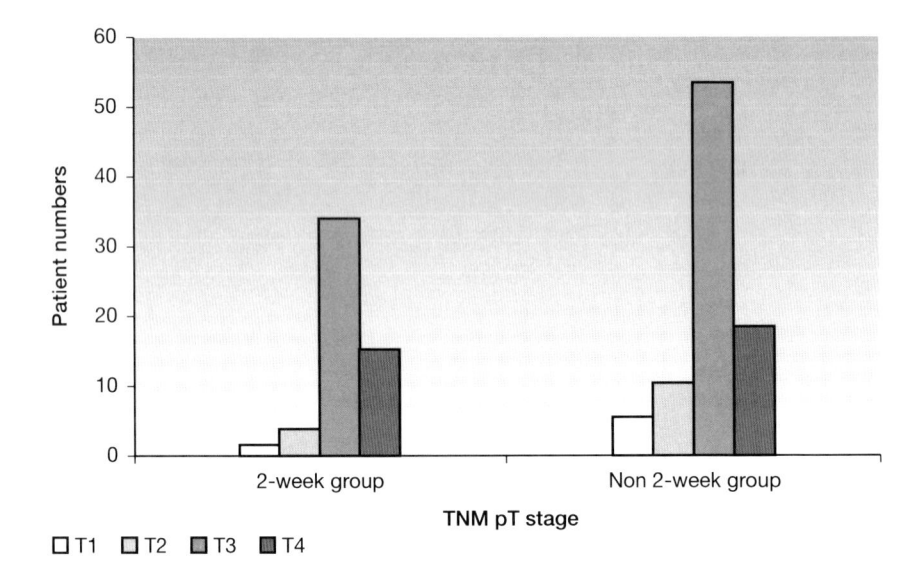

Figure 5.5 TNM pT stage two-week group and non-two-week group.

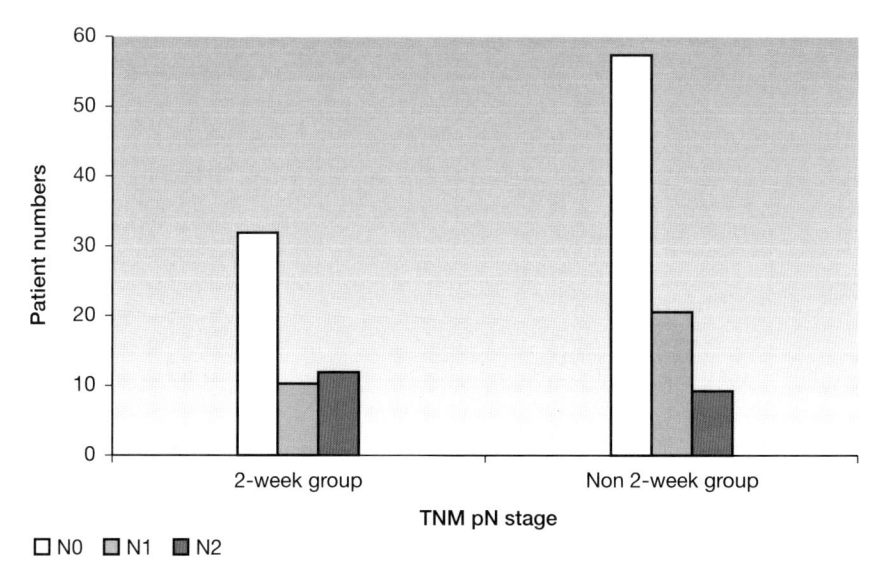

Clinical significance of the two-week pathway 69

Figure 5.6 TMN pN stage two-week group and non two-week group.

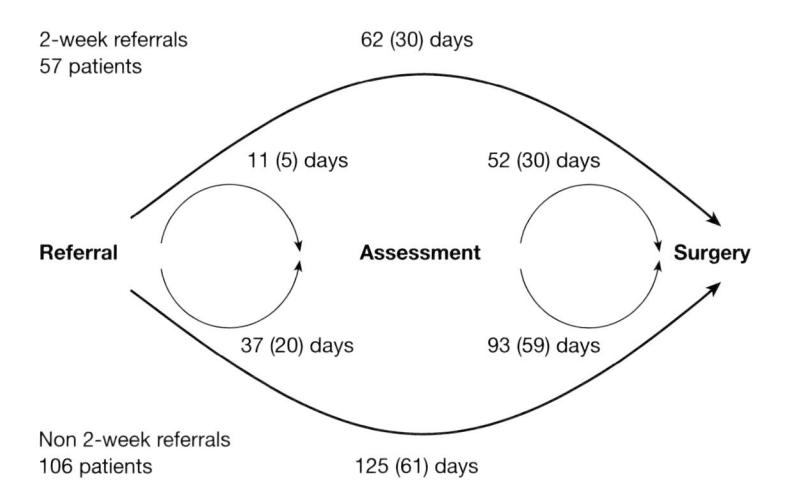

Figure 5.7 Timetable from referral to surgery by group. Values are means (SDs).

Table 5.5 Diagnosis to surgery by all referrals and colorectal team referrals.

	\multicolumn{3}{c}{Diagnosis to surgery, mean (SD) (days)}
	2-week clinic	Non-2-week clinic	p-value t-test
All referrals	37 (20)	45 (20)	0.02
Colorectal team referrals	37 (20)	48 (22)	0.008

Table 5.6 Timings by site

	Rectal days (SD)			Colonic days (SD)		
	2-week clinic	Non-2-week clinic	p-value t-test	2-week clinic	Non-2-week clinic	p-value t-test
Referral to appointment	11 (4)	36 (18)	> 0.0001	11 (6)	37 (20)	> 0.0001
Referral to surgery	67 (35)	111 (33)	0.002	60 (28)	129 (67)	> 0.0001
Diagnosis to surgery	39 (19)	51 (19)	0.048	34 (20)	43 (20)	0.0442

Table 5.7 Referral to diagnosis, study period vs period prior to two-week rule

	Referral to diagnosis mean (SD) days		p=0.89 t test
	2-week clinic	Non-2-week clinic	Overall
Study group	30 (23)	83 (64)	60 (59)
Control group	NA	NA	62 (57)

Discussion

Despite the introduction of two-week referral guidelines and considerable efforts to encourage awareness and uptake within primary care, a minority of patients referred for investigation of lower GI symptoms currently present through the two-week clinics (Heriot *et al.* 2001; Forster *et al.* 2002). While yields of cancers from these clinics can be high (Stone *et al.* 2001; Flashman *et al.* 2002) (16% in our series) only the minority of cancers present through this route (Hagger *et al.* 2001; Vieten *et al.* 2001; Bond *et al.* 2002). Like others we have shown that a large proportion of colorectal cancer patients referred through the non-two-week pathway had symptoms and signs that meet the DoH referral guidelines and therefore were eligible for the two-week clinics (Heriot *et al.* 2001; Clark *et al.* 2002). There is some evidence of poor uptake of this referral system in general practice (Forster *et al.* 2002) despite generally positive attitudes to guidelines within primary care (Watkins *et al.* 1999). Competition from the sheer volume of guidelines and difficulties accessing them when required may account for lack of use (Watkins *et al.* 1999; Delmothe 1993). A study from Portsmouth showed that most GPs found the two-week referral system useful and three-quarters were able to provide reasonable justification for not referring individual patients suitable for the two-week clinics (Basu *et al.* 2003). 'Inappropriate' referral rates to two-week clinics can also be high, with some centres reporting rates of over 50%, usually due to loose interpretation of the referral criteria (Coni *et al.* 2001; Eccersley *et al.* 2001; Warwick *et al.* 2002). It is clear that the colorectal cancer yield for the two-week clinics is proportional to the percentage of appropriate referrals and where inappropriate referrals are minimised yields of up to one in five patients with colorectal cancer may be achieved (Eccersley *et al.* 2001;

Coni, *et al.* 2001; MacDonald *et al.* (2002). Other studies have highlighted that the two-week referral pathway may also pick up several patients with significant benign colorectal pathology as well as patients with non-colorectal pathology including other pelvic malignancies (Vieten *et al.* 2002; Eccersley *et al.* 2001; Adeosum *et al.* 2002). This is an unintended but predictable benefit of the scheme.

Impact on waiting times and timing of surgery

The Department of Health has published quarterly results for time from referral to first clinic appointment. Nationally, trusts are seeing between 90% and 95% of two-week referrals for colorectal cancer within the designated time. During our study we managed 98% compliance; however, only 6% of our patients presenting by non-two-week clinics were seen within this time frame. We have shown that each step of the cancer journey from referral to surgery is quicker for patients presenting under the two-week rule despite standard investigation and staging for all and this is true of both colonic and rectal cancers. The advantage for two-week referrals is to be expected for times from referral to clinic, which then translates to an advantage for referral to surgery; however, we have also shown an unexpected advantage from diagnosis to surgery. Similar results have been shown in other studies (Soo *et al.* 2001; Smith *et al.* 2002). Significant delays have been reported when patients are referred to non-colorectal specialities (Wessex Cancer Intelligence Unit 1995; Carter & Winslet 1998; Potter & Wilson 1999) but our results do not support this as a major cause of delay at our trust.

There has been concern that the two-week rule may have an adverse effect on the non-two-week referrals (Thomas 2001; Jones *et al.* 2001); however, this has not been borne out in recent studies (Davies *et al.* 2001; MacDonald *et al.* 2002; Mihssin *et al.* 2001). In our current study the two-week referrals had faster times from referral to diagnosis compared with non-two-week referrals; however, overall, there has been no impact on delay from referral to diagnosis.

Impact on pathological stage

There is some evidence that sub-specialisation of colorectal cancer services and rapid access to investigation may alter disease stage (Shankar *et al.* 2001). However, we have failed to show any impact on either numbers of patients having curative resections or on pathological stage, which is in keeping with studies from Bedfordshire and Cambridge (Eccersley *et al.* 2003; Chohan *et al.* 2003). A study from Sheffield has also compared pathological stage (but for all elective patients presenting one year before and after the introduction of the two-week rule) and has also failed to show an impact (Arasaradnam *et al.* 2002). It is therefore unlikely that there will be significant influence of this rule on long-term survival or disease recurrence.

Impact of the two-week rule on colorectal services

The introduction of the two-week target has resulted in major reorganisation of services although there are few reports detailing specific measurable impacts. There have been examples of increased demand on endoscopy services (Davies *et al.* 2001; Stone *et al.* 2001), introduction of fast-track investigations (Glancy *et al.* 2002) and nurse lead clinics (Burke *et al.* 2002; Aldridge *et al.* 2001). Rapid referral clinics may have an impact on the numbers of emergency referrals (Shankar *et al.* 2001), and this may also be true of the two-week rule as Davies showed a non-significant reduction in the proportion of patients presenting as CRC emergencies from 35.7% to 25.9% ($p = 0.059$) (Davies *et al.* 2004).

Future trends and new targets

Attempts have been made to increase the diagnostic yields of referral criteria. Several studies have assessed scoring systems (Tekkis *et al.* 2002; Selvachandran *et al.* 2002; Bond *et al.* 2002). Selvachandran has developed a weighted numerical score from a patient questionnaire to prioritise patients referred by their GP. This can be set with a sensitivity to match the Department of Health referral criteria but with significantly fewer clinic referrals (Selvachandran *et al.* 2002). A *pro forma* referral system has been developed in Salisbury and Bath, which allows referral of all patients with potential symptoms of colorectal disease on one simple form. Patients are prioritised at hospital level and then directed to diagnostic services (barium enema, colonoscopy or flexible sigmoidoscopy) or to outpatient clinic for assessment (Thresher *et al.* 2002). Using this system, 23% of their workload were seen with the remit of the two-week target with cancer yields of 17% compared with 2.9% and 1.1% for 'soon' and 'routine' referrals, respectively. These referral tools provide modest improvements over the current Department of Health referral guidelines but are probably more complex to administer.

The next phase of targets for colorectal cancer allows only a two-month delay from referral to treatment and one-month delay from diagnosis to treatment for all patients. Currently, over half of our patients referred via the two-week pathway meet these targets. This contrasts starkly with referrals by traditional pathways where only 1 in 10 receives treatment within two months of referral, and this group comprises 60% of our elective cancer workload. It is therefore clear that diagnostic services and access to treatments will need to be improved to meet the next phase of targets.

We believe that the two-week referral pathway with the benefit of its accelerated cancer journey could provide a firm bases from which future targets could be meet and allow us to direct resources efficiently. However, to reach its full potential we will need to work with primary care so that a higher proportion of patients with high-risk symptoms are referred and 'inappropriate' referrals kept to a minimum.

Conclusion

The two-week target is the first of a series of phased targets culminating in a one-month delay from referral to the start of treatment for all patients with cancer. The Department of Health has produced referral guidelines with six referral criteria for colorectal cancers that have a 90% or greater sensitivity (NHS Executive 1999; Clark *et al.* 2002) and when used appropriately should identify one patient with cancer for every five elective referrals. Unfortunately, only a minority of patients with high-risk symptoms are referred on these guidelines via the two-week pathway and there is often a liberal interpretation of the referral categories. So far, patients referred to the two-week clinics are receiving treatment quicker, although there has been little demonstrable advantage in terms of disease stage at presentation. It is therefore unlikely that it will have a direct beneficial effect on survival rates for colorectal cancer with potential benefits restricted to reducing anxiety and symptom levels in patients waiting review. Setting national referral guidelines should also improve consistency of access to specialist care across regions and demographic groups.

If used to its full potential almost all elective cases of colorectal cancer could be identified using the Department of Health referral guidelines and referred through the two-week clinics with their accelerated cancer journey. This would go some way to meeting the next phase of cancer targets for colorectal cancer.

References

Adeosum, B. A., Wright, J., Ross, A. H. M. *et al.* (2002). A 2-week referral service for colorectal cancer has little impact on existing activity in the first year, *Colorectal Disease* **4** (Supplement 1), 50 (poster 030).

Airey, C., Becher, H., Erens, B. *et al.* (2002). *National Surveys of NHS Patients – Cancer: National Overview 1999/2000*. London: Department of Health.

Aldridge, A. J., Bundy, K., Parvanta, L. *et al.* (2001). Six month workload of a nurse practitioner-run rapid access colorectal clinic in a district general hospital, *Colorectal Disease* **3** (Supplement 1), 34.

Arasaradnam, R. P., Bhala, N., Shorthouse, A. J. *et al.* (2002). TNM&R staging in colorectal cancer: has the two week wait for patients made any difference? *Gut* **50**, poster 173.

Association of Coloproctology of Great Britain and Ireland (1996). *Guidelines for the Management of Colorectal Cancer*. London: The Royal College of Surgeons of England.

Basu, S., Flashman, K. G., O'Leary, D. P. *et al.* (2003). Why are patients with the Department of Health Higher Risk Criteria not referred to the '2-Week Standard Clinic'? *Colorectal Diseases* **5** (Suppl. 1), 42.

Berrino, F., Capocaccia, R., Esteve, J. *et al.* (1999). Survival of cancer patients in Europe: the EUROCARE study 11. Lyons: International Agency for Research on Cancer.

Bond, A., Murray, D. *et al.* (2002). Colorectal cancer – a simple scoring system to fast-track higher risk patients, *Colorectal Disease* **4** (Supplement 1), 49 (poster 026).

Burke, C. C., Smith, J. J., Mathur, P. *et al.* 2002). Colorectal specialist nurse: outpatient management of rectal bleeding and the 2-week rule. *Colorectal Disease* **4** (Supplement 1), 46.

Cancer Guidelines Sub-Group of the Clinical Outcomes Group (1997a). *Guidance on Commissioning Cancer Services: Improving outcomes in colorectal cancer: The Research Evidence*. Leeds: NHS Executive.

Cancer Services Collaborative (2001). *Bowel Cancer. Service Improvement Guide*. London: NHS Modernisation Agency.

Carter, S. & Winslet, M. (1998.) Delay in the presentation of colorectal carcinoma: a review of causation. *International Journal of Colorectal Disease* **13**, 27–31.

Chohan, D. P. K., Goodwin, K., Wilkinson, S. *et al.* (2003). How has the '2-week wait rule' affected colorectal cancer presentation? *Colorectal Disease* **5** (Suppl. 1) 40–41.

Clark, J. S., Williams, A. B. *et al.* (2002). Missing colorectal cancer – the 2-week wait. *Colorectal Disease* **4** (Supplement 1), 49 (poster 027).

Coleman, M. P., Babb, P., Damiecki, P. *et al.* (1999). *Cancer Survival Trends in England and Wales 1971–1995: Deprivation and NHS Region*. London: Stationery Office.

Coni, L., Flashman, K., Coleman, M. G. *et al.* (2001). Accuracy of referral to the 2 week standard clinic, *Colorectal Disease* **3** (Supplement 1), 33.

Davies, R. J., Welbourn, R., Collins, C. *et al.* (2001). A prospective study to assess the implementation of a fast track system to meet the two-week target for colorectal cancer. *Gut* **48** (Supplement 1), A53.

Davies, R. J., Collins, C. D., Vickery, C. J. *et al.* (2004). Reduction in the proportion of patients with colorectal cancer presenting as an emergency following the introduction of fast-track flexible sigmoidoscopy: a three-year propsective observational study. *Colorectal Disease* **6**, 265–267.

Delmothe, T. (1993). Wanted: guidelines that doctors will follow? *British Medical Journal* **307**, 218.

Department of Health (2001). *The NHS Cancer Plan: Making Progress*. 26059 1P. London: Department of Health.

Department of Health (2002). *Cancer Waiting Times. Guidance on making and tracking progress on cancer waiting times*. HSC 2002/005. London: Department of Health.

Eccersley, A. J. P., Wilson, E. M., Makris, A. *et al.* (2001). Referral guidelines for colorectal cancer. Do they work? *Colorectal Disease* **3** (Supplement 1), 34.

Eccersley, A. J., Wilson, E. M., Makris, A. *et al.* (2003). Referral guidelines for colorectal cancer – do they work? *Annals of The Royal College of Surgeons of England* **85**, 107–110.

Flashman, K., Faux, W., O'Leary, D. P. *et al.* (2002). Diagnostic yields of the six Department of Health (DOH) higher risk criteria for the 'two week standard' clinic (TWSC). *Colorectal Disease* **4** (Supplement 1), 48 (poster 024).

Forster, G., Lightfoot, T., Fitzgerald, P. (2002). Cancer fast track appointments: help or hindrance, *Colorectal Disease* **4** (Supplement 1), 48 (poster 023).

Glancy, D., Sylvester, P., Card, M. *et al.* (2002). The two-week wait for patients with suspected colorectal cancer: the role of fast-track barium enema. *Colorectal Disease* **4** (Supplement 1), 6.

Hagger, R., Ahmed, W., Scott, H. *et al.* (2001). Audit of the introduction of a 2 week rule scheme for colorectal cancer to a district general hospital. *Colorectal Disease* **3** (Supplement 1), poster 14.

Heriot, A. G., Chappell, B., Richardson, S. *et al.* (2001). A prospective study of the effect of the implementation of the 2 week rule for colorectal cancer referral in a district general hospital. *Colorectal Disease* **3** (Supplement 1), poster 12.

Jones, R., Rubin, G. & Hungin, P. (2001). Is the two week rule for cancer referrals working? *British Medical Journal* **322**, 1555–1556.

MacDonald, L., Mitchell, S. J. *et al.* (2002). Two-week wait colorectal cancer clinics: a prospective analysis of appropriateness of referral, *Colorectal Disease* **4** (Supplement 1), 47 (poster 021).

Mihssin, N., Debney, N., Pullan, R. D. *et al.* (2001). Prospective evaluation of introduction of 2 week referral pathway for colorectal patients in Torbay. *Colorectal Disease* **3** (Supplement 1), oral 33.

National Cancer Institute (1998). *SEER Stat-cancer Incidence Public Use Database 1973–95.* London: NCI.

NHS Executive (1997). *Guidance on Commissioning Cancer Services: Improving Outcomes in Colorectal Cancer: The Manual.* 97CV0119. London: Department of Health.

NHS Executive (1999 *Referral Guidelines for Suspected Cancer.* HSC 1999/241: 19. London: Department of Health.

NHS Executive (2000a).*The NHS Cancer Plan.* 22293. Leeds: NHS Executive.

NHS Executive (2000b). *NHS Plan. A Plan for Investment, a Plan for Reform.* London: Department of Health.

NHS Executive (2000c). *NHS Executives' Guidelines for Urgent Referral of Patients with Suspected Cancer.* London: Department of Health.

NHS Executive (2002). *Cancer Waiting Times: Guidance on Making and Tracking Progress on Cancer Waiting Times.* HSC 2002/005. London: Department of Health.

Potter, M. & Wilson, G. (1999). Diagnostic delay in colorectal cancer. *Journal of the Royal. College of Surgeons of Edinburgh* **44**, 313–316.

Selvachandran, S. N., Hodder, R. *et al.* (2002). Prediction of colorectal cancer by a patient consultation questionnaire and scoring system: a prospective study. *The Lancet* **360**, 278–283.

Shankar, P. J., Achuthan, R., Haray, P. N. (2001). Colorectal subspecialisation in a DGH. The way forward! *Colorectal Disease* **3**, 396–401.

Smith, J. A., Thompson, M. R., Lane, R. H. *et al.* (2002). The Wessex Colorectal Cancer Audit: 5 years outcome data suggest new standards of care, *Colorectal Disease* **4**, 21.

Soo, F. Y., Winterton, R. & Plusa, S. M. (2001). Impact of the 2 week rule on the treatment of colorectal cancer. *Gut* **48** (Supplement 1), A53.

Spurgeon, P., Barwell, F. & Kerr, D. (2000). Waiting times for cancer patients in England after general practitioners' referrals: retrospective national survey. *British Medical Journal* **320**, 838–839.

Stone, D., Hussaini, S. H., Mandel, A. *et al.* (2001). Audit of the two week cancer rule for gastrointestinal malignancy. *Gut* **48** (Supplement 1), abstract 175.

Tekkis, P. P., Savage, R. *et al.* (2002). Early symptomatic colorectal cancer detection by artificial neural networks. *Colorectal Disease* **4**, 13 (oral 037).

Thomas, S. (2001) Two week rule for cancer referrals. *British Medical Journal* **323**, 864.

Thompson, M. (2002). ACPGBI referral guidelines for colorectal cancer. *Colorectal Disease* **4**, 284.

Thresher, T., Linehan, J. D., Britton, D. C. *et al.* (2002). Success of a simple 'tick box' GP referral form for colorectal carcinoma and its impact on achieving the '2 week wait' target. *Gut* **50** (Supplement 2), abstract 360.

Vieten, D., Carney, L. J. *et al.* (2002). The 2-week referral pathway for colorectal cancer – potential to miss serious disease. *Colorectal Disease* **4**(Supplement 1), 50 (poster 029).

Vieten, D., Hollowood, A., Carney, L. *et al.* (2001). The 2-week colorectal referral pathway – is it effective? *British Journal of Surgery* **89**, 83.

Warwick, M., Watkinson, A. *et al.* (2002). Review of a rapid access service for colorectal cancer. *Colorectal Disease* **4** (Supplement 1), 49 (poster 028).

Watkins, C., Harvey, I., Langley, C. *et al.* (1999). General practitioners' use of guidelines in the consultation and their attitudes to them. *British Journal of General Practice* **49**, 11–15.

Wessex Cancer Intelligence Unit (1995). *Colorectal cancer in the South West.* Winchester: Institute of Public Health Medicine.

Chapter 6

The benefits of laparoscopic surgery in colorectal cancer

Polly M. King and Robin H. Kennedy

Introduction

The first description of laparoscopic colorectal resection for malignancy was in 1991 (Jacobs *et al.* 1991) but 12 years on controversy still surrounds the technique. In certain institutions throughout the world this surgery has reached an advanced level of sophistication and would be the method of choice in the majority of cancers. In Britain, however, its application is unfortunately only in approximately 1–2% of all colorectal cancer (CRC) resections. Controversy has prompted the National Institute for Clinical Excellence (NICE) to recommend that laparoscopic surgery for CRC should only be carried out as part of a randomised trial. Initial concerns centred on oncological outcomes. There were questions as to whether the same tumour clearance and lymph node yield could be obtained with the laparoscopic approach, but the unexpected appearance of metastases within the laparoscopic port sites also rang alarm bells. This chapter will discuss the evidence for and against laparoscopic surgery in the field of CRC and summarise some of the exciting possibilities now available to us in the treatment of this disease.

Current evidence

Oncological clearance and survival

Level one evidence from multicentre randomised trials looking at long-term oncological outcomes following laparoscopic resection for CRC is awaited. However, there is evidence from single centre randomised trials (Stage *et al.* 1997; Milsom *et al.* 1998; Lacy *et al.* 2002) and prospective cohort studies (Franklin *et al.* 1996; Psaila *et al.* 1998) that tumour clearance and lymph node yields are comparable between approaches. Local recurrence and cancer-related survival have also been examined in a number of studies. The Clinical Outcomes of Surgical Therapy (COST) Study Group performed a retrospective review of 372 patients who had received laparoscopic resection prior to embarking on a randomised controlled trial (Fleshman *et al.* 1996). They found that the three-year survival rates for these patients were similar to the reported figures for patients receiving open resection. Hartley's group (Hartley *et al.* 2000) performed a prospective non-randomised study examining the incidence of local and distant recurrence in 109 patients receiving either laparoscopic or open surgery. There was no difference in recurrence rates between the groups at a median follow-up of 42 months. Franklin *et al.* (2000) published recurrence rates in 50 patients with stage III disease at a mean follow up of 29 months. The fact that only three patients (6%) had local recurrence in the pelvis encouraged them to conclude that oncological outcomes were both satisfactory and comparable with reported rates for open surgery.

The most conclusive evidence to date has come from Lacy's group in Barcelona (Lacy *et al.* 2002). In a trial that randomised over 200 patients with colon cancer to either laparoscopic or open surgery, there was a significant improvement in cancer-related survival seen in the laparoscopic patients. This was a long-term study with a median follow-up of 43 months and interestingly the benefit was observed in those patients with stage III disease. This did not translate into a significant advantage in overall survival for the laparoscopic group, but there is a trend towards it and further large studies like this are clearly needed. One hypothesis for this unexpected finding is that the minimally invasive technique has a less suppressive effect on cell mediated immunity thus reducing tumour cell dissemination peri-operatively (Whelan *et al.* 2003).

There have been only occasional reports looking specifically at laparoscopic rectal surgery and the majority of these examine laparoscopic abdominoperineal resection. Morino *et al.* however, have published the results of a prospective study examining 100 consecutive patients treated with laparoscopic total mesorectal excision (TME) (Morino *et al.* 2003). The median follow-up was nearly four years and there was a single port site metastasis. The overall locoregional recurrence rate was 4.2%, which would seem to be an acceptable figure by comparison with studies of open TME for rectal cancer.

Port site metastases

When laparoscopic resection for CRC was in its infancy an unusual pattern of local wound recurrence was noted. This was occurring at sites of trocar insertion and was observed even in patients with Dukes' A lesions. Approximately 80% of such recurrences were within the first year. This led to concerns that the laparoscopic approach was causing a different pattern of recurrence as compared to open surgery. There have now been a number of studies that have looked at the issue of port site metastases. In three randomised controlled trials (Stage *et al.* 1997; Lacy *et al. 1998*; Milsom *et al.* 1998) port site recurrences were not observed in over 170 patients receiving laparoscopic surgery at a follow up of between 7 and 46 months. This is consistent with other prospective series in which the incidence of port site recurrences did not exceed 1.3% (Psaila *et al.* 1998; Pearlstone *et al.* 1999; Hartley *et al.* 2000). The development of port site metastases may therefore have more to do with the biology of the underlying tumour than the technique of laparoscopy, a theory supported by a similar wound recurrence rate in open surgery (Rickard *et al.* 2001).

In a total of 166 laparoscopic operations carried out at Yeovil for CRC since 1994, there have been no port site metastases so far.

In the early development of laparoscopic resection for CRC, port site metastases were seen as the real contraindication for this technique. It is difficult to explain these early recurrences but the evidence suggests that this is no longer a concern. Perhaps this now reflects a more meticulous approach to oncological principles in laparoscopic surgery: using techniques such as minimal handling of the tumour, fixation of the trocars to the abdominal wall, peritoneal cleansing with a tumouricidal agent and allowing all the gas to discharge before removal of the trocars.

Short-term outcome

Many studies have examined the short-term benefits of laparoscopic surgery and it is now clear that the laparoscopic approach can provide advantages in the immediate post-operative period with less pain, quicker restoration of bowel function, fewer post-operative complications and a shorter hospital stay (Lacy *et al.* 1995; Franklin *et al.* 1996; Stage *et al.* 1997; Milsom *et al.* 1998). It has been hypothesised that these improvements in short-term outcome are due to a reduced surgical stress response. After any major surgical procedure the patient is at risk of cardiopulmonary, thromboembolic and infectious complications not directly related to the surgical procedure. The pathogenesis of this post-operative morbidity, as well as the period of post-operative fatigue and convalescence, has been assumed to be secondary to changes in endocrine and metabolic functions – the surgical stress response (Kehlet 1999). The potential attenuation of this response by laparoscopic surgery could have a positive impact on the host – tumour relationship in colorectal malignancy, particularly micrometastatic disease, as well as allowing earlier recovery and reduced convalescence.

To date, there is no clear post-operative marker of the stress response and studies reveal conflicting results when comparing the immune and metabolic effects of laparoscopic surgery to those of the open approach. Braga *et al.* (2002) demonstrated that the post-operative inflammatory response was less pronounced with laparoscopic surgery in a randomised controlled trial, as demonstrated by lower levels of CRP. Further studies looking at interleukin-1 (IL-1) and interleukin-6 (IL-6) have reported similar results (Delgado *et al.* 2001). However, other authors have compared the systemic immunity in patients undergoing laparoscopic and open surgery and found no difference between the groups (Hewitt *et al.* 1998; Tang *et al.* 2001). It would appear, therefore, that the reduction in the surgical stress response associated with laparoscopic surgery is reflected in the decreased incidence of wound infections, fewer pulmonary complications and earlier recovery, rather than in a reproducible individual inflammatory marker.

Quality of life

Surgery for CRC may have a negative impact on many aspects of the patient's overall well-being. Quality of life (QOL) studies have emerged in recent years as a useful outcome measure when examining cancer surgery, and the maintenance of a high level of patient QOL should be a goal for any developing surgical technique. Two randomised studies comparing laparoscopic and open surgery for CRC have published QOL outcomes. One of these reports was from Weeks *et al.* who included 449 patients undergoing laparoscopic-assisted colectomy or open colectomy for colon cancer as part of the COST study (Weeks *et al.* 2002). Short-term outcomes of symptom distress, a single item global score and a QOL index were reported. Significantly better global QOL scores were observed two weeks after surgery in the laparoscopic group and a reduced requirement for parenteral analgesia was also noted. Schwenk *et al.* randomised 60 patients to laparoscopic or conventional open surgery and measured pain and fatigue QOL dimensions with visual analogue scores (Schwenk *et al.* 1998). Significant differences were reported in pain scores between the two groups and fatigue was worse in patients undergoing conventional open surgery. A further prospective study used the generic SF-36 QOL questionnaire to assess patients after laparoscopic and open surgery for CRC. Results showed a significant difference in favour of the laparoscopic group in the general health component of the questionnaire between the groups at two months post-operatively (Psaila *et al.* 1998). Ongoing multicentre randomised trials have included disease specific QOL assessments in the outcomes and results from these trials are awaited.

Disadvantages

The initial enthusiasm in the early 1990s for resecting certain cases of CRC laparoscopically was curbed by emerging oncological doubts. Now that these specific concerns have largely been disproved, studies are needed to clarify whether the improved efficacy seen following laparoscopic resection in single centre studies will translate into improved clinical effectiveness in multicentre research.

There is no doubt that laparoscopic colorectal procedures usually take longer than the corresponding open procedure during the learning curve (Schlachta *et al.* 2001), but it seems operative duration returns to normal after this period. There is also a trend towards an increased rate of conversion during this learning curve. Reports of conversion rates among those performing laparoscopic procedures vary wildly, ranging from 2% to 77%. There are certain patient-related and operative factors that make conversion more likely. These include patients with a high body mass index, rectal resection, previous surgery with resultant adhesions, and complicated benign disease. A large multicentre observational study in Europe examining conversion rates and subsequent morbidity looked at a total of 1658 laparoscopic operations (Marusch *et al.* 2001). The conversion rate was 5.2%. They found that both the mortality and morbidity rates were higher in the converted group. Slim *et al.* (1995)

in France described a higher morbidity rate of 50% for converted cases as compared with 21% for primary open cases, and other studies have shown an increase in hospital stay as well as the incidence of both minor and major complications after conversion. Randomised studies may clarify whether this increased morbidity is caused by conversion or whether the converted group just includes many of the more difficult cases who were predestined to have a more complicated recovery.

A further criticism levelled at laparoscopic surgery has been the use of expensive disposable equipment and the impact that this, in combination with prolonged theatre time, will have on health economics. Studies comparing the costs of open and laparoscopic surgery have produced conflicting results. Many of these have looked at a single procedure and few have looked at many patients. There is evidence that despite lengthened operating times and the use of disposable equipment, the overall cost of laparoscopic surgery is less than open surgery (Delaney *et al.* 2003). This is due to the fact that the hospital stay is usually decreased. Reducing hospital stay *per se* by a couple of days may not cover the increased operating cost, but the study by Delaney has shown that cost reductions are derived from economies in nursing care, pharmacy and laboratory costs. The patient requires less analgesia post-operatively, less nursing intervention and has a consequent earlier discharge. Other studies disagree with this finding and have found that the costs are similar between the approaches (Pfeifer *et al.* 1995) or that the laparoscopic group incur higher costs (Bokey *et al.* 1996). Until evidence from large multicentre randomised trials is available examining all aspects of post-operative recovery, including health economic evaluations, critics of the laparoscopic approach will not accept its use as the recommended standard for patients with CRC. Should such analysis prove that overall costs of the laparoscopic approach are increased, one has still to consider whether the benefits observed justify this expense.

Our current practice

In the last three years at Yeovil District Hospital, 158 patients have been operated on for CRC by the senior author. Of these, 85% have been elective operations and 15% followed unplanned admissions. During this time two randomised trials have been running consecutively, with all eligible patients being randomised on a 2:1 basis between laparoscopic and open surgery; 96% ($n = 86$) of those suitable for randomisation have been entered. In the 49 elective patients not randomised, the resection was attempted laparoscopically in all but 6. The reason for open resection in these 6 was, usually, either that a second organ also required resection or that they declined laparoscopic surgery.

The breakdown of results following surgery is shown in Table 6.1.

Table 6.1 Surgery for colorectal cancer at Yeovil District Hospital, 2000–2003

	n	Conversion (%)	Hospital and 30-day death (%)
Elective operation	135		4 (3)
Laparoscopic	102	12 (12)	2
Open: randomised	27		
Open: non-randomised	6		2
Operation after unplanned admission	23		5 (22)
Laparoscopic	2	0	
Open	21		5

Figure 1 demonstrates the proportion of elective patients currently suitable for laparoscopic surgery in our practice; those randomised to open surgery have been excluded from the analysis.

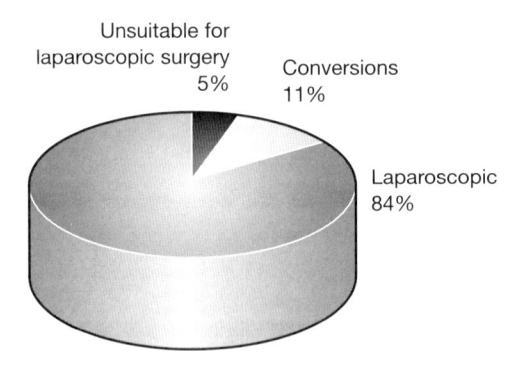

Figure 6.1 Elective surgery for colorectal cancer in Yeovil 2000–2003.

There have not been any port site recurrences observed but one wound recurrence occurred within a stoma following an R1 resection of rectal cancer. This has been successfully excised. Of the 49 patients undergoing rectal resection, positive margins have been present in 3 (6%), two open and one laparoscopic.

Conclusion

There is a lack of good-quality data from large randomised trials comparing laparoscopic and open surgery for CRC. Results from trials across Europe and North America, including the British CLASICC trial, are eagerly awaited. Overwhelming evidence exists, though, that an identical oncological clearance can be performed laparoscopically and that there are undoubted short-term benefits to this approach. There are now also reports that these benefits could be improved if the way patients are managed peri-operatively is optimised. Professor Kehlet's team in Copenhagen have developed a multimodal rehabilitation pathway aimed at enhancing post-operative recovery. Pre-operative counselling, optimal analgesia with neural blockade and minimal use of opiates, early enteral feeding and early mobilisation are the key features of this pathway. Kehlet's group have implemented this in cohorts of patients undergoing both laparoscopic and open colonic surgery and have reduced post-operative hospital stay to two or three days in both groups (Bardram *et al.* 2000; Basse *et al.* 2000). There is an associated earlier restoration of bowel function and less post-operative morbidity in both these groups of patients. Realising the potential of laparoscopic surgery may, therefore, require a change in management toward a multimodal rehabilitation pathway in order to reduce peri-operative stress responses. It is hoped that in combination with these techniques the full benefits of laparoscopic surgery will be demonstrated.

Acknowledgements

This work was undertaken by the authors, who received funding from the NHS Executive South West. The views expressed in this chapter are those of the authors and not necessarily those of the NHS Executive South West.

References

Bardram, L., Funch-Jensen, P. & Kehlet, H. (2000). Rapid rehabilitation in elderly patients after laparoscopic colonic resection. *British Journal of Surgery* **87**, 1540–1545.

Basse, L., Hjort, J. D., Billesbolle, P. *et al.* (2000). A clinical pathway to accelerate recovery after colonic resection. *Annals of Surgery* **232**, 51–57.

Bokey, E. L., Moore, J. W., Chapuis, P. H. *et al.* (1996). Morbidity and mortality following laparoscopic-assisted right hemicolectomy for cancer. *Diseases of Colon and Rectum* **39**, S24–S28.

Braga, M., Vignali, A., Zuliani, W. *et al.* (2002). Metabolic and functional results after laparoscopic colorectal surgery: a randomized, controlled trial. *Diseases of Colon and Rectum* **45**, 1070–1077.

Delaney, C. P., Kiran, R. P., Senagore, A. J. *et al.* (2003). Case-matched comparison of clinical and financial outcome after laparoscopic or open colorectal surgery. *Annals of Surgery* **238**, 67–72.

Delgado, S., Lacy, A. M., Filella, X. *et al.* (2001). Acute phase response in laparoscopic and open colectomy in colon cancer: randomized study. *Diseases of Colon and Rectum* **44**, 638–646.

Fleshman, J. W., Nelson, H., Peters, W. R. *et al.* (1996). Early results of laparoscopic surgery for colorectal cancer. Retrospective analysis of 372 patients treated by Clinical Outcomes of Surgical Therapy (COST) Study Group. *Diseases of Colon and Rectum* **39**, S53–S58.

Franklin, M. E., Kazantsev, G. B., Abrego, D. *et al.* (2000). Laparoscopic surgery for stage III colon cancer: long-term follow-up. *Surgical Endoscopy* **14**, 612–616.

Franklin, M. E. Jr, Rosenthal, D., Abrego-Medina, D. *et al.* (1996). Prospective comparison of open vs laparoscopic colon surgery for carcinoma. Five-year results. *Diseases of Colon and Rectum* **39**, S35–S46.

Hartley, J. E., Mehigan, B. J., MacDonald, A. W. *et al.* (2000). Patterns of recurrence and survival after laparoscopic and conventional resections for colorectal carcinoma. *Annals of Surgery* **232**, 181–186.

Hewitt, P. M., Ip, S. M., Kwok, S. P. *et al.* (1998). Laparoscopic-assisted vs open surgery for colorectal cancer: comparative study of immune effects. *Diseases of Colon and Rectum* **41**, 901–909.

Jacobs, M., Verdeja, J. C. & Goldstein, H. S. (1991). Minimally invasive colon resection (laparoscopic colectomy). *Surgical Laparoscopy, Endoscopy & Percutaneous Techniques* **1**, 144–150.

Kehlet, H. (1999). Surgical stress response: does endoscopic surgery confer an advantage? *World Journal of Surgery* **23**, 801–807.

Lacy, A. M., Delgado, S., Garcia-Valdecasas, J. C. *et al.* (1998). Port site metastases and recurrence after laparoscopic colectomy. A randomized trial. *Surgical Endoscopy* **12**, 1039–1042.

Lacy, A. M., Garcia-Valdecasas, J. C., Delgado, S. *et al.* (2002). Laparoscopy-assisted colectomy versus open colectomy for treatment of non-metastatic colon cancer: a randomised trial. *The Lancet* **359**, 2224–2229.

Lacy, A. M., Garcia-Valdecasas, J. C., Pique, J. M. *et al.* (1995). Short-term outcome analysis of a randomized study comparing laparoscopic vs open colectomy for colon cancer. *Surgical Endoscopy* **9**, 1101–1105.

Marusch, F., Gastinger, I., Schneider, C. *et al.* (2001). Importance of conversion for results obtained with laparoscopic colorectal surgery. *Diseases of Colon and Rectum* **44**, 207–214.

Milsom, J. W., Bohm, B., Hammerhofer, K. A. *et al.* (1998). A prospective, randomized trial comparing laparoscopic versus conventional techniques in colorectal cancer surgery: a preliminary report. *Journal of the American College of Surgeons* **187**, 46–54.

Morino M., Parini U., Giraudo G. *et al.* (2003). Laparoscopic total mesorectal excision: a consecutive series of 100 patients. *Annals of Surgery* **237**, 335–342.

Pearlstone, D. B., Mansfield, P. F., Curley, S. A. *et al.* (1999). Laparoscopy in 533 patients with abdominal malignancy. *Surgery* **125**, 67–72.

Pfeifer, J., Wexner, S. D., Reissman, P. *et al.* (1995). Laparoscopic vs open colon surgery. Costs and outcome. *Surgical Endoscopy* **9**, 1322–1326.

Psaila, J., Bulley, S .H., Ewings, P. *et al.* (1998). Outcome following laparoscopic resection for colorectal cancer. *British Journal of Surgery* **85**, 662–664.

Rickard, M. J. & Bokey, E. L. (2001). Laparoscopy for colon cancer. *Surgical Oncology Clinics of North America* **10**, 579–597.

Schlachta, C. M., Mamazza, J., Seshadri, P. A. *et al.* (2001). Defining a learning curve for laparoscopic colorectal resections. *Diseases of Colon and Rectum* **44**, 217–222.

Schwenk, W., Bohm, B. & Muller, J. M. (1998). Postoperative pain and fatigue after laparoscopic or conventional colorectal resections. A prospective randomized trial. *Surgical Endoscopy* **12**, 1131–1136.

Slim, K., Pezet, D., Riff, Y. *et al.* (1995). High morbidity rate after converted laparoscopic colorectal surgery. *British Journal of Surgery* **82**, 1406–1408.

Stage, J. G., Schulze, S., Moller, P. *et al.* (1997). Prospective randomized study of laparoscopic versus open colonic resection for adenocarcinoma. *British Journal of Surgery* **84**, 391–396.

Tang, C. L., Eu, K.W., Tai, B. C. *et al.* (2001). Randomized clinical trial of the effect of open versus laparoscopically assisted colectomy on systemic immunity in patients with colorectal cancer. *British Journal of Surgery* **88**, 801–807.

Weeks, J .C., Nelson, H., Gelber, S. *et al.* (2002). Short-term quality-of-life outcomes following laparoscopic-assisted colectomy vs open colectomy for colon cancer: a randomial trial. *Journal of the American Medical Association* **287**, 321–328.

Whelan, R. L., Franklin, M., Holubar, S. D. *et al.* (2003). Postoperative cell mediated immune response is better preserved after laparoscopic vs open colorectal resection in humans. *Surgical Endoscopy* **17**, 972–978.

Chapter 7

Progress towards total mesorectal excision as the new 'gold standard' for rectal cancer surgery

Bill Heald

Introduction

The fight to establish total mesorectal excision (TME) as the standard operation for rectal cancer surgery is providing an exciting new chapter in the textbook of medical education. For the first time the principal practical weapon is the video camera and the statistical objective is the meta-analysis of results from whole populations. Many years ago the distinguished American Professor Bill Silen made the following prescient observation in *The Lancet* (Silen 1993):

> *The likelihood that a proper prospective randomised controlled trial (PRCT) will ever be carried out to see whether TME provides an advantage over conventional surgery for rectal cancer is essentially nil. Possibly meta-analysis will help... In my view it is unconscionable to dismiss comparisons with retrospective controls when the procedure is SO superior in terms of both Local Recurrence and Survival.*

The impossibility of applying prospective randomised trial techniques to the detail of technical surgery has been a major impediment to its establishment as the new 'gold standard'. No PRCT has ever been successfully mounted to underpin a complex advance in surgical technique. Furthermore, significant confusion stems from the development of alternative basic technologies such as laparoscopic surgery. These are to some extent amenable to PRCT methods and trials are continuing. It is impossible, however, to compare optimal open with optimal laparoscopic cancer surgery because so few surgeons are optimal at both. It is important to understand that TME is an oncological principle that is theoretically achievable by either open or laparoscopic methods; these trials will add nothing to the most crucial controversy—the detail of the excision of the tumour.

TME is a system of cancer management that defines the block of tissue to be excised and describes the surgical detail of how this is to be achieved. It is now more readily comprehended by non-surgeons because of the development by specialist MRI radiologists of images that are far superior to anything so far achievable. These demonstrate, for the first time, the contours of the mesorectum and the distribution of the cancer within it. They will certainly in the future provide a rational basis for selecting those cases for radiotherapy or chemotherapy, where the mesorectal margin is in danger of being breached during surgery.

The TME concept can be extended now to embrace a multi disciplinary four-stage process:

1. Phased-array-coil fine slice MRI.
2. Pre-operative neoadjuvant therapy in selected cases.
3. Detailed precision surgery.
4. Detailed audit of the specimen after removal.

TME for the surgeon comprises five basic principles:

1. Perimesorectal 'Holy Plane' sharp dissection with diathermy and scissors under direct vision.
2. Specimen-orientated surgery and histopathology, of which the object is an intact mesorectum with no tearing of the surface and no circumferential margin involvement (CMI) – naked eye or microscopic. Quirke-style pathology audit for CMI as the principal outcome measure confirms the success or failure of the surgery.
3. Recognition and preservation of the autonomic nerve plexus, on which sexual and bladder function depend.
4. A major increase in anal preservation and reduction in the number of permanent colostomies.
5. Stapled low pelvic reconstruction, usually using Moran triple stapling technique plus short colon pouch anastomosed to low rectum or anal canal (Moran *et al.* 1994).

Professor John MacFarlane, from the University of British Columbia, published in August 1988 the second set of data from his independent audit of the results in Basingstoke where TME has been a surgical priority for over 20 years. These data comprised a personal series of 519 consecutive surgical cases with adenocarcinoma treated for cure or palliation (Heald *et al.* 1998). The largest group was 465 anterior resections (ARs) with low stapled anastomosis (407 TME), 37 abdominoperineal (AP) resections, 10 Hartmann resections, 4 local excisions and 3 laparotomy only. Pre-operative radiotherapy had been used in only 49 cases (7AP, 38 AR, 3 Hartmann, 1 laparotomy). Cancer-specific survival (CSS) rate of all surgically treated cases is 68% at 5 years and 66% at 10 years. There was a 6% local recurrence (LR) at 5 years (2–10% at 95% confidence interval (CI), 8% at 10 years (2–14% at 95% CI). In 405 'curative' resections the LR rate is 3% and 4% and the CSS rate 80% and 78% at 5 years and 10 years, respectively. All patients were followed regularly until death. The principal risk factors for recurrence include the necessity to perform AP as opposed to AR (for LR), Dukes' stage (for CSS) and extramural vascular invasion (EVI0 for LR and CSS).

Substantial improvements on all previously published, comprehensive, unselected consecutive series now appear confirmed beyond all doubts by these data. In addition, it becomes clear that low LR rates have a substantial effect on overall survival, ie that many LRs after conventional surgery are the result of regrowth of local mesorectal residues, which were the only residual disease present at the time of surgery. Thus, local control equates with cure in such cases and better local control with more cures.

Total mesorectal excision and precise perimesorectal plane dissection are being introduced in all the major countries of Europe. Increasingly the specimen is being audited by the detailed histopathology of Quirke and Dixon (1998). The most significant new evidence comes from joint publication from the Stockholm Colorectal Cancer Group and the Basingstoke Bowel Cancer Research Project. The first published report appeared in *The Lancet* in July 2000, showing a major impact of a teaching programme on cancer outcomes in a whole population. Both the permanent colostomy rate and the local recurrence rate have been more than halved for the entire population of Stockholm County (Lehander Martling *et al.* 2000). An interesting postscript to this study and to these video-based workshops was presented at a seminar in the Basingstoke Pelican Centre by Holm during 2001. The five most assiduous attendees at the 11 Stockholm workshops are now performing 48% of all the rectal cancer surgery in Stockholm – all with local recurrence rates below 5% in 'curative' cases. A major publication is awaited from Norway (Wibe, unpublished data) where a somewhat similar teaching programme was introduced, and a Danish study is close to completion. Individual series such as those already published in the USA by Enker and in New Zealand by Hill show strikingly similar results to those in Basingstoke. Hill called what is essentially an identical technique 'extra fascial excision' and also published similar results with 1.2% on all outcome parameters. Certainly the initial widespread dismissal of the early Basingstoke results with single figure local recurrence rates as inconceivable are now set aside by others achieving exactly the same. In all the individual surgeon series there is a significant improvement on the multi-surgeon series, as would be anticipated for a technique that is technically demanding and challenging.

It is now generally accepted in Europe and in many parts of the world that more precise surgery directed towards total mesorectal excision is the principal determinant of outcome and the principal hope for improvement. The author has undertaken over 200 television workshop demonstration operations in more than 22 countries. TME has become the national standard in Norway, Sweden, Denmark and The Netherlands. In the larger countries – Germany, France and the UK – official guidelines support the TME concept. In Germany, major studies are ongoing to introduce it and even embrace the specialisation and audit routines necessary to eliminate the surgeon variability that Hermanek *et al*. (1995) has so ably demonstrated.

Conclusion

For most of the 20th century it was simply accepted that the 'Miles operation' or abdominoperineal resection (APR) was so mutilating that it had to be as 'curative' or 'radical' as was possible. In reality the 'devil was in the detail'.

Until the TME controversy, almost nothing was published about dissection *around* a rectal cancer. The arbitrary 5 cm distal margin along the muscle tube, formally considered necessary for sphincter preservation, has long been abandoned, although the relevance or irrelevance of the internal iliac nodes provoked some controversy, which lingers on both in Japan and in Italy. Ten years ago local recurrence rates between 25% and 50% were standard, and recurrence within the pelvis was by far the most common presentation of recurrence and by far the cruellest mode of death. The early claims from Basingstoke of single figure local recurrence rates by TME were complemented by reports from Leeds that showed high positive predictive values of circumferential margin involvement (CMI) for local recurrence (LR) (Quirke & Dixon 1998). What has been difficult for many to comprehend is that this high predictive value applies only to series where the local recurrence rate is high, e.g. in Leeds at the time of the first CMI publication the overall local recurrence rate was 36%, whereas CMI was a much poorer predictor in Guildford where TME surgery was delivering a much lower LR rate (editorial in *The Lancet* 1990 (Anon. 1990)). Reports also appeared of wide variation in results between surgeons. The fact that three-quarters of the Leeds LRs had been predicted by CMI reflected a key reality, which went largely unnoticed; that most of these CMI cases could have been avoided by the wider circumferential clearance afforded by TME. Thus, the lower the local recurrence rate in any given series the less good a predictor CMI becomes, although it remains a predictor of cancer death. For the most part, margin involvement is a predictor of preventable local recurrence. In the future, CMI should almost never occur in a case that has *not* received pre-operative RT, which will have been selected in the planning stage because the risk had been recognised.

The real importance of CMI in the management of rectal cancer is, however, that it provides a key audit tool for better surgery. It is axiomatic that the margins of any surgical cancer specimen must be clear of cancer: low CMI rates reflect 'better' surgery and are an end in themselves; if TME surgeons deliver lower CMI rates then this is a self-evident benefit. Modern MRI provides the basis for a whole new discipline in prediction of the relationship of the outer tentacles of cancer to the mesorectal fascia and thus to the risk of an involved margin. Furthermore, those where the mesorectal fascia appears 'threatened' may prove to be those that require long-course pre-operative chemotherapy.

During 2001 by far the highest-profile published trial in the rectal cancer field came from Holland. Despite the initial determination to subject the actual surgical technique of TME to randomisation the planners of the Dutch study made two very interesting decisions. First, they recognised the impracticability of a PRCT of surgical technique and decided instead on a training protocol to *standardise* the surgery whilst *randomising* only short-course radiotherapy. Second, they decided that the value of chemotherapy in *rectal* cancer was so dubious that they omitted it altogether.

The first to appear from Leiden was in the *New England Journal of Medicine* (Kapiteijn 2001). No doubt it was ruthless editing that eliminated all but a single message – that short-course RT (Swedish-style 5 × 5 Gy in five days) reduced the local recurrence rate in *standardised TME surgery* from 8% to 2%. There are, however, caveats: the mean follow-up time is only two years; and the involved margin rate on Quirke-style histopathology audit is 18%. For mobile tumours this is really far too high and suggest that not all the surgeons were performing good-quality TMEs. This underlines the great difficulty of refining a surgical technique, although the audit practice and histopathology schedule introduced by Professor Quirke were exemplary demonstrations of 'logical best practice'.

Because the author was the primary TME 'workshop instructor' for this trial it is possible to predict that we will be hearing more interesting data from the 'Dutch TME Trial'. So far, as already indicated, the message is about RT, and this is already producing a large knock-on effect on British practice. In many parts of the country all patients are being given short-course RT without any attempt at pre-operative staging. The wisdom of this rapid change in practice must be questioned. The author's personal data, shortly to be published, do show that a combination of clinical assessment and fine-slice MRI make it possible, in a unit where precision TME is the priority, to select more than 75% of all referrals as being suitable for *no* RT and to deliver 2.5% local recurrence rate in this group.

RT is not without its own morbidity and it must surely be a priority for us to identify those patients where it is *not* required. Further analysis of the effect of RT (randomised) on a substantial number of patients with involved surgical margins will shortly be published and will still further fuel the confusion regarding short-course RT and the rationale for giving it. It is the author's opinion that *selection* is the key to future progress. The *selective* use of chemo-RT, almost invariably given *pre*-operatively, is surely the only efficient way to cut RT waiting times. The identification of a group requiring *no* RT is really urgent in the UK for this reason alone. Such chemo-irradiated cases are, however, at high risk for anastomotic leakage, especially when the long-course RT has been chosen.

Specialisation in deep pelvic surgery and the recognition that two consultants are sometimes optimal are key steps forward. Selection of the low or ultra-low anterior cancer in a difficult male for referral to such a team is a further logical step. In this most challenging malignancy selective use of neoadjuvants based on MRI, combined with improvements in surgery, mean that complete elimination of local disease is now a real possibility. This will also mean a substantial survival advantage and a real reduction in human suffering.

References

Anon. (1990). Breaching the mesorectum. *The Lancet* **335**, 1067–1068.

Heald, R. J. (1995). Total mesorectal excision is optimal surgery for rectal cancer: a Scandinavian consensus. *British Journal of Surgery* **82**, 1297–1299.

Heald, R. J. (1997). Total mesorectal excision: history and anatomy of an operation. In *Rectal Cancer Surgery: Optimisation – Standardisation – Documentation* (ed. O. Soreide & J. Norstein), pp. 203–219. Berlin: Springer-Verlag.

Heald, R. J., Husband, E. M. & Ryall, R. D. H. (1982). The mesorectum is rectal cancer surgery – the clue to pelvic recurrence? *British Journal of Surgery* **69**, 613–616.

Heald, R. J., Moran, B. J., Ryall, R. D. H., Sexton, R. & MacFarlane, J. K. (1998). Rectal cancer. The Basingstoke experience of total mesorectal excision, 1978–1997. *Archives of Surgery* **133**, 894–898.

Heald, R. J. & Ryall, R. D. H. (1986). Recurrence and survival after total mesorectal excision for rectal cancer. *The Lancet* **i**, 1479–1482.

Hermanek, P., Wiebelt, H., Staimmer, D. & Riedl, S. (1995). Prognostic factors of rectum carcinoma – experience of the German multicentre study SGCRC German Study Group Colo-Rectal Carcinoma. *Tumori* **8** (Supplement 3), 60–64.

Isbister, W. H. (1990). Basingstoke revisited. *Australia and New Zealand Journal of Surgery* **60**, 243–246.

Isbister, W. H. (1998). Food for thought – Basingstoke revisited again. *Australia and New Zealand Journal of Surgery*, in press.

Kapiteijn E. *et al.* (2001). Preoperative radiotherapy combined with total mesorectal excision for respectable rectal cancer. *New England Journal of Medicine* **345**, 638–646.

Lehander Martling, A., Holm, T. *et al.* (2000). Effect of a surgical training programme on outcome of rectal cancer in the County of Stockholm. *The Lancet* **356**, 93–96.

Moran, B. J., Docherty, A. & Finnis, D. (1994). Novel stapling technique to facilitate low anterior resection for rectal cancer. *British Journal of Surgery* **81**, 1230.

Quirke, P. & Dixon, M. F. (1998). The prediction of local recurrence of rectal adenocarcinoma by histopathological examination. *International Journal of Colorectal Disease* **3**, 127–131.

Silen, W. (1993). Mesorectal excision for rectal cancer. *The Lancet* **341**, 1279–1280.

Chapter 8

Optimising sphincter-sparing surgery in rectal cancer

Rob Glynne-Jones and Marina Wallace

Introduction

Radical surgery for rectal cancer requires the complete removal of the primary cancer with all the associated lymph nodes. The importance of meticulous sharp dissection of the mesorectum (total mesorectal excision) has been recognised not only in terms of reducing local recurrence but also maximising sphincter-sparing surgery (SPSS). For optimal results it is also vital for the surgeon to understand the pattern of tumour spread and how the anal sphincter works. Several different surgical options are possible.

Controversy arises for a cancer that is close to, but does not involve, the anal sphincter mechanism. Should these patients have their anus removed with an abdominoperineal resection, or are there alternative methods that allow the sphincter to be preserved, thereby avoiding a permanent stoma? Most surgeons consider the low position of some rectal cancers will inevitably require an abdominoperineal resection particularly if the sphincter is invaded. In addition, bulky anterior tumours in obese men with a narrow pelvis may prove technically demanding to achieve sphincter-sparing surgery. However, the varying skills, training and philosophy of each surgeon mean that a unanimous and consistent approach is difficult. For this reason it seems clear that there is no accepted practice for a cancer 3–6 cm from the anal verge.

A further issue is the role of combining chemotherapy and/or radiotherapy with surgery to shrink and hence facilitate sphincter-saving surgery. Despite a dramatic increase in the use of radiotherapy in rectal cancer over the last decade, there has not been a marked increase in the number of patients whose sphincter is preserved. It appears obvious that sphincter preservation is likely to be achieved more frequently with pre-operative as opposed to post-operative radiotherapy, and the addition of chemotherapy to achieve more effective downsizing may contribute further.

Over the past decade non-randomised studies have confirmed that pre-operative treatment with radiotherapy (Wagman 1998) can facilitate sphincter-sparing options. A study from Lyon compared immediate and delayed surgery after pre-operative radiotherapy (Francois *et al*. 1999). Sphincter preservation was achieved in 79% of patients with a long interval (4–6 weeks) following radiotherapy, compared with 69% of patients where the interval was only short (2 weeks). A further report (Glehen *et al*. 2003) documents that with a median follow-up of 6.3 years no differences were found in the degree of local control, overall survival, morbidity, anal function or surgical complications between the two groups. The local recurrence rate was 13 of 99 in the short interval (13%) and 10 of 102 in the long interval group (10%). Interestingly, patients who underwent sphincter-saving surgery where the distal resection margin was <1.5 cm appeared to have a higher local recurrence rate, ie 9 out of 43 (21%) compared with 7 out of 76 (9%) in patients where the distal resection margin was in excess of 1.5 cm. This data suggest that a delay between pre-operative radiotherapy and surgery increases downstaging and may be helpful to optimise response rates and sphincter preservation, but does not improve survival.

The addition of chemotherapy to radiotherapy (chemoradiation) can be used to shrink the primary tumour further and facilitate sphincter-sparing options. Impressive results appear to have been achieved in phase II studies with chemoradiation (Grann *et al.* 1997; Rullier *et al.* 2001) and long-term follow-up has confirmed an excellent outcome if there is marked shrinkage of the primary tumour (Ruo *et al.* 2002).

The aim of this article is to discuss neoadjuvant chemoradiotherapy in rectal cancer and the evidence for its role in downstaging, or more accurately, downsizing the tumour with a view to facilitating sphincter-sparing surgery. We have not chosen to explore the role of local excision following or preceding chemoradiation.

Surgery: the role of the distal margin

Little information has been published on the ideal distal margin needed when making a decision to perform sphincter-preserving surgery. Originally the accepted distal margin was 5 cm (Goligher 1951), and in the 1970s and 1980s surgeons continued to recommend this minimum distance. Many authors since have questioned whether less than this is sufficient. A 2 cm margin was advocated by Paty (1994) and supported by other authors (Shirouza 1995; Vernava 1992). Paty suggested that in practice very few rectal cancers extend more than 1–2 cm distally in terms of intramural spread and that narrow distal margins do not appear to compromise either local control or survival. Currently, most surgeons consider a 2 cm distal margin acceptable. There is some evidence that in more locally advanced rectal cancers there is a higher likelihood of distal spread beyond 1 cm. The Lyon study (*vide supra*) shows that after radiotherapy a 1.5 cm distal resection margin may be important in reducing local recurrence.

A recent study (Moore *et al.* 2003) assessed the effect of a distal margin of 1 cm or less on both local control and survival in a large series of patients with rectal cancer treated with pre-operative chemoradiation and undergoing sphincter-sparing procedures in the context of sharp mesorectal excision. One hundred and seventeen consecutive patients were treated with pre-operative chemoradiation between 1991 and August 2000 followed by low anterior resection, and in the case of complete pathological responses the distal margin was reported as the distance between the residual scar and the distal cut margin. This study clearly suggests that distal resection margins of less than 1 cm do not seem to adversely affect local recurrence or survival if chemoradiation has been given first, despite the fact these patients will have been selected for pre-operative chemoradiation because of more advanced disease (Shibata *et al.* 2002). In the light of such data, many surgeons now consider 1 cm as an adequate distal margin following chemoradiation (Kuvshinoff *et al.* 2001).

The role of pre-operative chemoradiation

It seems logical to presume, therefore, that if tumour size can be reduced pre-operatively, local recurrence rates may be reduced and sphincter-sparing surgery performed.

Several surgical series have reported results of patients with clinically resectable rectal cancer, in whom clinical assessment by their surgeon categorised height of the cancer from the anal verge as requiring an abdominoperineal resection. These patients then received pre-operative radiotherapy and were subsequently reassessed before definitive surgery. Three of the studies used radiotherapy alone (Francois *et al.*; Wagman *et al.*; 1998; Rouanet 1995) and five have used synchronous chemoradiation (NSABP R-O3 (Hyams 1997; Roh *et al.* 2001); Valentini *et al.* 1998; Grann *et al.* 2001; Maghfoor *et al.* 1997; Sauer *et al.* 2003). At first glance pre-operative chemoradiation appears to offer a 10% (Roh *et al.* 2001) or even a 20% (Sauer *et al.* 2003) higher chance overall in achieving SPSS. Although it is not clear how these patients have been selected as the rate of sphincter preservation is only 23% in the NSABP R-03 series compared with 42% in the German study and approximately 70% in some phase II chemoradiation trials. Patients with very low rectal cancers infiltrating the levator muscles and responding to pre-operative chemoradiation therapy were treated with sphincter-sparing procedures instead of an abdominoperineal excision. The risks of local recurrence appear low, and functional results seem satisfactory (Fucini *et al.* 2002).

Surgical complications after chemoradiation

Luna-Perez *et al.* (2003) examined the role of chemoradiation in rectal cancers located between 3 and 6 cm from the anal verge and the feasibility, morbidity and functional results of sphincter-sparing surgery with coloanal anastomosis following pre-operative treatment. Thirty-three patients (17 males, 15 females) with tumours located a mean of 4.7 cm above the anal verge were studied. Coloanal anastomosis and J-pouch was performed in 22 patients, and a straight anastomosis in 10, with a mean distal surgical margin of 1.3 cm. Surgical complications were not insignificant, with pelvic abscess in three patients, rectovaginal fistulae in two (unsuccessfully repaired) and a coloanal anastomotic dehiscence in one patient. Diverting stomas were finally closed in 30 patients after a median follow-up of 25 months. Local recurrence occurred in only one patient where a positive lateral circumferential resection margin was observed histopathologically. This study also examined anal sphincter function using the Kirwan classification. Five patients had grade 3 gastrointestinal toxicity and three patients had grade 4 toxicity. Continence appeared better for patients who underwent J-pouch anastomosis rather than a straight coloanal anastomosis. Many authors suggest that the potential problems after pre-operative chemoradiation include sepsis in the perineal surgical scar when an AP excision of the rectum is performed; a delay of wound healing and also an increased rate of anastomotic leaks in restorative procedures (Janjan *et al.* 1998; Pucciarelli *et al.* 1999; Shumate *et al.* 1993). However, there seems little increase in the incidence of major intra-abdominal sepsis or post-operative ileus. Many surgeons still have anxieties that pre-operative chemoradiation increases the risks of both post-operative surgical morbidity and increases mortality.

Pucciarelli *et al.* (1999) reported on 71 patients treated at the University of Padua who underwent an anterior resection: 41 patients received pre-operative chemoradiotherapy and 30 did not receive any pre-operative treatment. Anastomotic leaks were considered major complications if they were associated with the production of pus or a faeculent discharge from the drain. In contrast, minor anastomotic leaks were defined as clinically negligible leaks or leaks discovered as an unexpected finding at follow-up. Although non-randomised, the two groups with and without pre-operative chemoradiation did not have a statistically significant difference either in the duration of surgery or the amount of inter-operative blood loss. An anastomotic leak was discovered in 11 of 41 patients receiving pre-operative chemoradiotherapy (24%) compared with 4 out of 29 in the surgery alone group (13.7%), although this is only defined as a major anastomotic leak for 3 patients in each group. More complications were observed for those who did not have a diverting stoma.

Finally, evidence from the German randomised CAO/ARO/AIO-94 trial demonstrates an identical anastomotic leak rate (12%) for patients treated with pre-operative chemoradiation and those proceeding directly to surgery (Sauer *et al.* 2003).

The role of randomised controlled trials

Clearly, the question of whether pre-operative chemoradiation really does facilitate sphincter-sparing procedures or just offers the surgeons confidence to carry them out should be answered. It is not clear to these authors why, in some series, very distal tumours close to the ano-rectal ring can be resected with sphincter preservation (Crane *et al.* 2003a) where in other series (Valentini 2001), this is not the case. Hopefully the results of the Polish study (Bujko *et al.* 2002)—which randomises between 25 Gy in 5 fractions followed by immediate surgery, and 50 Gy in 25 fractions in combination with 5-fluorouracil (5-FU) followed by surgery after six weeks have elapsed to allow response to the tumour – will answer this question.

Inevitably, randomised controlled trials in this arena will be very difficult to accomplish. Given the choice of two different procedures; one conservative and one more mutilating and with the potential for a permanent colostomy, most patients will refuse to be randomised even if it remains unclear which of these two procedures will have the better outcome in oncological terms. Despite recent data from Germany (Grumann *et al.* 2001) on the quality of life when an AP excision of the rectum is compared with an anterior resection, most patients in Europe have an almost pathological terror of the prospect of a colostomy (Rouanet *et al.* 2002).

In addition, there is a wide variety of approaches between surgeons, from the very conservative where the APR rate may be up to 30%, to the much more aggressive with an APR rate in the region of 10%. Every surgeon will have an individual judgement as to the advisability of sphincter-sparing surgery in any particular patient. Therefore, it seems odd that it could be possible to give a prospective assessment regarding the objective feasibility of sphincter-sparing surgery. This decision is often made per operatively.

Late functional results

As well as ensuring complete resection of rectal cancers with low local recurrence rates, functional results are also an important factor in deciding whether the sphincter mechanism should be saved. Tumours above the peritoneal reflection are excised and an end-to-end anastomosis performed with good functional results. Total mesorectal excision (TME), taking the cancer with the entire mesorectum to the pelvic floor, is performed for tumours below the peritoneal reflection. These can be anastomosed with per anal staples or hand sutured endoanal anastomosis, straight or colo-pouch anal anastomosis. Functional results depend on the distance of the anastomosis from the anal canal and type of reconstruction. The use of a J-pouch reconstruction reduces stool frequency, decreases incontinence, and improves compliance and ambulatory manometric findings when compared with straight colo-anal anastomosis. This benefit seems to last for at least two years after surgery.

For this reason, functional outcome in rectal cancer following treatment is determined by: the level of anastomosis; the type of reconstruction, i.e. whether there is a pouch; whether pre-operative or post-operative radiotherapy or chemoradiation has been used; and finally the age of the patient. These factors vary between surgeons, and depend on case-mix.

The results will also change over time. Radiation effects generally start to be expressed after one year, worsen over time and are accepted to be more prominent at five years following surgery than at two. In contrast, after a surgical procedure, function will usually continue to improve for up to two to three years. However, there is little evidence to clarify the late results of surgery alone and pre-operative radiotherapy chemoradiation in surgery with similar surgical techniques (Shibata *et al.* 2000). Only when adequate data are available will we be able to balance the use of neoadjuvant chemoradiation against the operative technique to gain optimal tumour control and maintain ideal functional outcome.

Functional results have been assessed in a recent report (Dehni *et al.* 2002) by a standardised questionnaire which asked questions about the number of bowel movements/nocturnal defecation/anal irritation/the need to wear a protective pad/ regular use of loperamide or laxative and finally if the patients considered they had diarrhoea or constipation compared with their usual bowel habits before surgery. Urgency was defined as the inability to defer defecation for more than 15 minutes.

The results showed that in terms of long-term functional results, nocturnal defecation was significantly commoner for patients who had pre-operative radiotherapy (36% versus 15% for those who did not). Diarrhoea is similarly more common (39% versus 13%). Otherwise, no significant differences were found. This study would suggest that pre-operative radiation therapy in rectal cancer has little in the way of adverse effects on function if the patient has a J-pouch. It is only diarrhoea and nocturnal defecation that were significantly different. However, it is not possible to say whether the lack of differences relates to more meticulous surgery and the J-pouch or whether this study employed smaller volumes /more accurate radiotherapy.

Is the degree of clinical response important?

Crane recently published a thought-provoking paper from the M. D. Anderson Hospital, Houston, Texas (Crane 2003a). The aim was to determine whether objective tumour response increased the possibility of performing sphincter-preserving surgery in low rectal cancers. They reviewed the records of 238 patients with T3/T4 adenocarcinoma of the rectum treated between December 1989 and December 2000 with pre-operative chemoradiation and either TME or local excision where the lower border was 6 cm or less from the anal verge. Patients received 45 Gy in 25 fractions over five weeks with continuous infusion 5-FU at a dose of 300 mg/m^2 Monday–Friday.

Because it is well recognised that definitions of response are difficult and inaccurate following chemoradiation, the authors chose to use a definition of complete clinical response, ie cases of either no residual tumour cells or only microscopic tumour cells in the resected specimen. The results showed that 47% of patients achieved a complete clinical response, 49% in T3 and 32% in T4 cases.

The surgeons achieved sphincter preservation in 102 patients by performing a coloanal anastomosis and in 15 patients performing a local excision; 113 patients had an AP excision of the rectum and 8 underwent a total pelvic exenteration.

In total, 49% of patients with tumours less than 6 cm from the anal verge achieved sphincter-sparing surgery. Distance of tumour from anal verge, the year of treatment (evaluated as a continuous variable) and a complete clinical response appeared independently significant. The overall five-year actuarial rate of pelvic recurrence was 13% in patients who underwent sphincter-sparing surgery compared with 14% who underwent AP excision of the rectum. Despite a significant increase in sphincter-sparing surgery over the three time periods in the study, the rate of local recurrence did not rise. None of the 15 patients who had a local excision experienced pelvic recurrence, with a median follow-up of 34 months (range 8–96 months).

A further recent paper from the M. D. Anderson Cancer Center, examining retrospective results from two centres in the USA over a 17-year period, also suggests that the addition of 5FU to pre-operative radiotherapy in locally advanced rectal cancer improves tumour response and thereby increases the chance of SPS in low rectal cancer (Crane *et al*. 2003b).

The questions for the surgeon remain

It remains unclear which of the following four reasons account for why surgeons may increase the rate of sphincter-sparing surgery after pre-operative chemoradiation particularly where there is significant tumour regression:

1. That tumour regression will allow the surgeon to take a *narrower* distal margin.
2. That tumour regression will allow the surgeon more easily to perform sharp dissection particularly in males with a narrow pelvis.
3. That the surgeons would have greater *confidence* in dividing the colon close to the distal margin after the use of pre-operative radiotherapy.
4. That tumour regression may allow a surgeon divide where tumour clearly and unequivocally existed before neoadjuvant chemoradiation.

The final point is arguably the most contentious. Without doubt surgeons will sometimes cut through areas of tumour regression in the circumferential plane, for example where tumour regression has occurred in a pre-treatment radiologically defined T4 tumours extending beyond the CRM, or tumours previously fixed to the pelvic side-wall or sacrum. Should we also extend this to the distal 'regression' margin?

Conclusion

Response to pre-operative chemoradiation does seem to influence surgeons in performing sphincter-sparing procedures. The authors feel that the main advantage of pre-operative chemoradiation is that surgeons with experience of this technique will gain the confidence to take a narrower distal resection margin when they see that patients are not at higher risk of local recurrence. However, it takes time and experience to change surgical philosophy and techniques.

The authors believe that large studies with much longer follow-up than is conventionally undertaken are required to accurately assess the long-term results of pre-operative chemoradiation and sphincter-sparing surgery. It is possible that local recurrence is delayed by radiotherapy and chemoradiation rather than prevented (Merkel *et al*. 2002). It is also recognised that the late effects of radiotherapy are still evolving even at 10 years (Eifel *et al*. 1995). As specialisation and multimodality treatment ensures that more patients survive longer, it is important to know the late effects and functional outcome of the above approach.

Even for the enthusiasts, pre-operative chemoradiation provokes many questions, which remain unanswered. What is the role of chemoradiation for the master surgeon who performs TME? Which patients will benefit most from neoadjuvant chemoradiation? What is the role of the new drugs in the neoadjuvant setting? What is the optimal sequence of drugs? What is the optimum interval between chemoradiation and definitive surgery? Should all borderline resectable tumours where the surgeon is unsure of performing sphincter-sparing surgery receive pre-operative chemoradiation? Should surgeons perform a frozen section analysis of the distal margin to ensure there is no microscopic evidence of residual disease at or close to the resection margin?

Finally, what is the late function if a surgeon performs an ultra-low anterior resection after full-dose pre-operative chemoradiation? Is the quality of life really better than that experienced by patients who underwent an APER (Grumann *et al.* 2001)? Only randomised studies will give us the answers.

References

Bujko, K., Nowacki, M., Bebenek, M. *et al.* (2002). Randomized trial comparing high dose per fraction preoperative radiotherapy with immediate surgery versus conventional pre-operative radiochemotherapy with delayed surgery for patients with low rectal cancer. *Radiotherapy and Oncology* **64**, S1–S47.

Crane, C. H., Skibber, J. M., Feig, B. W. *et al.* (2003a). Response to preoperative chemoradiation increases use of sphincter-preserving surgery in patients with locally advanced low rectal cancer. *Cancer* **97**, 517–524.

Crane, C. H., Skibber, J. M., Birnbaum, E. *et al.* (2003b). The addition of continuous infusion 5-FU to pre-operative radiation therapy increases tumour response, leading to increased sphincter preservation in locally advanced low rectal cancer. *International Journal of Radiation Oncology, Biology, Physics* **57**, 84–89.

Dehni, N., McNamara, D., Schlegal, R. D. *et al.* (2002). Clinical effects of pre-operative radiation therapy on anorectal function after proctectomy and colonic J-pouch anal anastomosis. *Diseases of the Colon and Rectum* **45**, 1635–1640.

Eifel, P. J., Levenback, C., Wharton, J. T., Oswald, M. J. (1995). Time course and incidence of late complications in patients treated with radiation therapy for FIGO stage IB carcinoma of the uterine cervix. *International Journal of Radiation Oncology, Biology, Physics* **32**, 1289–1300.

Francois, Y., Nemoz, C. J., Baulieux, J., Vignal, J., Grandjean, J. P., Partensky, C., Souquet, J. C., Adeleine, P. & Gerard, J. P. (1999). Influence of the interval betweenpre-operative radiation therapy and surgery on downstaging and the rate of sphincter-saving surgery for rectal cancer: the Lyon R90-01 randomized trial. *Journal of Clinical Oncology* **17**, 2396–2402.

Fucini, C., Elbetti, C. *et al.* (2002). Excision of the levator muscles with external sphincter preservation in the treatment of selected low T4 rectal cancers. *Diseases of the Colon and Rectum* **45**(12), 1697–1705.

Glehen, O., Chapet, O., Adham, M. *et al.* (2003). Long-term results of the Lyons R90-01 randomized trial of pre-operative radiotherapy with delayed surgery and its effect on sphincter-saving surgery in rectal cancer. *British Journal of Surgery* **90**, 996–998.

Goligher, J. C., Dukes, C. E., Bussey, H. J. R. (1951). Local recurrence after sphincter saving excisions for carcinoma of the rectum and rectal sigmoid. *British Journal of Surgery* **39**, 199–211.

Grann, A., Minsky, B. D. & Cohen, A. M. (1997). Preliminary results of pre-operative 5-fluorouracil, low dose leucovorin and concurrent radiation therapy for clinically resectable T3 rectal cancer. *Diseases of the Colon and Rectum* **40**, 414–522.

Grann, A., Feng, C. et al. (2001). Pre-operative combined modality therapy for clinically resectable uT3 rectal adenocarcinoma. *International Journal of Radiation Oncology, Biology, Physics* **49**, 987–995.

Grumann, M. M., Noack, E. M., Hoffmann, I. A. & Schlag, P. M (2001). Comparison of quality of life in patients undergoing abdominoperineal extirpation or anterior resection for rectal cancer. *Annals of Surgery* **233**, 149–156.

Hyams, D. M., Mamounas, E. P., Petrelli, N. et al. (1997). A clinical trial to evaluate the worth of pre-operative multimodality therapy in patients with operable cancer of the rectum. *Diseases of the Colon and Rectum* **40**, 131–139.

Kuvshinoff, B., Maghfoor, I., Miedena, B. et al. (2001). Distal margin requirements after preoperative chemoradiotherapy for distal rectal carcinomas: Are ≤1 cm distal margin sufficient? *Annals of Surgical Oncology* **8**, 163–169.

Janjan, N. A., Khoo, V. S, Rich, T. et al. (1998). Advanced rectal cancer: surgical complications after infusional chemotherapy and radiation therapy. *Radiology* **206**, 131–136.

Luna-Perez, P., Rodgrigues-Ramirex, S., Hernandez-Pachedo, F. et al. (2003). Anal sphincter preservation in locally advanced low rectal adenocarcinoma after preoperative chemoradiation therapy in coloanal anastomosis. *Journal of Surgical Oncology* **82**, 3–9.

Maghfoor, I., Wilkes, J., Kuvshinoff, I. et al. (1997). Neoadjuvant chemoradiotherapy with sphincter sparing surgery for low lying rectal cancer. *Journal of Clinical Oncology* **16**, 274 (abstract).

Merkel, S., Meyer, T., Gohl, J. et al. (2002). Late loco-regional recurrence in rectal carcinoma. *European Journal of Surgical Oncology* **28**, 716–722.

Moore, H. G., Riedel, E., Bruce, D. et al. (2003). Adequacy of 1 cm distal margin after restorative rectal cancer resection with sharp mesorectal excision and preoperative combined modality therapy. *Annals of Surgical Oncology* **10**, 80–85.

Moore, H. G., Riedel, E., Minsky, B. D. et al. (2003). Adequacy of 1 cm distal margin in rectal cancer following chemoradaition *Annals of Surgical Oncology* **10**, 80–85.

Paty, B. B., Enker, W. E., Cohen, A. M. et al. (1994). Treatment of rectal cancer by low anterior resection with colo-anal anastomosis. *Annals of Surgery* **219**, 365–373.

Pucciarelli, S., Toppan, P., Friso, M. L. et al. (1999). Preoperative combined radiotherapy and chemotherapy for rectal cancer does not affect early post operative morbidity and mortality in low anterior resection. *Diseases of the Colon and Rectum* **42**, 1276–1284.

Roh, M., Petrelli, N., Wieand, H. et al. (2001). Phase III randomised trial of preoperative versus postoperative mutimodality therapy in patients with carcinoma of the rectum (NSABP R-03). *Journal of Clinical Oncology Proc ASCO* **20**, abstract 123.

Rouanet, P., Fabre, J. M., Dubois, J. B. et al. (1995). Conservative surgery for low rectal carcinoma after high-dose radiation. Functional and oncologic results. *Annals of Surgery* **221**, 67–73.

Rouanet, P., Aubert, B., Lemanski, C. et al. (2002). Restorative and non-restorative surgery for low rectal cancer after high dose radiation – long term oncological functional results. *Diseases of the Colon and Rectum* **45**, 305–313.

Rullier, E., Goffre, B., Bonell, C. et al. (2001). Preoperative radio chemotherapy and sphincter saving resection in T3 carcinomas of the lower third of the rectum. *American Surgeon* **234**, 633–640.

Ruo, L., Tikoo, S., Klimstra, D. et al. (2002). Long term prognostic significance of extended rectal cancer response to pre-operative radiation and chemotherapy. *American Surgeon* **236**, 75–81.

Sauer, R., Fietkau, R., Wittekind, C. *et al.* (2003). Adjuvant vs neoadjuvant radiochemotherapy for locally advanced rectal cancer: the German Trial CAO/ARO/AIO-94. *Colorectal Disease* **5**, 406–415.

Shibata, D., Guillem, M., Lanouette, B. *et al.* (2002). Functional and quality-of-life outcomes in patients with rectal cancer after combined modality therapy, intraoperative radiation therapy and sphincter preservation. *Diseases of the Colon and Rectum* **43**, 752–758.

Shirouza, K., Isomoto, H. & Kakegawa, T. (1995). Distal spread of rectal cancer and optimal margin of resection for sphincter preserving surgery. *Cancer* **76**, 388–392.

Shumate, C. R., Rich, T. A., Skibber, J. M. *et al.* (1993). Preoperative chemotherapy and radiation therapy for locally advanced primary and recurrent rectal carcinoma. *Cancer* **71**, 3690–3696.

Valentini, V., Rosetto, M. E., Fares, C., Mantini, G., Salvi, G. & Turriziani, A. (1998). Radiotherapy and local control in rectal cancer. *Rays* **23**, 580–585.

Valentini, V., Coco, C., Cellini, N. *et al.* (2001). Ten years of preoperative chemoradiation for extraperitoneal T3 rectal cancer: acute toxicity, tumor response, and sphincter preservation in three consecutive studies. *International Journal of Radiation Oncology, Biology, Physics* **51**(2), 371–83.

Vernava, A. M. & Moran, M. (1992). A prospective evaluation of distal margins in carcinomas of the rectum. *Surgical Gynaecology and Obstetrics* **175**, 333–336.

Wagman, R., Minsky, B. D., Cohen, A. M. *et al.* (1998). Sphincter preservation in rectal cancer with pre-operative radiation therapy and coloanal anastomosis: long term follow-up. *International Journal of Radiation Oncology, Biology, Physics* **42**, 51–57.

Chapter 9

Intensive follow-up after colorectal cancer: recent successes and future challenges

Andrew G. Renehan, Matthias Egger, Mark P. Saunders, David K. Whynes and Sarah T. O'Dwyer

Introduction

Colorectal cancer is the second most common cause of cancer-related mortality in Europe (Pisani *et al.* 1999). This burden of disease means that colorectal cancer follow-up is of major clinical, social, and economic importance. The rationale for follow-up after initial curative resection for colorectal cancer is 3-fold: psychological support, facilitation of audit, and an opportunity for the potential early detection and treatment of recurrent disease and/or metachronous (second colorectal primary) disease, with concomitant improvement in survival (Scholefield & Steele 2002). The merits of the latter role of follow-up have been debated for many years. This lack of consensus is reflected in current UK guidelines for the management of patients with colorectal cancer, stating that there is 'no evidence' (ACPGBI 2001), or that intensive follow-up is 'not worth while' (SIGN 1997). In the USA, there are no guidelines on follow-up strategies per se; rather the recommendations are based on the relative merits of individual surveillance tools in the detection of recurrent disease (Desch et al. 1999; Berman et al. 2000). We know, from a survey based on practice five years ago, that some form of routine testing during follow-up is offered by almost 90% of surgeons (Mella *et al.* 1997), but not surprisingly, there is wide variation in follow-up practice (Mella *et al.* 1997; Bruinvels *et al.* 1995; Virgo *et al.* 1995). Among these many different protocols, the costs to health services are considerable and need to be justified with evidence.

To estimate the benefits from intensive follow-up, investigators often work from a starting point of 100% of patients undergoing initial primary treatment, and undertake calculations based on the number of recurrences, numbers offered re-operations, numbers salvaged, and so on (Weiss & Cook 1998; Kievit 2002). This approach is very imprecise. For each estimate (e.g. recurrence rates), there is an associated variance that needs to be considered when calculating the next estimate. Thus, as one reaches the 'numbers salvaged', the confidence intervals are very large and, indeed, include negative numbers. Because of the uncertainty of 'fit' with each ascending estimate, we have referred to this approach as the 'Russian-Doll' phenomenon (see Figure 9.1). This approach also assumes that if there is a benefit from follow-up, this is solely through the detection and successful salvage of recurrent disease. We will discuss later that non-salvage benefit may also be relevant.

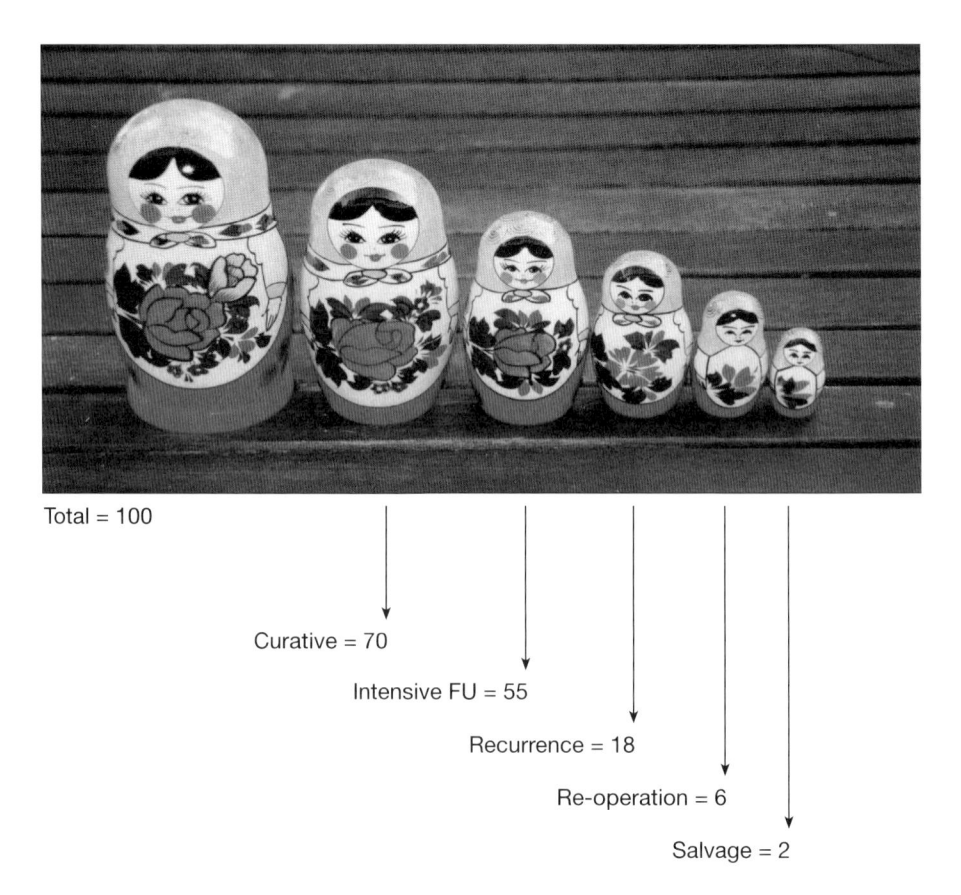

Total = 100
↓
Curative = 70
↓
Intensive FU = 55
↓
Recurrence = 18
↓
Re-operation = 6
↓
Salvage = 2

Figure 9.1 'Russian Doll' phenomenon. Each successive doll fits loosely into the end – i.e. the 'fit' is imprecise.

The only systematic approach to evaluating follow-up is through randomised controlled trials. To date, a number of trials have addressed this issue, but none had sufficient statistical power. Until recently, two meta-analyses on colorectal cancer follow-up have been published – one was entirely based on non-randomised data (Bruinvels *et al.* 1994), and the other on combined randomised trials with cohort studies (Rosen *et al.* 1998). Against this background, we performed an up-dated systematic review and meta-analysis of randomised controlled trials only to examine the evidence on the benefit, or otherwise, of intensive follow-up strategies after curative resection for colorectal cancer. This study, published in the *British Medical Journal* (Renehan *et al.* 2002), demonstrated a survival benefit with intensive follow-up, and is presented here in a shortened form. We believe that our study stands at a crossroads in the research field of colorectal cancer follow-up. A number of international investigators posted responses to this study on the BMJ website (www.bmj.com/ cgi/content/abstract/324/7341/813#responses), but these have never been published, despite the *British Medical Journal* editorial board being urged to do so. In pursuit of a transparent debate, we have included summarised versions of these responses. Owing to pressures of space, some text within each response has been shortened but without amendments to the major points.

The systematic approach to the review identified many limitations, as well as merits and, thus, the final part of the chapter deals with the challenges of future trials.

Efficacy, effectiveness and efficiency

Before considering the evidence of the merits of colorectal cancer follow-up, it is worth examining the terms used to describe the utility of any intervention: efficacy, effectiveness, and efficiency. These were originally defined by a WHO Expert group in 1970 (White 2000) as follows:

Efficacy. The benefit or utility to the individual of the service, treatment regimen, drug or prevention or control measure advocated or applied.
Effectiveness. The effect of the activity and the end-results, outcomes or benefits for the population achieved in relation to the stated objectives.
Efficiency. The effects or end-results achieved in relation to the effort expended in terms of money, resource and time.

Cochrane (1972) subsequently defined efficacy as the extent to which an intervention does more good than harm *under ideal circumstances* of healthcare practice, whereas effectiveness assesses the same when provided *under usual circumstances*. Most clinical trials attempt to measure efficacy. However, clinical trials are analysed on an intention-to-treat basis, and in the context of post-resection colorectal cancer surveillance, the ability to measure efficacy is affected by uptake rates and dropout rates during follow-up. Specifically in colorectal cancer surveillance studies, there are also problems with concealment of outcome assessment and major risks of bias in treatment decision making, post-detection of recurrent disease. More importantly, the assessment and treatment of these secondary outcomes may impact on the primary outcome, mortality. Thus, in terms of particular follow-up strategies after curative resection for colorectal cancer, it is more appropriate to speak of *effectiveness* rather than *efficacy*. These issues will be addressed again later in this chapter.

Meta-analysis of randomised controlled trials
Methodology

The methodological details have been reported elsewhere (Renehan *et al.* 2002). In brief, we undertook a comprehensive search of published and grey literature using Cochrane methodology (Lefebrve & Clarke 2001). Studies were considered for inclusion in the meta-analysis on the basis of four criteria: study design (randomised controlled trial); target population (patients with colorectal cancer treated surgically with curative intent); timing of randomisation (at or shortly after surgery), and availability of cancer-related survival data. We included studies comparing intensive follow-up strategies with control follow-up regimens, as defined by the individual trials. The primary outcome was all-cause mortality at five years. Secondary outcomes included the total number of recurrences, any type of local recurrences, isolated local recurrences, any hepatic metastases, isolated hepatic metastases, lung metastases, intra-luminal recurrences, and metachronous (second primary colorectal) cancers. Importantly, we assessed the following quality aspects: adequacy of concealment of patients' allocation to treatment groups, double-blinding, and withdrawals (Juni *et al.* 2001).

As different diagnostic tests were used during follow-up in different trials, we made an important *a priori* hypothesis and subsequently performed subgroup analyses based on this. The hypothesis was that the early detection of extramural recurrent disease (namely local pelvic recurrences and solitary hepatic metastases), with investigations such as computed tomography and frequent measurements of serum carcinoembryonic antigen, or both, was more likely to be effective in improving cancer-related survival than strategies directed only at the detection of intra-luminal disease (such as the use of colonoscopy).

A variety of robust statistical analyses were performed and results were expressed as combined risk ratios using both the fixed-effects and the random-effects methods. Sources of heterogeneity were evaluated through statistical tests for heterogeneity and subgroup analyses. The presence of publication bias was examined in funnel plots and related statistical tests (Egger *et al.* 1997).

Results

Five randomised trials (Makela *et al.* 1995; Ohlsson *et al.* 1995; Schoemaker *et al.* 1998; Pietra *et al.* 1998; Kjeldsen *et al.* 1997) met the inclusion criteria for the meta-analysis. These comprised 1,342 participants, 666 assigned to intensive follow-up and 676 assigned to controls. The baseline characteristics of the participants enrolled in these trials are shown in Table 9.1. The tests and the frequency of their use varied considerably, and importantly, no study directly compared specific tests. However, in four trials (Makela *et al.* 1995; Ohlsson *et al.* 1995; Schoemaker *et al.* 1998; Pietra *et al.* 1998) both computed tomography and frequent measurements of serum CEA were limited to the intensive arms. These trials were categorised as the *extra-mural* detection group. The Danish study (Kjeldsen *et al.* 1997) focused heavily on the increased detection of intra-luminal disease, and thus formed the *intra-mural* detection group.

Data on all-cause mortality were available in all studies. At five years, 197 of 666 patients (30%) allocated to intensive follow-up and 247 of 676 (37%) allocated to control groups had died. By the fixed-effects method, the combined risk ratio was 0.81 (95% confidence interval 0.70–0.94, $p = 0.007$) in favour of intensive follow-up

Intensive follow-up after colorectal cancer 105

Table 9.1 Detailed characteristics of surveillance programmes used in the five randomised trials

Study	Surveillance regimens	
	Intensive	Control
Makela et al.[17]	Seen in clinic 3 monthly for first 2 years, then 6 monthly: physical examination, FBC, FOBT, CEA levels, and CXR. Yearly colonoscopy. Sigmoidoscopy 3 monthly for rectal and sigmoid cancers. US liver 6 monthly. CT scan yearly. Proportion followed-up to 5-years = 100%.	Seen in clinic 3 monthly for first 2 years, then 6 monthly: physical examination, FBC, FOBT, CEA levels, and CXR. Yearly barium enema. Rigid sigmoidoscopy 3 monthly for rectal cancers. Proportion followed-up to 5-years = 100%.
Ohlsson et al.[18]	Seen in clinic 3 monthly for the first 2 years, then 6 monthly: physical examination, rigid proctosigmoidoscopy, LFTs, CEA levels, FOBT, CXR. Colonoscopy at 3, 15, 30 and 60 months, CT scan after APR at 3, 6, 12, 18, and 24 months. Proportion followed-up to 5-years = 100%.	No systematic follow-up. Patients were instructed to leave faecal samples for FOBT testing every third month during the first two years and then every year. Proportion accounted for to 5-years = 100%.
Shoemaker et al.[19]	Seen in clinic 3 monthly for first 2 years, then 6 monthly for 5 years; physical examination, FBC, LFTs, and Haemoccult II. Yearly CXR. Yearly CT liver. Yearly colonoscopy. CEA measurements were performed but not used to trigger further examinations. Proportion followed-up to 5-years = 94%.	Seen in clinic 3 monthly for first 2 years, then 6 monthly for 5 years; physical examination, FBC, LFTs, CEA levels, and Haemoccult II. CEA measurements were performed but not used to trigger further examinations. Proportion followed-up to 5-years = 95%.
Pietra et al.[20]	Seen in clinic 3 monthly for first 2 years, then 6 monthly for next 3 years, thereafter yearly; physical examination, USS liver, CEA levels. Yearly colonoscopy, CXR, and CT scan. Proportion followed-up to 5-years = 100%.	Seen in clinic 6 monthly for first year, then yearly; physical examination, US liver, CEA levels. Yearly colonoscopy and CXR. Proportion followed-up to 5-years = 100%.
Kjeldsen et al.[21]	Physical examination, digital rectal examination, gynaecological examination, Haemoccult-II, colonoscopy, CXR, FBC, ESR, LFTs, at 6 monthly in first 3 years, then 12 monthly for next 2 years, then 5 yearly. Proportion followed-up to 5-years = 79%.	Physical examination, digital rectal examination, gynaecological examination, Haemoccult-II, colonoscopy, CXR, FBC, ESR, LFTs, at 5 and 10 years. Proportion followed-up to 5-years = 73%.

FU: follow-up. FBC: full blood count. LFTs: liver function tests. ESR: erythrocyte sedimentation rate. CEA: carcinoembryonic antigen. FOBT: faecal occult blood test. CXR: chest x-ray. CT scan: computerised tomography scan. US: ultrasonography. APR: abdominoperineal resection.

(see Figure 9.2). Similar values for risk ratios were estimated by the random-effects method. The five-year mortality in the control group ranged from 32% to 50%, which translates into an absolute reduction in mortality of 6–9% ((0.50) × (1–0.81), and so on).

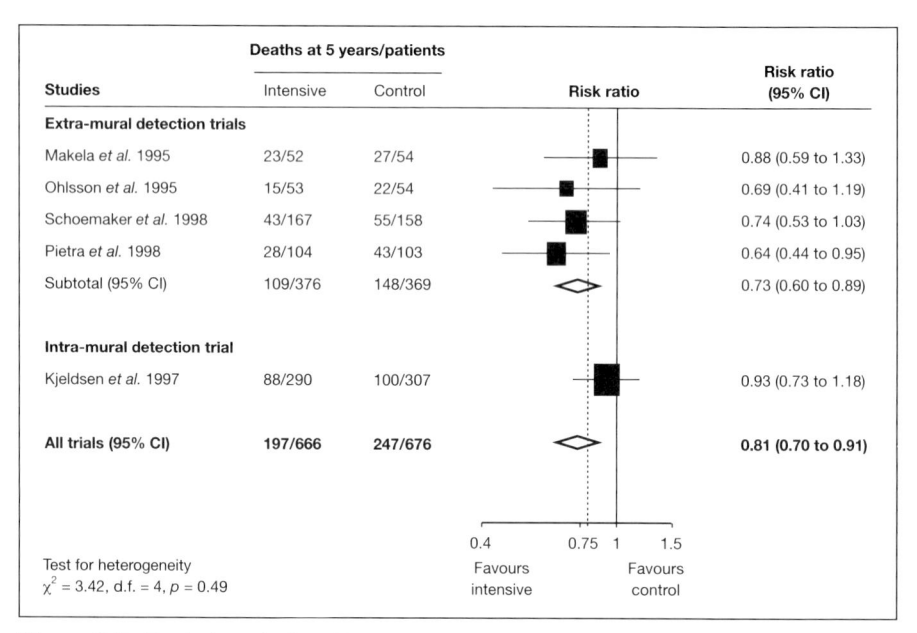

Studies	Deaths at 5 years/patients Intensive	Control	Risk ratio	Risk ratio (95% CI)
Extra-mural detection trials				
Makela et al. 1995	23/52	27/54		0.88 (0.59 to 1.33)
Ohlsson et al. 1995	15/53	22/54		0.69 (0.41 to 1.19)
Schoemaker et al. 1998	43/167	55/158		0.74 (0.53 to 1.03)
Pietra et al. 1998	28/104	43/103		0.64 (0.44 to 0.95)
Subtotal (95% CI)	109/376	148/369		0.73 (0.60 to 0.89)
Intra-mural detection trial				
Kjeldsen et al. 1997	88/290	100/307		0.93 (0.73 to 1.18)
All trials (95% CI)	197/666	247/676		0.81 (0.70 to 0.91)

Test for heterogeneity
$\chi^2 = 3.42$, d.f. = 4, $p = 0.49$

Favours intensive   Favours control

Figure 9.2 Pooled analysis with summary estimates (fixed effects method) for five-year all-cause mortality: data categorised into detection groups in accordance with a priori hypothesis. (Note: there were minor corrections in the 95% confidence interval bars as depicted in the originally published plots in the *British Medical Journal* – these have been amended for this figure.)

The effect on mortality was most pronounced in the four extra-mural detection trials that used computed tomography and frequent measurements of serum CEA (combined risk ratio 0.73, 0.60 to 0.89, $p = 0.002$). The absolute reduction in mortality of 9–13% or a number needed to treat (the number of patients needed to prevent one death) of 8–11.

The results for the secondary outcomes can be summarised as follows. There were no differences in rates of recurrence in all sites between the two groups: 212/666 (32%) for intensive versus 224/676 (33%) for control follow-up. However, recurrences were detected 8.5 months earlier with intensive follow-up. The detection rates for all local recurrences and all hepatic and lung metastases were also similar in the two groups, but based on data from three trials, intensive follow-up was associated with a significantly increased detection of isolated local recurrences (15% versus 9%: risk ratio 1.61, 1.12 to 2.32, $p = 0.011$). Intensive follow-up was also associated with a small non-significant increase in hepatic metastasis detection. Overall, intra-luminal recurrences and metachronous cancer detection rates were low (3.2% and 1.3%, respectively), and there were no differences between follow-up regimens.

Strongest evidence so far

The findings of our meta-analysis (Renehan *et al.* 2002) support the view that intensive follow-up after curative resection for colorectal cancer improves survival at five years. Independently, the Cochrane review group reported their review at the same time (Jeffrey *et al.* 2002). They identified and included the same five studies in their analysis, and using slightly difference statistics (Peto's odds ratio), they also demonstrated a significant improvement in all-cause mortality in patients followed intensively. A small randomised trial has subsequently been published supporting these findings (Secco *et al.* 2002).

In terms of grading of evidence (ACPGBI 2001), these data fulfil level Ia criteria (highest level of evidence) and thus are the strongest indication to date that intensive follow-up has a survival benefit. For the purpose of discussing colorectal cancer follow-up, we refer to these trials as first generation (see Conclusion), as they prove a point of principle.

Our analysis, in particular, demonstrated that using modern follow-up regimens (including computed tomography and frequent measurements of serum CEA) there was an absolute reduction in mortality of 9–13%. This improvement compares favourably with, for instance, the 5% benefit observed for adjuvant chemotherapy in Dukes' C disease (Dube *et al.* 1997) and is applicable to a wider range of clinical stages of colorectal cancer (Renehan & O'Dwyer 2000). In addition, the trials included in our analysis predated multidisciplinary approaches to the treatment of colorectal cancer, including the wider practice of hepatic resections for metastases, pelvic exenterations for recurrent pelvic disease, and the use of combined therapies for advanced disease. These approaches influence survival, and hence the potential survival benefits from intensive follow-up may be even greater than those expressed in the present analysis.

We acknowledged in our discussion that there were potential inadequacies in the quality of studies included. Specifically, no trial reported adequate concealment of allocation or comprehensive blinding of outcome assessment, and only two studies stated that randomisation was stratified for major prognostic factors. These problems need to be addressed in future trials (see later). Other issues were further discussed in correspondences to the *British Medical Journal* website as follows.

Letters in response to *British Medical Journal* paper

Response from Cochrane group

The results of this meta-analysis are very similar to our Cochrane review (Jeffrey *et al.* 2002). There are, however, some errors in the description and interpretation of the data which require comment. Renehan *et al.* (2002) state that 'in four trials computed tomography and frequent measurements of CEA were limited to the intensive arms'. In fact in three studies, CEA was measured with equal frequency in both arms. Only in the study by Ohlsson *et al.* (1995) (which showed no difference in mortality) was CEA measurement limited to the intensive arm. Therefore, the conclusion that there is an absolute reduction in mortality of 9–13% 'using modern follow up regimens' is not justified.

The review divided the five trials into those designed to look for 'intramural recurrences' or 'extramural recurrences'. This division seems somewhat arbitrary and leads to the exclusion (from a subgroup analysis on mortality) of the Danish trial (Kjeldsen *et al.* 1997), which contributed 45% patients included in the overall meta-analysis. The Danish trial included measures designed to look for distant metastases (physical examination, CXR, ESR, liver function tests) and it was the intent of the study investigators to look for all types of recurrences, not just 'intramural' disease (personal communication with Ole Kronberg). We need reassurance that the exclusion from analysis of this study was not a post-hoc decision.

The final conclusion in Renehan's paper is that 'we believe that clinical guidelines should be revised'. Given the varied components and intensity of follow-up (different tests and frequency of tests) across the five trials, it is impossible to deduce which aspect of follow-up is responsible for the survival benefit. The conclusions of our Cochrane review were more cautious and more accurately reflect the validity of the data: 'The results of this review support the general principle of clinical follow-up for patients with CRC after curative treatment. The exact details of the optimal follow-up regimen still need clarification.'

G. M. Jeffery, B. E. Hickey, P. Hider
on behalf of the Cochrane Colorectal Cancer Group Review

Response from the GILDA group

The authors (Renehan *et al.* 2002), claim that the survival benefit was more evident in trials designed to compare follow-up regimens having major differences in extramural recurrences detection power. While dividing trials into such categories is not always straightforward, the expected differences in the number of isolated local recurrences (23/156 – 10/157 = 13 cases) and isolated liver metastases (20/323 – 15/315 = 5 cases) seem far from conclusive. Thus, while we welcome this new piece of evidence, we also feel encouraged to continue our randomised clinical trial (GILDA – Gruppo Italiano di Lavoro per la Diagnosi Anticipata). Both the Renehan study and the Cochrane review call for new trials to assess the role of individual investigations and underscore the importance of adding psychological well-being and cost-effectiveness as outcome measures. The GILDA trial is a project we launched after publishing the results of the GIVIO study on early breast cancer patients follow-up.

GILDA is aimed at testing the impact on survival, health-related quality of life and costs of two follow-up regimens – with rather balanced differences in both extramural and intramural diagnostic intensity – in patients with colorectal carcinoma. The details of the follow-up schedules are shown on the website (www.bmj.com/cgi/content/abstract/324/7341/813#responses). Thirty-seven centres, mostly in Italy, are participating in this trial. Trial recruitment started in April 1998 and by March 2002, 670 patients have been enrolled into the study. GILDA is the largest randomised trial conducted in this field up to now and is the only protocol where health-related quality of life and economic aspects of follow-up besides the usual clinical end points are being addressed. The trial is still ongoing.

G. Apolone, P. Mosconi, R. Fossati
on behalf of GIVIO and GILDA Investigators

Response from Audisio and colleagues

Renehan *et al.* (2002) have performed a *state of the art* meta-analysis on the basis of five trials published between 1995 and 1998, and have found that intensive follow-up reduces five-year overall mortality. Convincing though this may seem, in our opinion several issues remain to be resolved. The authors suggest that gains in survival are primarily generated through the increased curative treatment of isolated local recurrences. This is not convincing for three reasons. First, the differentiation between the one intramural and four extramural trials generates the opposite finding – mortality reduction is only found in the pooled extramural detection trials. In the intramural detection trial, where diagnosis is primarily aimed at local recurrence, no mortality difference is found. Second, the survival gains from treatment of local recurrence are heavily influenced by the Pietra (1998) study, a study that reports such high local recurrence rates (15% for colon cancer and 37% for rectal cancer) that one may doubt the quality of the primary cancer surgery on which this study is based. Thirdly, both surgical oncological clinical practice, and the majority of the literature on follow-up suggests that gains can primarily be achieved from the treatment of liver metastases, and not from the treatment of local recurrences (treatment of liver recurrences being reported 5–10 times more often), and contributes to far more patients with five-year survival after recurrence, than treatment of local recurrence.

In all five trials, to our knowledge, there was no blinding of follow-up. This leaves the majority of the decision-making and subsequent care with respect to cancer recurrences to the discretion of the non-blinded clinician. One cannot ignore the gains that may in part be the result of unobserved and unreported differences in post-detection care, and thereby produce an inappropriately positive picture of follow-up effectiveness.

R. A. Audisio, Liverpool, United Kingdom
J. Kievit, Leiden, The Netherlands
T. Wiggers, Groningen, The Netherlands
K. S. Virgo, St Louis, USA
F. E. Johnson, St Louis, USA

Authors' reply

Our objective was to compare two broad strategies of surveillance after curative resection for colorectal cancer: a more intensive strategy with less intensive or no follow-up. We found a significant reduction in *all-cause mortality* with intensive follow-up and suggested that this survival benefit was *in part* attributable to the early detection of all recurrences and the increased detection of isolated recurrent disease. We agree that at present it is difficult to identify which aspects of intensified follow-up are responsible for the benefit observed and we acknowledged this in the discussion section of our paper. We called for trials that are specifically designed to address this issue. The ongoing GILDA trial is to be applauded for its large recruitment to date, but we have concerns that the study design, while balancing diagnostic intensity with extramural and intramural detection, has the disadvantage that no single test is directly compared between the two arms.

In response to Jeffery and colleagues, we performed our subgroup analysis based on the *a priori* hypothesis that the *early* detection of extramural recurrent disease was more likely to be effective in improving survival related to cancer than strategies directed only at the detection of intraluminal disease. Within this definition, we included the potential to salvage both local pelvic recurrences and solitary hepatic metastases. While the Danish study was the largest trial within the meta-analysis, it had distinct characteristics. It may have been designed to detect distant metastases (e.g. chest radiograph), but these diagnostic tools were unlikely to contribute to the *early* detection of recurrences. While no trial directly compared a specific diagnostic tool, all four extramural studies included computed tomography and frequent measurements of serum CEA. Computed tomography and frequent measurements of CEA are the only tests that are reasonably sensitive for the detection of either hepatic metastases or local recurrences. Thus, considering these two tests together is justified.

Audisio and colleagues may have misunderstood the distinction between extra- and intra-luminal detection studies. Intra-luminal detection tools infrequently diagnose early local recurrence as these are typically outside the large bowel lumen. These authors are correct to point out that results of the meta-analysis must be interpreted in light of the period when the included studies were performed. This reinforces the need for continuing research in this area.

While it is important that clinical guidelines are prescriptive, it is equally important that they are embracing. We believe that it would be inappropriate if guidelines simply ignored the available evidence that intensifying follow-up can improve survival. By implication, the practice of no follow-up is no longer acceptable. Clearly, further trials are required to identify the specific components of follow-up that are most beneficial, and until then, we cannot be prescriptive.

Challenges for future trials and recommendations

It is clear from the above debate that the majority of interested groups recognise the need for further trials. We list here a number of issues that we believe are important in designing future trials. Additional views can be found in other reviews (van den Hout *et al.* 2002; Kievit 2002; Audisio & Robertson 2000).

General principles

Before embarking on the specific questions of proposed trials, there are a number of issues specific to randomised trials in colorectal cancer follow-up, some already alluded to:

- Randomisation is clearly an obligatory prerequisite. Randomisation consists of two parts: generation and concealment of allocation (Juni *et al.* 2001). An important component of generation is stratification. For colorectal cancer follow-up, stratification by stage is relevant, as stage remains the main predictor of mortality. In a large trial, subgroup analysis by stage of cancer based on *a priori* hypotheses would be appropriate. Stratification by age is equally relevant as all-cause mortality is a primary endpoint, and in economic evaluations, life years (LY) gained is the preferred unit of outcome. Finally, stratification by site is important as rates and patterns of recurrence vary between rectum and colon.
- Of equal importance is standardisation of treatments. Increasingly, evidence suggests that the quality of a surgical procedure has a major influence on trial outcome. The importance of quality assurance and standardisation of surgical practice has been exemplified by the Dutch Rectal Cancer Trial (Landheer *et al.* 2002). For surgical procedures, this requires specialised training (Martling *et al.* 2000). Standardisation of indications for adjuvant therapies using uniformly applied regimens is also required.
- Specific attention should be given to the problems of blinding of the follow-up clinician in the assessment and treatment of recurrences.
- Power calculations need to take account of the observation that modern therapies are associated with lower local recurrence rates – for instance rectal cancer, compared with historical data –reducing the potential for survival gain through salvage.
- Equally, power calculations need to consider the potential gains in survival through non-salvage mechanisms – for example, improved general well-being and enhanced treatment of unrelated medical conditions. These are referred to as *non-salvage benefits*.
- In our meta-analysis, we estimated that among patients with recurrences undergoing salvage therapies, the failure rate at five years after initial treatment was approximately 50% (unpublished data). It is likely that second recurrences and delayed cancer-related deaths will present after this time such that trial periods beyond five years may need to be considered.

Efficacy of individual surveillance tools

The aforementioned two meta-analyses have demonstrated the *effectiveness* of intensive follow-up after curative resection for colorectal cancer. We urge that second generation trials now address the *efficacy* of individual surveillance tools – for example, a trial with identical arms except that one includes abdomino-pelvic computer tomography, and the other none. This type of study is referred to as a *single question design*. Single question designs reduce 'contamination' due to non-salvage benefits of intensive follow-up.

Table 9.2 summarises several ongoing and proposed trials in colorectal cancer follow-up. Detailed analysis of each trial proposal is beyond the scope of this chapter, but a glance at the summary table demonstrates that most designs are complex (further details on our website: www.christie.nhs.uk/profinfo/departments/surgery/research_activity.htm). We have concerns that in many of these proposals, there are temptations to address too many simultaneous questions with inevitable lack of focus. Again, this emphasises the importance of single question designs.

Having demonstrated that intensifying follow-up can improve survival, by implication the practice of no follow-up is not acceptable. By a similar rationale, there are major ethical concerns if a proposal includes a 'no-follow-up' arm. Control arms should, therefore, include 'standard' practice follow-up regimens, but this may vary between cultures and countries (Audisio & Robertson 2000).

Trial designs based on risk-stratification (Secco *et al.* 2002) appear at first glance to be a logical way forward. Thus, for example, an intensive regimen of frequent computer tomography is evaluated in Dukes' C cancers only. However, although recurrence rates may be lower in lower stage cancers, it is conceivable that the latter are more salvageable (lower biological aggression). Equally, a risk-stratification approach may exclude low-risk patients from the non-salvage benefits of follow-up.

Colonoscopy surveillance may be a special case for consideration. Our meta-analysis reported that the rate of metachronous cancers at five years was 1.3% (Renehan *et al.* 2002). In a recent SEER (Surveillance Epidemiology and End Results) survey, with follow-up ranging up to 17 years (median 4.2 years), the rate of second primary tumours was 1.9% (4,202 out of 217,705 between 1979 and 1996) (Shureiqi *et al.* 2001). These data suggest that intensive efforts directed at the detection of metachronous disease are probably of low benefit and unsuitable to evaluate by randomised trial. However, there may be merit in pursuing a risk-stratified approach in this case, analogous to low- and high-risk adenomatous polyps (Atkin & Saunders 2002). For the great majority of patients with colorectal cancer, multi-stage modelling suggests that there is no underlying genetic instability, and by implication their tumour is a rare sporadic event highly unlikely to occur again (Luebeck & Moolgavkar 2002). In the future, we may see colonoscopic surveillance prescribed accordingly. Interesting, the SEER data (Shureiqi *et al.* 2001), and a second population-based study in the south-west of England (Evans *et al.* 2002), reported high risk ratios for men under 60 years and women under 65 years, whereas risk ratios

Intensive follow-up after colorectal cancer 113

Table 9.2 Randomised trials in preparation or ongoing

	Status	Design summary	Target
GILDA Trial: A randomised trial of intensive versus minimalist follow-up of patients with resected Dukes' B–C colorectal cancer. *Source:* www.bmj.com/cgi/content/abstract/324/7341/813#responses accessed Sept 2002	Ongoing	Two-arm muli-centered international study designed to evaluate the efficacy of increased frequency of testing with extraluminal (US/CT) and intraluminal (colonoscopy) tools. Includes quality of life and health economic assessments.	670 recruited March 2002
FACS Trial: A randomised controlled trial to assess the cost-effectiveness of intensive versus no scheduled follow-up in patients who have undergone resection for colorectal cancer with curative intent. *Source:* www.nern.org.uk/portfolio/data.asp?ID=762 accessed Feb 2003	Pilot study	A four-arm multi-centered national (England) 2 x 2 factorial design. No follow-up as control arm (arm A), with increasing levels of follow-up intensity in remaining arms. Emphasis on high-quality liver surgery for hepatic metastasis. Includes cost-effectiveness analysis.	N_e = 4890 with 5 years FU
UKCCCR Colorectal Cancer Group: To compare the value of intensive versus minimalist follow-up following apparently curative resection for colorectal cancer on disease-free and overall survival *Source:* ukcccr.icnet.uk/groups/colohome.html, accessed Feb 2002; and McArdle C. 2000.	Proposal	A four-arm multi-centered national (England) 2 x 2 design comparing minimal versus intensive follow-up with randomisation to with or without CEA monitoring, and in the settings of hospital versus community. Similar to FFCD protocol.	
FFCD Group: To evaluate the frequency of follow-up monitoring in patients with Dukes' C colorectal cancer. *Source:* Audisio and Robertson 2000	Proposal	Two-arm multi-centered national study designed to evaluate frequency of CXR, US and rectal US, with further randomisation to with or without CEA in intensive arm.	N_e = 2750 with 3 years FU
EORTC-GITCG Group: To evaluate intensive follow-up versus a minimalist intervention control group with overall and disease-free survival as endpoints. Source: Audisio and Robertson, 2000	Proposal	A four-arm multi-centered internal study design. No follow-up as control arm (arm A), with increasing levels of follow-up intensity in remaining arms: Arm B, frequent CT scan; Arm C as arm B plus CEA; Arm D as arm C plus colonoscopy.	N_e = 4300 with 5 years FU

GILDA: Gruppo Italiano di Lavoro per la Diagnosi Anticipata. UKCCCR: United Kingdom Colorectal Cancer Collaborative Group (superseded by National Cancer Research Network). FFCD: Foundation Francaise de Cancerologie Digestive. EORTC-GITCG: European Organisation for Research in the Treatment of Cancer - Gastrointestinal Tract Co-operative Group. N_e = estimated numbers need. Other abbreviations as in Table 1.

above these ages overlapped with those for the general population. However, these data represent relative risk estimates only, and before prescribing different colonoscopic surveillance stratified by age group, there is a need to convert these data to absolute risks and numbers needed to treat (NNT).

Economic issues

Previous studies have examined health economic issues related to colorectal cancer follow-up (Virgo *et al*. 1995; Norum & Olsen 1997; Edelman *et al*. 1997; Beart 2000) but as these pre-dated the effectiveness data provided by the two aforementioned meta-analyses, they were not truly cost-effectiveness analyses. As a natural extension of our interests, we undertook a cost-effectiveness analysis based on the data from our meta-analysis, which has now been published in the *British Medical Journal* (Renehan *et al*. 2004) and its abstract is included as the Appendix. The results, expressed as ICER (incremental cost-effectiveness ratio), demonstrate that intensive follow-up is cost-effective within the margin of NHS cost acceptability. Notably, calculations remain robust after extremity sensitivity analyses including maximum costs for surveillance and treatment. Within this study, we identified several issues for consideration in future trials:

- There is a need to consider costs beyond five years (for the reasons mentioned above).
- The analysis demonstrated that surveillance rather than treatment costs were the greater predictor of ICER.
- When recurrent disease occurs, it is important to appreciate that palliative therapy (more usual for control patients) is not inexpensive and partially offsets the costs of salvage therapy (which is more prevalent among patients intensively followed).
- Ideally, the economic evaluation should address societal perspectives. For instance, there is evidence that travel and time off work are important in colorectal cancer screening (Frew *et al*. 1999) and may also be relevant to colorectal cancer surveillance.
- Economic evaluation needs to include capital costs for additional laboratory, radiological and/or clinical capacity.

Quality of life

There is currently a paucity of data on quality-of-life-related issues and colorectal cancer follow-up. Moreover, the specific question of whether or not the earlier detection of recurrent disease affects quality of life is complex. The Leiden group adapted the MOS-SF20 assessment for use in colorectal cancer follow-up and failed to demonstrate increased anxiety associated with frequent monitoring (Stiggelbout *et al*. 1997). A sub-study of the Danish randomised trial (Kjeldsen *et al*. 1999), using the Nottingham Health Profile, demonstrated a small benefit in health-related quality of life in those intensively followed. These preliminary data suggest that intensive follow-up is not deleterious in terms of quality of life. However, there are still unexplored issues, of which two examples are worth mentioning. First, with ever increasing sensitivity among surveillance tools, there will be inevitable increases in false positive tests. Second, our meta-analysis showed that intensive follow-up brings forward the date of recurrence detection by on average eight months – we do not know the consequences of this on quality of life. There is a need to develop innovative approaches to assessing the anxieties associated with these side effects of intensive follow-up.

Conclusion

This chapter has summarised the current evidence on colorectal cancer follow-up and convincingly demonstrated the effectiveness of intensifying follow-up. This evidence can be considered as that derived from first generation trials (see Table 9.3). There is now an urgent need to evaluate the efficacy of individual investigative tools used in colorectal cancer surveillance through second-generation trials. We have emphasised the importance of single question designs. Parallel economic evaluation and quality of life assessment will be essential prerequisites of these proposed trials. Our cost-effectiveness data suggest that such trials are justified economically. Beyond these trials, there are third generation studies that will embrace novel diagnostic modalities (e.g. PET scan) and molecular markers (e.g. DNA microarrays). There is a continual need to approach this complex area of colorectal cancer management through systematic research, for ultimately, many patients will benefit.

Table 9.3 Colorectal cancer follow-up – generations of trials

First generation trials
- RCT: intensive versus controls
- Two meta-analysis proving point of principle

Second generation trials
- Single question trials (eg identical arms except for with and without CT scan)
- Non-randomised data for rare events (eg second primary colorectal cancers)
- Economic evaluation
- Quality of life studies

Third generation trials
- Risk-stratification (based on efficacy date from 2nd generation trials)
- Novel surveillance tools/tumour predictors (eg PET scan, DNA microassays)

RCT: randomised controlled trial. CT: computer tomography. PET: positron emission tomography.

Appendix

Objective: To determine the cost-effectiveness of intensive follow-up in colorectal cancer patients compared with conventional follow-up as controls.

Design: Incremental cost-effectiveness analysis recognising differences in follow-up strategies, based on effectiveness data from a meta-analysis of five randomised trials.

Setting: United Kingdom.

Main outcome measures: Taking a health service perspective, incremental costs-effectiveness ratios (ICERs) per patient followed were estimated, and reported for all five trials and for the four trials that were designed for early detection of extramural recurrences (targeted surveillance).

Results: Based on 5-year follow-up, the numbers of LYs gained by intensive follow-up were 0.73 and 0.82 for the five and four trial models. For all five trials, the adjusted net (extra) cost per patient was £2,479 and per life gained was £3,402, substantially lower than the current threshold of NHS cost acceptability (£30,000). The corresponding values for the four trial model were £2,529 and £3,077, suggesting that targeted surveillance is more cost effective. The main predictor of ICER was surveillance rather than treatment costs. Judged against the NHS cost acceptability, the predicted incremental cost threshold was ninefold and the effectiveness threshold was three percent.

Conclusions: Based on the available data and current costs, the strategy of intensive follow-up after curative resection for colorectal cancer is economically justified and should be normal practice. There is a continuing need to evaluate the efficacy of specific surveillance tools: this study forms the basis for economic evaluations in such trials.

References

Association of Coloproctology of Great Britain and Ireland (ACPGBI) (2001). *Guidelines for the Management of Colorectal Cancer*. London: ACPGBI.

Audisio, R. A. & Robertson, C. (2000). Colorectal cancer follow-up: perspectives for future studies. *European Journal of Surgical Oncology* **26**, 329–337.

Atkin, W. S. & Saunders B. P. (2002). Surveillance guidelines after removal of colorectal adenomatous polyps. *Gut* **51**, V6–V9.

Beart, R. W. Jr (2000). Follow-up: does it work? Can we afford it? *Surgical Oncology Clinics of North America* **9**, 827–834.

Berman, J. M., Cheung, R. J. & Weinberg, D. S. (2000). Surveillance after colorectal cancer resection. *The Lancet* **355**, 395–399.

Bruinvels, D. J., Stiggelbout, A. M., Kievit, J., van Houwelingen, H. C., Habbema, J. D. & van de Velde, C. J. (1994). Follow-up of patients with colorectal cancer. A meta-analysis. *Annals of Surgery* **219**, 174–182.

Bruinvels, D. J, Stiggelbout, A. M., Klaassen, M. P., Kievit, J., Dik, J., Habbema, F. & van de Velde, C. J. (1995). Follow-up after colorectal cancer: current practice in The Netherlands. *European Journal of Surgery* **161**, 827–831.

Cochrane, A. (1972). *Effectiveness and Efficiency: Random reflections on health services*. London: Nuffield Provisional Hospital Trust.

Desch, C. E., Benson, A. B. III, Smith, T. J., Flynn, P. J., Krause, C., Loprinzi, C. L., Minsky, B. D., Petrelli, N. J., Pfister, D. G. & Somerfield, M. R. (1999). Recommended colorectal cancer surveillance guidelines by the American Society of Clinical Oncology. *Journal of Clinical Oncology* **17**, 1312.

Dube, S., Heyen, F. & Jenicek, M. (1997). Adjuvant chemotherapy in colorectal carcinoma. Results of a meta-analysis. *Diseases of the Colon and Rectum* **40**, 35–41.

Edelman, M. J., Meyers, F. J. & Siegel, D. (1997). The utility of follow-up testing after curative cancer therapy: a critical review and economic analysis. *Journal of General and Internal Medicine* **12**, 318–331.

Egger, M., Davey Smith, G., Schneider, M. & Minder, C. (1997). Bias in meta-analysis detected by a simple, graphical test. *British Medical Journal* **315**, 629–634.

Evans, H. S., Moller, H., Robinson, D., Lewis, C. M., Bell, C. M. & Hodgson, S. V. (2002). The risk of subsequent primary cancers after colorectal cancer in southeast England. *Gut* **50**, 647–652.

Frew, E., Wolstenholme, J. L., Atkin, W. & Whynes, D. K. (1999). Estimating time and travel costs incurred in clinic based screening: flexible sigmoidoscopy screening for colorectal cancer. *Journal of Medical Screening* **6**, 119–123.

Jeffery, G. M., Hickey, B E. & Hider, P. (2002). Follow-up strategies for patients treated for non-metastatic colorectal cancer (Cochrane Review). In: *The Cochrane Library*, issue 1. Oxford: Update Software.

Juni, P., Altman, D. G. & Egger, M. (2001). Systematic reviews in health care: assessing the quality of controlled clinical trials. *British Medical Journal* **323**, 42–46.

Kievit, J. (2002). Follow-up of patients with colorectal cancer: numbers needed to test and treat. *European Journal of Cancer* **38**, 986–999.

Kjeldsen, B. J., Kronborg, O., Fenger, C. & Jorgensen, O. D. (1997). A prospective randomized study of follow-up after radical surgery for colorectal cancer. *British Journal of Surgery* **84**, 666–669.

Kjeldsen, B. J., Thorsen, H., Whalley, D. & Kronborg, O. (1999). Influence of follow-up on health-related quality of life after radical surgery for colorectal cancer. *Scandinavian Journal of Gastroenterology* **34**, 509–515.

Landheer, M. L., Therasse, P. & van de Velde, C. J. (2002). The importance of quality assurance in surgical oncology. *European Journal of Surgical Oncology* **28**, 571–602.

Lefebrve, A. & Clarke, M. (2001). Identifying randomised trials. In *Systematic Reviews in Health Care: Meta-analysis in Context* (ed. M. Egger, G. Davey-Smith & D. G. Altman), pp. 69–86. London: BMJ Books.

Luebeck, E. G. & Moolgavkar, S. H. (2002). Multistage carcinogenesis and the incidence of colorectal cancer. *Proceedings of the National Academy of Science of the United States of America* **99**, 15,095–15,100.

Makela, J. T., Laitinen, S, O. & Kairaluoma, M. I. (1995). Five-year follow-up after radical surgery for colorectal cancer. Results of a prospective randomized trial. *Archives of Surgery* **130**, 1062–1067.

Martling, A. L., Holm, T., Rutqvist, L. E., Moran, B. J., Heald, R. J. & Cedemark, B. (2000). Effect of a surgical training programme on outcome of rectal cancer in the County of Stockholm. Stockholm Colorectal Cancer Study Group, Basingstoke Bowel Cancer Research Project. *The Lancet* **356**, 93–96.

Mella, J., Datta, S. N., Biffin, A., Radcliffe, A. G., Steele, R. J. & Stamatakis, J. D. (1997). Surgeons' follow-up practice after resection of colorectal cancer. *Annals of the Royal College of Surgeons of England* **79**, 206–209.

Norum, J. & Olsen, J. A. (1997). A cost-effectiveness approach to the Norwegian follow-up programme in colorectal cancer. *Annals of Oncology* **8**, 1081–1087.

Ohlsson, B., Breland, U., Ekberg, H., Graffner, H. & Tranberg, K. G. (1995). Follow-up after curative surgery for colorectal carcinoma: Randomized comparison with no follow-up. *Diseases of the Colon and Rectum* **38**, 619–626.

Pietra, N., Sarli, L., Costi, R., Ouchemi, C., Grattarola, M. & Peracchia, A. (1998). Role of follow-up in management of local recurrences of colorectal cancer: a prospective, randomized study. *Diseases of the Colon and Rectum* **41**, 1127–1133.

Pisani, P., Parkin, D. M., Bray, F. & Ferlay, J. (1999). Estimates of the worldwide mortality from 25 cancers in 1990. *International Journal of Cancer*, **83**, 18–29.

Renehan, A. G. & O'Dwyer, S. T. (2000). Surveillance after colorectal cancer resection [letter]. *The Lancet*, **355**, 1095–1096.

Renehan, A. G., Egger, M., Saunders, M. P. & O'Dwyer, S. T. (2002). Impact on survival of intensive follow up after curative resection for colorectal cancer: systematic review and meta-analysis of randomised trials. *British Medical Journal* **324**, 813–817.

Renehan, A. G., O'Dwyer, S. T. & Whynes, D. K. (2004). Cost effectiveness analysis of intensive versus conventional follow up after curative resection for colorectal cancer. *British Medical Journal* **328**, 81–86.

Rosen, M., Chan, L., Beart, R. W. Jr, Vukasin, P. & Anthone, G. (1998). Follow-up of colorectal cancer: a meta-analysis. *Diseases of the Colon and Rectum* **41**, 1116–1126.

Schoemaker, D., Black, R., Giles, L. & Toouli, J. (1998). Yearly colonoscopy, liver CT, and chest radiography do not influence 5-year survival of colorectal cancer patients. *Gastroenterology* **114**, 7–14.

Scholefield, J. H. & Steele, R. J. (2002). Guidelines for follow up after resection of colorectal cancer. *Gut* **51** (Supplement 5), V3–5.

Secco, G. B. Fardelli, R., Gianquinto, D., Bonfante, P., Baldi, E., Ravera, G., Derchi, L. & Ferraris, R. (2002). Efficacy and cost of risk-adapted follow-up in patients after colorectal cancer surgery: a prospective, randomized and controlled trial. *European Journal of Surgical Oncology* **28**, 418–423.

Shureiqi, I., Cooksley, C. D., Morris, J., Soliman, A. S., Levin, B. & Lippman, S. M. (2001). Effect of age on risk of second primary colorectal cancer. *Journal of the National Cancer Institute* **93**, 1264–1266.

Scotland Intercollegiate Guidelines Network (SIGN) (1997). *Clinical guidelines for colorectal cancer*. (www.sign.ac.uk/guidelines/published/index.html, accessed February 2002).

Stiggelbout, A. M., de Haes, J. C., Vree, R., van de Velde, C. J., Bruijninckx, C. M., van Groningen, K. & Kievit, J. (1997). Follow-up of colorectal cancer patients: quality of life and attitudes towards follow-up. *British Journal of Cancer* **75**, 914–920.

van den Hout, W. B., van den Brink, M., Stiggelbout, A. M., van de Velde, C. J. H. & Kievit, J. (2002). Cost-effectiveness analysis of colorectal cancer treatments. *European Journal of Cancer* **38**, 953–963.

Virgo, K. S., Vernava, A. M., Longo, W. E., McKirgan, L. W. & Johnson, F. E. (1995). Cost of patient follow-up after potentially curative colorectal cancer treatment. *Journal of the American Medical Association* **273**, 1837–1841.

Weiss, N. S. & Cook, L. S. (1998). Evaluating the efficacy of screening for recurrence of cancer. *Journal of the National Cancer Institute* **90**, 1870–1872.

White, K. (2000). Cochrane may not have been the first to define efficacy and effectiveness. *British Medical Journal* **320**, 121.

PART 3

Evidence and opinion for medical intervention

Chapter 10

Evidence and opinion for chemotherapy in the management of early disease

Robert Wade and Clare Topham

The last fifteen years have seen significant changes in adjuvant chemotherapy for colon cancer. Moertal *et al.* (1990) demonstrated that 5-fluorouracil (5FU) in conjunction with levamisole (an antihelminthic agent) produced an improvement in 5yr disease free survival (63% vs 47% p<0.0001) and a similar improvement in overall survival (71% vs 55% $p = 0.0007$) in stage III disease. In addition, a final report by Moertal *et al.* (1995) demonstrated significant reductions in recurrence (40% ($p < 0.0001$)) and mortality (33% $p = 0.0007$)). Wolmark *et al.* (1993) treated 1083 stage II/III patients with either lomustine, vincristine, 5-fluorouracil or 5FU and its cofactor for thymidylate synthase, leucovorin. This demonstrated an overall survival advantage and improved disease free survival in the 5FU leucovorin group.

Since then there has been much interest in determining the most appropriate 5-fluorouracil regime and how best to modulate 5FU with either levamisole or leucovorin (for reviews see Chau *et al.* (2003); Michael and Zalcberg (2000)). A number of trials set out to address this question. US intergroup Int 0089 (O'Connell *et al.* (1998)) compared 5FU and levamisole with or without leucovorin over a six or twelve month period in 891 stage II/III patients. They concluded that there was no difference in survival for six months or twelve months and that the addition of leucovorin in addition to levamisole was superior to levamisole alone (70% vs 60% $p< 0.01$).

Wolmark *et al.* (1999) in NSABP C-04 randomised 2151 stage II and stage III patients to receive either 5FU leucovorin, 5FU levamisole or 5FU leucovorin and levamisole. This showed a significant improvement in disease free survival (65% vs 60% $p = 0.04$) in favour of the 5FU leucovorin group and demonstrated that the addition of levamisole provided no further benefit.

The Quasar 1 (Quick and simple and reliable) trial recruited 4927 patients with colorectal cancer (Quasar collaborative group (2000)). They received 370mg/m^2 5FU and either high or low dose folinic acid with either levamisole or placebo. Survival at 3 years was similar for both the high and low dose arms (70.1 vs 71.0 % $p = 0.43$) and levamisole showed no benefit. In addition further analysis of the dose of 5FU administered (the trial allowed either 5FU 370mg/m^2 weekly for 30 weeks or 370mg/m^2 for 5 days every 4 weeks) showed that the weekly dose was better tolerated and did not affect outcome (Kerr *et al.* (2000)). These were, however, non randomised data.

Six months of bolus 5FU leucovorin chemotherapy remains the standard of care for adjuvant stage III colorectal carcinoma at present in the United Kingdom, with expected survival benefit of between 10–14% at 5 years and a reduction in the risk of relapse of 33%.

Do combination therapies offer an advantage over 5-FU alone?

Metastatic colorectal cancer has benefited from two treatments, the third generation platinum compound oxaliplatin and the topoisomerase 1 inhibitor irinotecan. It has been postulated that there may also be benefits to using these treatments in the adjuvant setting.

Oxaliplatin

Andre et al. (2004) have recently published the results of the MOSAIC (multicentre international study of oxaliplatin/5-fluorouracil/leucovorin in the adjuvant treatment of colon cancer) trial. 2246 patients were recruited and allocated to have 5FU leucovorin with or without oxaliplatin. Oxaliplatin was given on day 1 (85mg/m^2) followed by leucovorin 200mg/m^2, bolus 5FU (400mg/m^2) with infusional 5FU, 600mg/m^2 over 22 hours for two days, repeated two weekly (FOLFOX4). The primary endpoint was disease-free survival.

The main dose limiting side effect of oxaliplatin was peripheral sensory neuropathy. 12.4% of patients suffered grade III sensory neuropathy with only 1% affected after one year of cessation of treatment and only 0.5% affected at 18 months. Although 41.1% of patients also developed neutropenia, only 1.8% developed febrile neutropenia. Other toxicities included diarrhoea (10.4%), stomatitis (2.7%) and vomiting (5.9%). There was also an increase in allergic reactions in the oxaliplatin arm. All cause mortality in both arms was 0.5%.

Addition of oxaliplatin to 5FU leucovorin provided a benefit in disease free survival at 3 years (78.2% vs 72.9% $p = 0.002$), see Figure 10.1. The hazard ratio for recurrence was 0.77 $p = 0.02$. The 4-year disease-free survival was 75.9% vs 69.1%, Hazard ratio 0.76 $p = 0.0008$. Therefore addition of oxaliplatin is superior to 5FU leucovorin alone. This improvement in disease free survival was carried over in stage II disease, (3 year disease free survival in FOLFOX 4 arm 87 % vs 84.3%). These data are summarised in Figure 10.2. Cox-model analysis showed that the reduced risk of recurrence with 5FU and oxaliplatin was similar in those with stage II and stage III disease ($p = 0.77$). The hazard ratio of relapse was 0.79 (Confidence Interval 0.57-1.09). A small benefit was also confirmed for stage II disease.

A parallel trial in the US (NSABP C-07) compared bolus 5FU (Roswell Park regime 5FU weekly × 4 then 2wks off, 24 weeks total treatment) with or without oxaliplatin 85mg/m^2 in stage II and III patients. Results were presented at ASCO 2005 for oxaliplatin/FU/LV 3 yr DFS 76.5% compared to 71.6%, for FU/LV $p = 0.004$, HR 0.79, 95% CI [0.67–0.93]. (Wolmark et al. 2005)

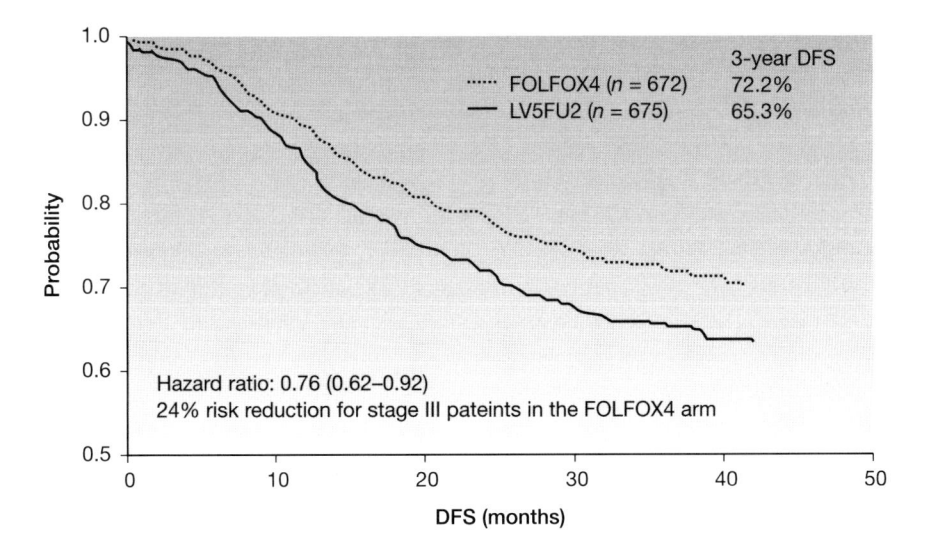

Evidence and opinion for chemotherapy in the management of early disease 123

Figure 10.1 Kaplan Meier plot showing Disease-Free Survival in Stage III Colorectal cancer patients (De Gramont, *et al.*, ASCO (2003)).

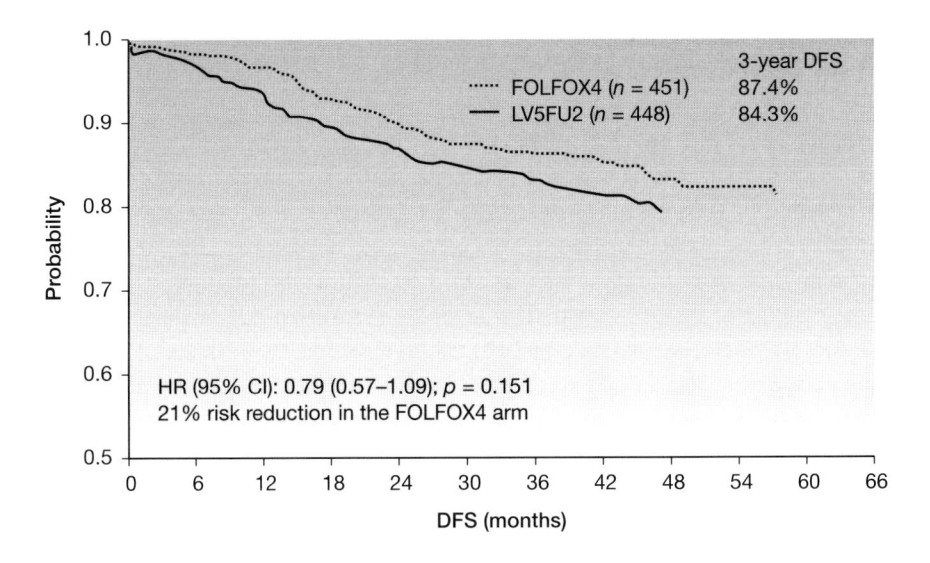

Figure 10.2 Kaplan Meier Plot showing Disease Free Survival in Stage II colorectal cancer patients treated with either 5FU leucovorin or 5FU oxaliplatin leucovorin (Hickish, T. *et al.*, ESMO (2004)).

Irinotecan

The role of irinotecan in the adjuvant setting is currently being investigated. Saltz *et al.* (2004) recently published the results of CALGB C89803. In this trial 1263 stage III colorectal cancer patients received either bolus 5FU or bolus 5FU and irinotecan. Initial safety data demonstrated an excess of early deaths in the irinotecan arm (0.8% vs 2.2%). Furthermore, irinotecan did not offer any benefit over 5FU alone in either overall survival or failure free survival. This was a completely negative trial. The PETACC3 trial compared continuous infusional 5FU with or without irinotecan in either the AIO or FOLFIRI regimen (IF vs F). This study randomised 2094 stage III patients and the results were presented at ASCO 2005. The primary endpoint was 3 year DFS which was defined as relapse, second primary colon cancer, second primary other tumour or death from other cause. Three year DFS for IF vs F was 63.3% compared to 60.3%, HR 0.89, 95% CI [0.77–1.11] *p* 0.091 (Van Cutsen *et al.* 2005). Therefore, at the current time, there appears to be no advantage for the use of irinotecan in the adjuvant setting. However, long term follow-up of PETACC3 is awaited.

Is there any benefit to treating Stage II colorectal cancer patients?

Adjuvant treatment of T3N0 and T4N0 colorectal cancer patients has been the subject of much research and debate. The IMPACT B2 investigators (1999) pooled together data from 5 different clinical trials to assess this very question. They analysed 1016 patients with Dukes B2 (T4) carcinoma of the colon. Hazard ratios for 5 year survival and event free survival did suggest a trend towards clinical benefit to treating these patients although the results were not significant (EFS 0.83 90% CI 0.72 – 1.07; OS 0.86 90% CI 0.68 to 1.07).

Gill *et al.* (2004) performed a further meta-analysis of seven trials and accrued 3302 patients. 44% were node negative and 42% had one to four nodes positive. 51% received 5FU based chemotherapy and 49% received no treatment. For all patients 5 year disease free survival improved with 5FU based chemotherapy from 55% to 67% with a corresponding 30% reduction in risk of recurrence (Hazard ratio 0.70 (0.65–0.78)). There were 1440 patients with node negative disease and their univariate analysis suggested a significant benefit of chemotherapy in node negative patients for disease free survival (DFS) but not overall survival (OS) (DFS 72% vs 76%, *p* = 0.0490, OS 80% vs 81%, *p* = 0.1127).

The QUASAR 1 trial addressed this issue by including an uncertain arm in the original trial where there was an uncertainty about benefit from chemotherapy. Patients were randomised to observation or to receive chemotherapy with 5FU/leucovorin (Gray *et al.* (2004)). This suggested a small but definite (3–4%) survival benefit (*p* = 0.04)) for chemotherapy in stage II disease. These data are tabulated in Figure 10.3.

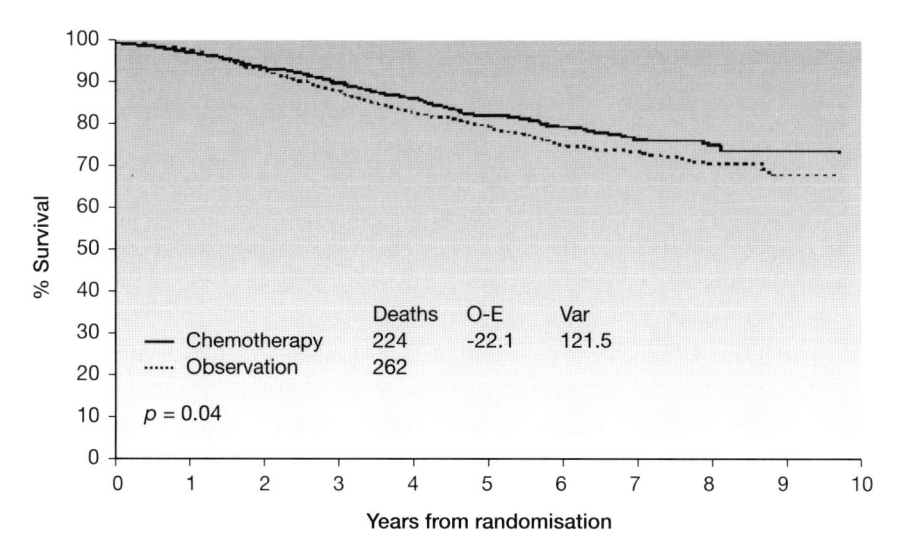

Figure 10.3 Kaplan Meier plot of disease free survival from Quasar uncertain arm for stage II colorectal cancer comparing 5FU leucovorin chemotherapy to placebo (Gray et al., ASCO (2004)).

The MOSAIC trial also looked at combination chemotherapy with 5FU/Oxaliplatin in Stage II disease as described earlier in this chapter, suggesting an additional benefit for adjuvant treatment with oxaliplatin 5FU of 2.7% (Andre et al. (2004)).

Some stage II patients will be at higher risk of recurrence. This has sparked considerable interest in the use of prognostic factors to identify subsets of patients who may have an additional benefit to chemotherapy. High risk factors for recurrence include young age, perforation, intestinal obstruction, presence of vascular/lymphatic invasion, T4 tumours and poorly differentiated tumours (Compton et al. (2000)). Hickish et al. (2004) presented subset data for high risk stage II disease from the MOSAIC trial. These demonstrated a trend toward improved disease free survival in the FOLFOX 4 high risk arm of 28% (HR 0.72 (95% CI 0.48–1.08)). These data are summarised in Figure 10.4.

Other predictive markers have also been investigated in colorectal cancer. DNA microsatellite instability (an end result of defective DNA mismatch repair) has been used as a prognostic marker in colorectal cancer. Tumours with high frequency microsatellite instability appear to have a better prognosis and not respond to adjuvant 5FU chemotherapy as compared to tumours which are microsatellite stable or with low frequency microsatellite instability (Ribic et al. (2003)).

Thymidylate synthase expression and expression of the putative tumour suppressor gene Deleted in Colorectal Cancer (DCC) are currently being investigated as predictive markers. Aschele et al. (2004) analysed DCC expression in 42 metastatic patients retrospectively following treatment with bolus 5FU modulated with

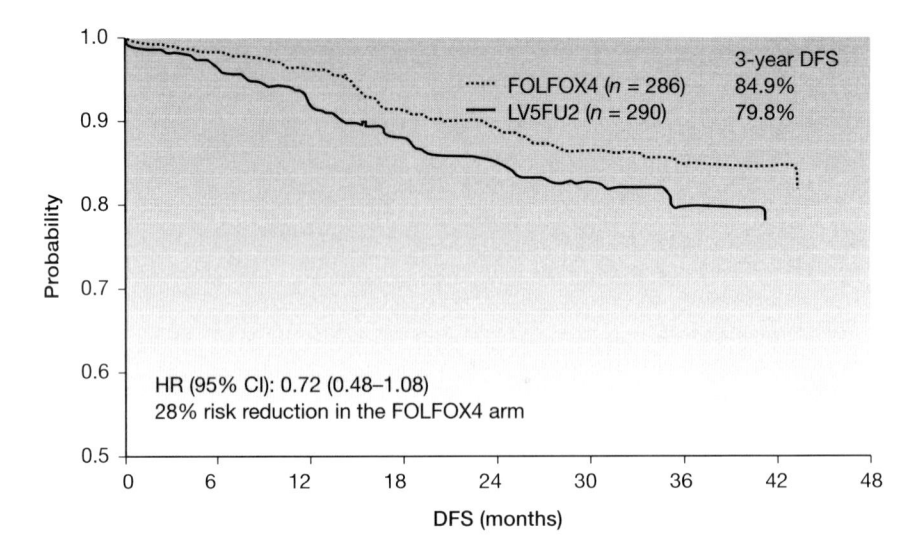

Figure 10.4 Kaplan Meier plots for disease free survival of high risk stage II patients from the Mosaic trial. The FOLFOX 4 arm is in grey and the 5FU leucovorin arm is in black (Hickish, T. et al. (2004)).

methotrexate or infusional 5FU modulated with leucovorin. Although the patient numbers were small, DCC expression was correlated with an improvement in survival (21.4 months for DCC positive tumours versus 14.3 months without DCC (log rank test, $p = 0.04$)).

Thymidylate synthase (TS) polymorphisms and expression may predict for response to 5FU chemotherapy and overall survival in the adjuvant setting. High levels of thymidylate synthase expression appear to correlate with worse survival in both the adjuvant and metastatic setting (Popat et al. (2004)), but due to heterogeneity between trials and possible publication bias the magnitude of benefit was not clear.

Further studies should clarify the significance of microsatellite instability, deleted in colorectal cancer and thymidylate synthase expression in colorectal cancer and help to further identify patient groups that may benefit from chemotherapy.

The American Society of Clinical Oncology has published comprehensive guidelines for the use of chemotherapy in stage II disease (Benson et al. (2004)). Ultimately, the clinical decision as to whether or not to treat the patient should be based on discussions with the patient about the relevant evidence, likelihood of benefit, associated risk factors and possible co-morbidities. These patients should all be considered for clinical trials.

Can convenience in administration be improved?

Capecitabine and uracil tegafur are oral fluoropyrimidines which have the advantage that they obviate the need for central venous catheters.

The uracil tegafur/leucovorin versus 5FU leucovorin is currently being assessed in the NASBP C-06 trial.

Capecitabine has the advantage that its metabolising enzyme thymidine phosphorylase is expressed in higher levels in tumours which allows for targeted therapy.

The X-act trial compared 1250mg/m^2 capecitabine bd days 1–14 with 5FU/leucovorin (MAYO regimen). Capecitabine caused significantly more palmar plantar erythema but less diarrhoea, stomatitis, neutropenia, nausea, vomiting and alopecia (Scheithauer *et al.* (2003), Cassidy *et al.* (2004)).

This trial had disease free survival as the primary end point and relapse free survival as one of the secondary endpoints. Relapse free survival included all relapses, those who developed a new primary colon cancer and all those who died from colon cancer treatment. Disease free survival data included the relapse free survival data and deaths from other causes.

Capecitabine showed a trend towards superior disease free survival as demonstrated in Figure 10.5 and superior relapse free survival as demonstrated in Figure 10.6 (hazard ratio 0.86 (95% CI 0.704–0.99, $p = 0.407$)). Figure 10.7 illustrates a trend towards improved overall survival (81.3% vs 77.6%, hazard ratio 0.84 (95% CI 0.69–1.01, $p = 0.0706$)) and disease free survival (64.2% vs 60.7%, HR 0.87 (CI 0.75–1.00, $p = 0.0528$)) although these results were not significant.

Protracted venous infusional regimes seem to be comparable to treatment with 5FU alone and may allow for shorter treatment times. Saini *et al.* (2003) compared continuous 300mg/m^2/day 5FU over 12 weeks vs a 6 month bolus 5FU/leucovorin

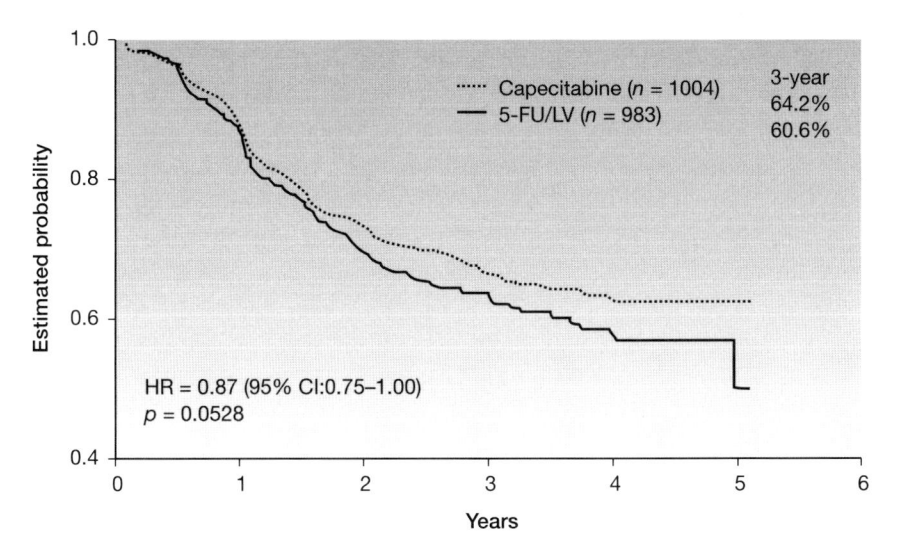

Figure 10.5 Kaplan Meier Curve Comparing disease free survival with capecitabine verses 5FU in the adjuvant treatment of Dukes C colorectal cancer (Cassidy, J. *et al.* (2004)).

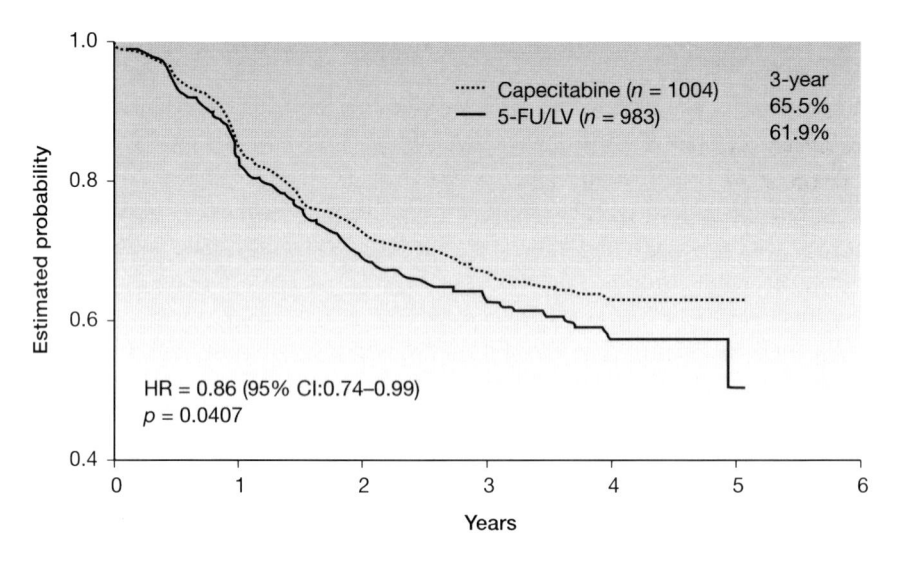

Figure 10.6 Kaplan Meier curve showing improved relapse free for capecitabine as opposed to 5FU/leucovorin (Cassidy, J. et al. (2004)).

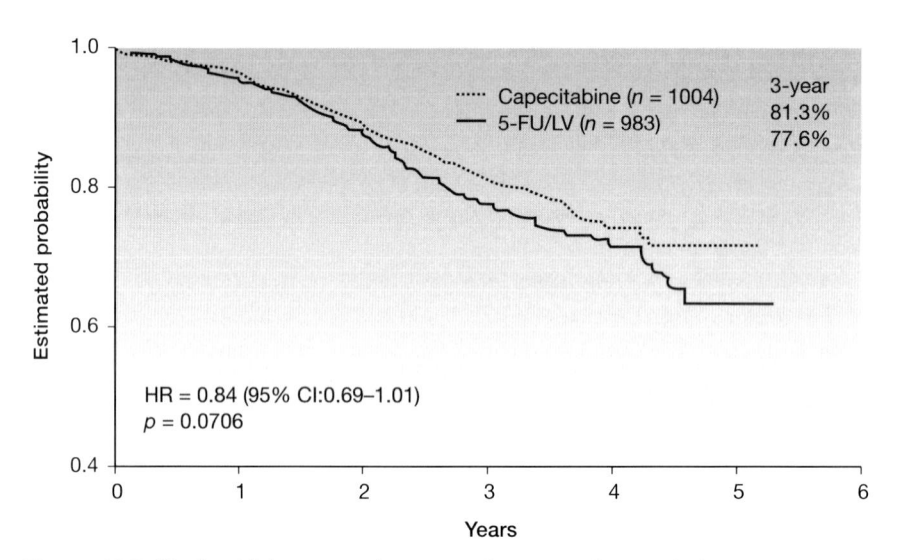

Figure 10.7 Kaplan Meier curve demonstrating a trend towards improved overall survival (ITT) for capecitabine verses 5FU (Cassidy, J. et al. (2004)).

Mayo regime in 716 stage II/III colorectal cancer patients. There was no difference in overall survival, but PVI patients had an improved relapse free survival (80% vs 68%, $p = 0.023$) and significantly less toxicity. In addition, those patients with rectal cancer treated in the bolus 5FU arm had a trend towards worse survival ($p = 0.08$) and shortened time to relapse ($p = 0.043$). This was however a small trial and will require confirmation in larger studies.

There are several recent chemotherapy trials exploring combination therapy with capecitabine. NO16968 compared capecitabine and oxaliplatin to bolus 5FU/leucovorin (stage III, $n = 1950$). This trial has finished recruitment. Quasar II aims to treat 2400 high risk stage II/III patients with either capecitabine or capecitabine irinotecan with a further randomisation to receive the vascular endothelial growth factor receptor bevacizumab.

We can however conclude that capecitabine is at least as effective as bolus 5FU and that when one considers its ease of administration and toxicity, our view is that capecitabine should replace 5FU completely in the adjuvant setting.

Do the 'biologicals' have a clinical role in the adjuvant setting?

Cetuximab

The epithelial growth factor receptor expressed on 80% of colonic tumours can be blocked by the chimeric anti-EGFR antibody cetuximab. Cunningham *et al.* (2003) treated 470 EGFR positive patients who had previously relapsed on irinotecan with either cetuximab and irinotecan or cetuximab alone. The latter arm had the option of receiving irinotecan and cetuximab on relapse. This study demonstrated an improved time to progression and response rate in the metastatic setting on treating irinotecan refractory patients with cetuximab and irinotecan as opposed to cetuximab alone. This did not translate into an overall survival benefit due to crossover. These compelling results have stimulated considerable interest in cetuximab in the adjuvant setting.

NCCTG N0147 plans to recruit stage III colorectal cancer patients into three arms. The patients will either receive 6 months 5FU, leucovorin and oxaliplatin, with or without cetuximab. The irinotecan arms were withdrawn following PETACC3.

Bevacizumab

Bevacizumab is a chimeric monoclonal antibody which binds to vascular endothelial growth factor (VEGF). This factor is required to support angiogenesis in tumours. Bevacizumab has been used in the metastatic setting with some degree of success. Hurwitz *et al.* (2003) compared irinotecan with irinotecan plus bevacizumab as first line metastatic treatment. 925 patients were enrolled into this study. The combination of bevacizumab and irinotecan improved objective response, median survival and progression free survival. Trials are now planned to see whether there is an adjuvant role for this agent.

The NSABP C-08 trial aims to recruit 2500 patients with stage II or III disease. One arm will receive 5FU, leucovorin and oxaliplatin. The other arm will receive leucovorin, oxaliplatin, 5FU and bevacizumab.

MOSAIC 2 aims to recruit 4500 patients into one of three arms, 5FU, leucovorin, oxaliplatin or 5FU, leucovorin oxaliplatin and bevacizumab, capecitabine, oxaliplatin and bevacizumab.

Conclusion

Considerable progress has been made in extending the boundaries for the adjuvant treatment of early stage colorectal cancer. We know that combination treatment with oxaliplatin offers a survival benefit over 5FU alone. We think that this combination treatment should be the standard of care for the adjuvant treatment of stage III colorectal cancer.

There appears to be an extra benefit in stage II disease with combination treatment. We would advise at present that stage II patients considered for combination treatment should be carefully selected on the basis of accompanying risk factors and entered into clinical trials where possible. With the advent of further predictive markers we may in the future be able to predict subgroups of patients who are most likely to benefit.

We know that we can replace 5FU with capecitabine, providing further benefit for patients in terms of convenience and safety with no loss of efficacy.

The biological agents herald the future for chemotherapy, and coupled with further understanding of the genome and the genetic drivers behind colon cancer, hold great promise. Current clinical trials will help elucidate their place in the adjuvant setting.

References

Aschele, C., Debernardis, D., Lonardi, S., Bandelloni, R., Casazza, S., Monfardini, S., Gallo, L. (2004). Deleted in Colon Cancer Protein Expression in colorectal cancer metastasis: A major predictor of survival in patients with unresectable metastatic disease receiving palliative fluorouracil-based chemotherapy. *Journal of Clinical Oncology* **22**(18), 3758–3765.

André, T., Boni, C., Mounedji-Boudiaf, L., Navarro, M., Tabernero, J., Hickish, T., Topham, C., Zaninelli, M., Clingan, P., Bridgewater, J., Tabah-Fisch, I., de Gramont, A. (2004). Oxaliplatin, fluorouracil and leucovorin as adjuvant treatment for colon cancer. *New England Journal of Medicine* **350**, 2343–2351.

Benson, A., Schrag, D., Somerfield, M., Cohen, A., Figueredo, A., Flynn, P., Kryzanowska, M., Maroun, J., McAllister, P., Cutsem, E., Brouwers, M., Charette, M., Haller, D. (2004). American Society of Clinical Oncology Recommendations on adjuvant chemotherapy for stage II colon cancer. *Journal of Clinical Oncology* **22**(16), 3408–3419.

Cassidy, J., Scheithauer, W., McKendrick, J., Kroning, H., Nowaki, M., Seitz, J., Twelves, C., Van Hazel, G., Wong, A., Diaz-Rubio, E. (2004). Capecitabine vs bolus 5FU/leucovorin as adjuvant therapy for colon cancer (the XACT study) positive efficacy results of a phase III trial. *Proceedings of the American Society of Clinical Oncology* **22**(14S), Abstract 3509.

Chau, I., Chan, S., Cunningham, D. (2003). Overview of preoperative and postoperative therapy for colorectal cancer: The European and United States Perspectives. *Clinical Colorectal Cancer* **3**(1), 1–15.

Compton, C., Fielding, L., Burgart, C. *et al.* (2000). Prognostic factors in colorectal cancer. College of American Pathologists Consensus Statement 1999. *Archives Pathology Laboratory Medicine* **124**, 979–994

Cunningham, D., Humblet, Y., Siena, S., Khayat, D., Bleiberg, H., Santoro, A., Bets, D., Muerser, M., Harstrick, A., Van Cutsem, E. (2003). Cetuximab alone or in combination with irinotecan in patients with epidermal growth factor receptor (EGFR) positive, irinotecan-refractory metastatic colorectal cancer. *Proceedings of the Society of Clinical Oncology* **252**, Abstract 1012.

De Gramont, A., Banzi, M., Navarro, M., Taberno, J., Hickish, T., Bridgewater, J., Rivera, F., Figer, A., Fountzilas, G., Andre, T. (2003). Oxaliplatin/5FU/LV in adjuvant colon cancer: Results of the international randomized mosaic trial. *Proceedings of the American Society of Clinical Oncology*, Abstract 1015.

Gill, S., Loprinzi, C., Sargent, D., Thome, S., Alberts, S., Haller, D., Benedetti, J., Francini, G,. Shepherd, L., Seitz, J., Labianca, R., Chen, W., Cha, S., Heldebrant, M., Goldberg, R. (2004). Pooled analysis of fluorouracil based adjuvant chemotherapy for stage II and III colon cancer: Who benefits and by how much? *Journal of Clinical Oncology* **22**(10), 1797–1806.

Gray, R., Barnwell, J., Hills, R., McConkey, C., Williams, N., Kerr, D. (2004). Quasar: A Randomised study of adjuvant chemotherapy vs observation including 3238 patients. *Journal of Clinical Oncology* **22**(14S), 3501.

Hickish, T. *et al.* ESMO 04 abstract 284, poster presentation.

Hurwitz, H., Fehrenbacher, L., Cartwright, T., Hainsworth, J., Heim, W., Berlin, J., Griffing, S., Novotny, W., Holmgren, E., Kabbinavar, F. (2003). Bevacizumab (a monoclonal antibody to vascular endothelial growth factor) prolongs survival in first-line colorectal cancer (CRC): Results of a phase III trial of bevacizumab in combination with bolus IFL (irinotecan, 5-fluorouracil, leucovorin) as first-line therapy in subjects with metastatic CRC. *Proceedings of the American Society of Clinical Oncology*, Abstract 3646.

International Pooled analysis of B2 colon cancer trials Investigators (IMPACT) (1999). Efficacy of adjuvant fluorouracil and folinic acid in B2 colon cancer. *Journal of Clinical Oncology* **17**, 1356–1363.

Kerr, D. J., Gray, R., McConkey, C., Barnwell, J. for the QUASAR Colorectal Cancer Study Group (2000). Adjuvant chemotherapy with 5-fluorouracil, L-folinic acid and levamisole for patients with colorectal cancer: Non-randomised comparison of weekly verses four –weekly schedules – less pain, some gain. *Annals of Oncology* **11**, 947–955.

Michael, M. & Zalcberg, J. R. (2000). The optimal 5-fluorouracil regimen for the adjuvant therapy of colon cancer: Where to from here? *Annals of Oncology* **11**, 915–918.

Moertal, C., Fleming, T., Macdonald, J., Haller, D., Laurie, J., Tangen, C., Ungerleider, J., Emerson, W., Tormey, D. C., Glick, J., Veeder, M., Mailliard, J. (1995). Fluorouracil plus levamisole as effective therapy after resection of stage III colon carcinoma: A final report. *Annals of Internal Medicine* **122**(5), 321–326.

Moertal, C., Fleming, T., Macdonald, J. *et al.* (1990). Levamisole and fluorouracil for adjuvant therapy of resected colon cancer. *New England Journal of Medicine* **322**, 352–358.

O'Connell, M., Laurie, J., Kahn, M., Fitzgibbons, R., Erlichman, C., Shepherd, L., Moertel, C., Kocha, W., Pazdur, R., Wieand, S., Rubin, J., Vukov, A., Donohue, J., Krook, J., Figueredo, A. (1998). Prospectively randomised trial of postoperative adjuvant chemotherapy in patients with high – risk colon cancer. *Journal of Clinical Oncology* **16**(1), 295–300.

Quasar Collaborative Group (2000). Comparison of fluorouracil with additional levamisole, higher-dose folinic acid, or both, as adjuvant chemotherapy for colorectal cancer: A randomised trial. *Lancet* **355**, 1588–96.

Popat, S., Matakidou, A., Houlston, R. (2004). Thymidylate synthase expression and prognosis in colorectal cancer: A systemic review and meta-analysis. *ASCO Gastrointestinal Cancers Symposium*, Abstract 208.

Ribic, C., Sargent, D., Moore, M., Thibodeau, S., French, A., Goldberg, R., Hamilton, S., Laurent-Puig, P., Gryfe, R., Shepherd, L., Tu, D., Redston, M., Gallinger, S. (2003). Tumour microsatellite-instability status as a predictor of benefit from fluorouracil based adjuvant chemotherapy for colon cancer. *New England Journal of Medicine* **349**, 247–257.

Saini, A., Norman, A. R., Cunningham, D., Chau, I., Hill, M., Tait, D., Hickish, T., Iveson, T., Lofts, F., Jodrell, D., Ross, P. J., Oates, J. (2003). Twelve weeks of protracted venous infusion of 5 fluorouracil is as effective as 6 months of bolus 5FU folinic acid as adjuvant treatment in colorectal cancer. *British Journal of Cancer* **88**, 1859–1865.

Saltz, L., Niedzwiecki, D., Hollis, D., Goldberg, R., Hantel, A., Thomas, J., Fields, A., Carver, G., Mayer, R. (1994). Irinotecan plus fluorouracil/leucovorin verses fluorouracil/leucovorin alone in stage III colon cancer (intergroup trial CALGB C89803). *Journal of Clinical Oncology* **22**(14S), Abstract 3500.

Scheithauer, W., McKendrick, J., Begbie, S., Borner, M., Burns, W., Burris, H., Cassidy, J., Jodrell, D., Koralewski, P., Levine, E., Marschner, N., Maroun, J., Garcia-Alfonso, P., Tujakowski, J., Van Hazel, G., Wong, A., Zaluski, J., Twelves C. (2003). Oral capecitabine as an alternative to iv 5-fluorouracil based adjuvant therapy for colorectal cancer: Safety results of a randomised, phase III trial. *Annals of Oncology* **14**, 1735–1743.

Van Cutsem, E., Labianca, R., Hossfeld, D. *et al.* (2005). Randomised phase III trial comparing infused irinotecan/5-FU (5-FU-folinic acid) (IF) versus 5-FU/FA (F) in stage III colon cancer patients (PETACC3). *Proceedings of the American Society of Clinical Oncology*, **23**, Abstract 8

Wolmark, N., Wieand, S., Kuebler, J. P. *et al.* (2005). A phase III trial comparing FULV to FULV + oxaliplatin in stage II or III carcinoma of the colon: results of NSABP protocol C-07. *Proceedings of the American Society of Clinical Oncology*, **23**, Abstract 3500

Wolmark, N., Rockette, H., Mamounas, E., Jones, J., Wieand, S., Wickerham, D., Bear, H., Atkins, K., Dimitrov, N., Glass, A., Fisher, E., Fisher, B. (1999). Clinical trial to assess the relative efficacy of fluorouracil and leucovorin, fluorouracil and levamisole, and fluorouracil, leucovorin and levamisole in patients with Dukes' B and C carcinoma of the colon: results from National Surgical Adjuvant Breast and Bowel project C-04. *Journal of Clinical Oncology* **17**(11), 3553–3559.

Wolmark, N., Rockette, H., Fisher, B. *et al.* (1993). The Benefit of Leucovorin – modulated fluorouracil as postoperative adjuvant therapy for primary colon cancer: results from National Breast and Bowel Project C-03. *Journal of Clinical Oncology* **11**, 1879–1887.

Chapter 11

Evidence and opinion for combination therapy in the management of advanced disease

Ashita Waterston and Jim Cassidy

Introduction

Colorectal cancer is a major cause of morbidity and mortality in the developed World. In the USA it is the second commonest cancer with 106,000 people diagnosed with colon cancer in 2004 (American cancer society facts and figures). In the UK in 2000 the incidence was 35,300, which is 13% of the cancer population (Cancer Research UK figures). Despite advances in therapy, only 40–50% of these patients will survive 5 years, most succumbing to metastatic disease. For the purpose of this review advanced disease will be taken as that which is beyond the scope of potential cure by original complete resection.

Colorectal cancer reaches a peak incidence in the 7th decade of life, so patients often have co-morbidities and a reduced expectation of life. Since metastatic disease is incurable there is a major emphasis on controlling symptoms and the prolongation of life is to some extent a secondary issue. Consequently, for large Phase III trials of metastatic colon cancer a quality of life study is often incorporated into the trial. It is very important to ensure that treatment toxicities do not have a detrimental effect on quality of life.

Up until the 1990s, most oncologists considered colorectal cancer untreatable as it had a reputation for being chemo-resistant. Patients were thus offered nothing more than palliative care in the majority of institutions. This has now changed. A number of randomised controlled trials demonstrated an improvement in the quality of life as well as survival benefit when chemotherapy was compared to best supportive care or delayed therapy (Nordic Gastrointestinal Tumour Adjuvant Therapy Group 1992; Scheithauer *et al.* 1993; Glimelius *et al.* 1995; Berretta *et al.* 1997). In general, with the use of therapy based on 5FU/FA, there has been an increase in median survival from 6 months to 1 year. Following the establishment of overall benefit from 1st line chemotherapy in the metastatic setting, the use of chemotherapy as second line was also examined. Cunningham et al in 1998 showed an additional benefit of 3 months median survival (Cunningham *et al.* 1998). Consequently, patients with metastatic disease are living longer on chemotherapy but the challenge is now finding the most suitable combinations of treatments and the optimum scheduling.

In the past ten years significant new drugs, some with novel mechanisms of action, have been developed and are now on the market in many countries. The most significant of these are oxaliplatin and irinotecan. The introduction of oral fluoropyrimidines is also worthy of note. Capecitabine, with its tumour selective activation pathway, has at least a theoretical advantage over its main competitor, UFToral. There is also a rapidly expanding field of biological and small molecule agents that in theory are targeted to the signalling pathways of cancerous cells. The most advanced in terms of assessment in the clinical setting are two monoclonal antibodies: bevacizumab (anti-VEGFR) and cetuximab (anti-EGFR).

Progress with 5FU agents

A number of patients respond to first line chemotherapy with 5FU and duration of therapy is not constrained by dose limiting toxicities. There is no consensus on how long patients responding to 5FU and folinic acid should remain on treatment. In a randomised controlled trial 176 patients on continuous infusional 5FU and folinic acid were compared to 178 patients who stopped treatment after 12 weeks and then restarted with the same regime on progression. There was no difference in overall survival (OS) and patients in the intermittent group had fewer toxic effects. This indicates that it is safe to stop treatment after 12 weeks and restart the same treatment on progression (Maughan *et al.* 2003).

5FU has been used in the clinic for over 40 years and has remarkably low anti-cancer effect when administered in a low dose bolus regimen. A better understanding of the mechanism of action of 5FU and a deeper understanding of its biochemical action has lead to the development of infusional regimens. A number of these infusional regimes have been developed in Europe and have demonstrated a better response with less toxicity (Meta-Analysis Group In Cancer 1998a; Meta-Analysis Group In Cancer 1998b; de Gramont *et al.* 1997). However, the early studies did not shown any difference in overall survival. Consequently, from the American perspective, it was felt that the inconvenience and expense of using infusional regimens outweighed any benefit in contrast to the European perspective where the response and its reduced toxicity are considered to be of great benefit. This has been reflected in the choice of standard therapy and combination with newer agents that have been developed for trials on either side of the Atlantic. In the USA, bolus 5FU and folinic acid have until recently represented standard therapy while in Europe, infusional 5FU and folinic acid based on the de Gramont regimen is more commonly used.

Capecitabine

5-fluorouracil is one of the oldest chemotherapy agents used regularly in the treatment of cancer and has formed part of the standard treatment for metastatic and adjuvant therapy for colon cancer for several decades. The development of oral fluoropyrimidines marks an important milestone in the treatment of colon cancer. Patients may benefit from the convenience of an orally administered drug with reduced hospital stays and the avoidance of central catheterisation. There are many drugs for administration via the oral route being tested in clinical trials. These include UFT (uracil and tegafur), UFToral (UFT and leucovorin) and capecitabine (Xeloda). The latter is the most advanced in terms of its clinical use in a wide variety of solid tumours. It is a third generation activated fluoropyrimidine. In two large randomised trials comparing oral capecitabine to bolus 5FU and leucovorin (the MAYO regimen) in metastatic colon cancer there were greater tumour response rates in the oral capecitabine group and time to disease progression and survival were equivalent. (Hoff *et al.* 2001; Van Cutsem *et al.* 2001). Furthermore, capecitabine was better tolerated and more convenient to administer. In Europe, however, the standard schedule for ACRC receiving LV/5FU is infusional treatment and there has not been a direct comparison of capecitabine with modified de Gramont.

Newer cytotoxics

Both 5FU and capecitabine have now been used in combination with the newer agents irinotecan and oxaliplatin and these are discussed below.

Irinotecan

This is an inhibitor of the enzyme topoisomerase 1 responsible for relieving torsional stress in DNA. It is over expressed in colorectal cancers and thus makes an ideal drug target. Irinotecan is a camptothecin derivative, which is metabolised *in vivo* to the more active compound SN38. SN38 is excreted in bile and then is reabsorbed from the gut into the blood (undergoing enterohepatic recirculation). It is believed that SN38 in the large intestine is the major cause of dose-limiting diarrhoea. The use of anti-diarrhoeals appears to enhance the entero-hepatic recirculation and may potentiate neutropaenia (the other dose-limiting side-effect of this compound) (Kawato *et al.* 1991; Slatter *et al.* 2000). Current interest is thus focused on agents which may bind or inactivate SN38 in the gut and thus counteract the diarrhoea.

First Line Therapy

Initially, many investigators proceeded with caution when combining irinotecan with 5FU because of fears of enhanced toxicity, particularly diarrhoea, but there have now been 3 large studies which have failed to show increased diarrhoea with the combination (See Table 11.1). Two studies combined irinotecan with infusional 5FU which was also used in the standard arm (Douillard *et al.* 2000; Köhne *et al.* 2003) and one study used bolus 5FU (the MAYO regimen) as the standard arm (Saltz *et al.* 2000). The addition of irinotecan increased responses by approximately 20%. The progression free survival (PFS), which was a primary endpoint also increased by 2 months in both the trials using infusional 5FU while the PFS in the Saltz trial showed an increase by 3 months months. However, all the trials extended the PFS to around

Table 11.1 Phase III first line studies on ACRC using irinotecan and 5FU/LV

Author	Protocol	RR (%)	PFS (mos)	OS (mos)
Saltz et al. 2000	FU/LV bolus (Mayo)	21	4.3	12.6
	FU/LV bolus + Irinotecan IFL	39	7.0	14.8
	p-value	<0.001	0.004	0.04
Douillard et al. 2000	FU/LV inf.	31	4.4	14.1
	FU/LV inf. + Irinotecan	49	6.7	17.4
	p-value	<0.001	<0.001	0.031
Koehne et al. 2003	FU/LV inf.	31.5	6.4	16.9
	FU/LV inf. + Irinotecan	54.2	8.5	20.1
	p-value	0.0001	0.0001	NS

7 months. These findings translated into a significant increase in overall survival (OS) from 17.4 versus 14.1 months in the Doullard trial and 14.8 versus 12.6 months in the Saltz trial, in favour of the combination. In the Köhne trial, OS was 20.1 versus 16.9 months, which did not reach significance although the results were compounded by a cross over of 62% in the 5FU alone arm to further irinotecan. The quality of life of these patients was not compromised by irinotecan. Although there was more grade 3 diarrhoea in the irinotecan arm the grade 4 diarrhoea was similar in both arms for the Saltz trial while in the Doullard trial there was greater grade 3/4 diarrhoea in the irinotecan arm. The degree of neutropaenia also differed in the two trials with greater febrile neutropaenia in the bolus 5FU compared to the combination for the Saltz trial but more febrile neutropaenia in the combination arm compared to infusional 5FU alone for the Doullard trial. This may reflect differences in toxicity with infusional versus bolus 5FU. Irinotecan combinations can cause severe diarrhoea and these patients need to be managed carefully. In the adjuvant setting the trial of combination of irinotecan and 5FU versus 5FU caused significantly greater treatment related deaths in the combination arm (Rothenberg et al. 2001). Irinotecan alone has also been examined as second line therapy in ACRC. The studies of second line therapy compared to either BSC or 5FU alone have showed an improvement in overall survival with irinotecan (Cunningham et al. 1998; Rougier et al. 1998). Furthermore, in both these studies quality of life was also examined and found to improve with irinotecan treatment.

Oxaliplatin

The other new chemotherapy agent being used in ACRC is oxaliplatin, which belongs to the diaminocyclohexane (DACH) platinum family. It is believed that this DACH group makes DNA adducts less susceptible to DNA repair mechanisms, explaining the relative lack of cross-resistance with the parent molecule. In addition, preclinical synergy was demonstrated with 5FU.

First Line Therapy

Three phase III trials have been reported using the combination of 5FU and oxaliplatin first line in advanced colon cancer (See Table 11.2). The trials differed in the scheduling of 5FU. The Giachetti study used chronotherapy, a technology based on the use of circadian biological rhythm to modulate the rate of drug administration and thereby reduce toxicity while maximising the delivered dose intensity (Giacchetti *et al.* 2000). The de Gramont study used infusional LV5FU2 (fortnightly regime of 5FU 400mg/m^2 bolus, D1 and D2, 600mg/m^2 22 hour infusion, D1 and D2; leucovorin 200mg/m^2 in a 2-hour intravenous infusion, D1 and D2) and added fortnightly oxaliplatin (de Gramont *et al.* 2000). The third study by Grothey *et al.* used bolus 5FU with the Mayo regimen (arm B-5FU 425mg/m^2 D1–D5, folinic acid 20mg/m^2 D1–D5, every 4 weeks), for the standard arm and compared this to weekly oxaliplatin and 5FU/FA (arm A-OXA 50mg/m^2 2 hour infusion, 5FU 2000mg/m^2, folinic acid 500mg/m^2) (Grothey *et al.* 2002). The response rates for the standard 5FU arms were 16–22% with a significant additional benefit of oxaliplatin giving a response rate of 50%. The PFS was 6 months for the 5FU control arm and the combinations gave a PFS of 9 months for the infusional combinations and 7.8 months for the bolus combination, these differences were all significantly in favour of the combination. Unfortunately this did not translate into a significant overall survival benefit despite both the de Gramont and Grothey studies showing an approximate increase in survival of 2 months compared to 5FU alone. The reason for this lack of a statistically significant survival advantage may be explained by the numbers of patients in the control arm either crossing over to receive oxaliplatin/5FU or receiving irinotecan which is known to give a survival benefit. When these studies were planned there were

Table 11.2 Phase III first line studies of ACRC using oxaliplatin and 5FU/LV

Author	Protocol	RR (%)	PFS (mos)	OS (mos)
Giacchetti *et al.* 2000	FU/LV inf.	16	6.1	19.9
	FU/LV inf. + Oxaliplatin	53	8.7	19.4
	p-value	<0.0001	0.048	n.s.
de Gramont *et al.* 2000	FU/LV inf.	22.3	6.2	14.7
	FU/LV inf. + Oxalipl. FOLFOX4	50.7	9.0	16.2
	p-value	0.0001	<0.0001	n.s.
Grothey *et al.* 2002	FU/LV Bolus (Mayo)	22.6	5.3	16.1
	FU/LV inf. + Oxaliplatin	49.1	7.8	19.7
	p-value	<0.0001	0.0001	n.s.

no second line treatments known to give a survival benefit so this was not considered a crucial variable in the design of the study. A more recent study published in abstract form comparing infusional 5FU and oxaliplatin as developed by de Gramont to the chronomodulated 5FU and oxaliplatin combination showed no difference in response rates, PFS or OS with a >18 month median survival in both arms; however there was significantly less grade 3/4 neutropaenia and diarrhoea in the chronomodulated arm (Giachetti *et al.* 2004). Based on the lack of survival benefit in the Phase III trials the FDA delayed approving this combination for metastatic colorectal cancer and it was reserved for patients with operable liver metastases which require down staging. The FDA has now approved oxaliplatin for the treatment of metastatic colorectal cancer. The LIFE study was designed to provide definitive evidence of benefit for first line oxaliplatin in ACRC with all patients planned to receive second line irinotecan. The study has 4 arms with continuous infusion 5FU 350mg/m^2/day with or without oxaliplatin day 1 at 85mg/m^2 versus bolus LV 5FU with or without oxaliplatin at 85mg/m^2 every 14 days. 725 patients were recruited with the aim of showing an OS benefit of 10% absolute improvement in 2-yr survival with the addition of oxaliplatin in first line to 5-FU followed by irinotecan sequence in advanced colorectal cancer. Results were presented at ASCO 2005. Overall response rate was 54% for the oxaliplatin arm versus 30% $p< 0.0001$, PFS 7.9 months vs 5.9 months $p< 0.0001$. However, this did not translate into an overall survival advantage (15.9 vs 15.2 months). A possible explanation for the OS results was a low number of patients receiving second line irinotecan therapy in the oxaliplatin arm (41%). That is, only a small proportion were exposed to all three active agents (Pluzanska *et al.* 2005).

What is the optimum schedule and dose?

From the trials published so far it is clear that there is an increase in time to progression with oxaliplatin or irinotecan combined with 5FU. We therefore have two combinations that produce similar responses when given as first line therapy, so which should we choose? At present, studies are ongoing to examine the dose and scheduling of combinations. We should, however, also be aware of the toxicities induced by both combinations. Oxaliplatin can induce a sensory neuropathy which initially presents as a cold induced dysaethesia in the hands and feet. A short-lived laryngo-pharyngeal syndrome can also occur, which usually does not require any treatment. For the majority of patients the neuropathy is short-lived and reverses on cessation of treatment. The OPTIMOX study was designed to determine whether an alteration of scheduling could modify the dose-limiting problem of sensory neuropathy (de Gramont *et al.* 2004). Patients were randomised to standard FOLFOX 4 (85mg/m^2 oxaliplatin day 1, 200mg/m^2 LV, bolus 5FU 400mg/m^2 and 22 hours 600mg/m^2 days 1 and 2 with the cycles repeating every 2 weeks.) In the FOLFOX 7 arm patients were allowed a break from oxaliplatin while still being exposed to high doses of oxalipatin on either side of the break. The regimen consisted of 400mg/m^2

LV and 130mg/m² oxaliplatin administered from hours 0–2 on day 1 followed by 2400mg/m² 5FU administered over 46 hours. This was given for 6 cycles followed by a simplified regime of LV5FU2 for 12 cycles which consisted of 400mg/m² of LV over 2 hours followed by bolus 5FU 400mg/m² and then 2400mg/m² to 3000mg/m² 5FU over 46 hours, with the cycles repeating every 2 weeks. Following the 12 cycles of simplified 5FU another 6 cycles of FOLFOX 7 were re-introduced. The initial results were presented at ASCO 2004 and showed no difference in the response rates, PFS and OS. In terms of toxicities in the FOLFOX 7 arm there was greater thrombocytopenia ($p = 0.0006$) but less neutropaenia ($p = 0.13$), less hand and foot syndrome ($p = 0.04$) and less neurotoxicity ($p = 0.117$). Interestingly, there was no increase in neuropathy in the subpopulations in which oxaliplatin was reintroduced. The same proportion of patients had second line irinotecan (58.3%) in both arms. The reintroduction of oxaliplatin was 42% in the FOLFOX 7 and 8.4% in the FOLFOX 4 arm. There was a wide variation in reintroduction in the different centres. The Kaplein Meier plot suggested a possible improvement in survival in centres with higher reintroduction rates. An OPTIMOX 2 study is planned using lower oxaliplatin dose intensity to improve reintroduction rates.

What is the optimum combination?

Goldberg et al undertook a large randomised trial (N9741) to compare FOLFOX 4 versus irinotecan and 5FULV (IFL) versus a combination of irinotecan and oxaliplatin (IROX) (Goldberg *et al.* 2004). An imbalance in early deaths lead to temporary closure of the trial followed by a reduction in the dose of IFL from 125mg/m² to 100mg/m² of irinotecan and from 400mg/m² of bolus 5FU to 300mg/m². The results of the trial were published this year. Patients receiving FOLFOX 4 showed an increase in time to progression of 8.7 months, response rates of 45% and median survival time of 19.5 months which was significantly superior to IFL for all end points (6.9 months, 31%, and 15 months respectively) or for IROX (6.5 months, 35% and 17.4 months respectively). There was significantly greater febrile neutropaenia, mucositis, nausea, vomiting, dehydration and diarrhoea in the IFL arm with only parasthesia significantly greater in the oxaliplatin containing arms. The authors concluded that oxaliplatin and infusional 5FU should be first line therapy of choice in metastatic colorectal cancer. Interestingly 60% of patients received second line irinotecan after the study finished while only 24% received second line oxaliplatin. This may have therefore affected the overall survival results. Following on from these trials with more than one combination appearing to be beneficial in ACRC the role of sequential therapy needs to be investigated to try and elucidate the optimum sequence of treatment. A few studies have been undertaken to answer this question. A trial of 220 patients with untreated metastatic disease compared FOLFOX6 (using 100mg/m² oxaliplatin unlike FOLFOX 4 which uses 85mg/m²) versus FOLFIRI (irinotecan 180mg/m² combined with infusional LV/5FU), which then crossed over to the alternative arm (Tournigand *et al.* 2004). This showed a similar overall survival of 21.5 months for those treated with FOLFIRI followed by FOLFOX versus 20.6 months in patients treated with FOLFOX followed by FOLFIRI. The PFS and response rates after first line treatment were similar for both arms (8–8.5 months and 55% respectively). After second line treatment PFS was 2.5 months and RR 4% in those that were given FOLFIRI while those given FOLFOX second line had a PFS of 4.2 months and achieved a RR of 15%. Comparing FOLFIRI to historic data on single agent irinotecan the survival benefit is no different and therefore the addition of LV/5FU may not be necessary for second line treatment of metastatic colon cancer. Interestingly, 21% of patients initially treated with FOLFOX 4 underwent hepatic resection and only 9% of patients treated initially with FOLFIRI underwent hepatic resection. Since inoperability criteria were not provided it is difficult to compare the combinations in terms of ability to alter operability between regimens. The toxicity profile did differ between FOLFIRI and FOLFOX with greater grade 3/4 mucositis, nausea and vomiting and greater grade 2 alopecia in the FOLFIRI arm and greater grade 3/4 neutropaenia and neurosensory toxicity in the FOLFOX arm. This is clinically useful since in discussions between the physician and patient it would be possible to offer alternative choices with similar activity but different toxicity profiles. Comparing median survivals in the more recent randomised trials it appears that the use of all three drugs in 60% or more of patients increased over all survival to around 20 months (see Table 11.3) (Grothey *et al.* 2004). The recent FOCUS trial, which has 5 arms, compares patients with metastatic disease who had previous MAYO adjuvant chemotherapy (Figure 11.1). The preliminary results have shown a similar PFS for those receiving combination therapy (arms C and E) as those receiving sequential therapy (arms A, B and D).

Table 11.3 Median survival correlates with all 3 active drugs.

Study	1st line regimen	Number of pts	% of pts 3 drugs	median OS
Saltz 2000	IFL	231	5	14.8
Douillard 2000	FOLFIRI	198	15.7	17.4
Koehne 2003	FUFIRI	214	54	20.1
de Gramont 2000	FOLFOX	210	29.5	16.2
Grothey 2002	FUFOX	123	67.5	19.7
Tournigand 2001	FOLFOX	111	62	20.5
	FOLFIRI	109	74	21.5
	IROX	264	50	17.4
Goldberg 2002	IFL	264	24	14.8
	FOLFOX	267	60	19.5

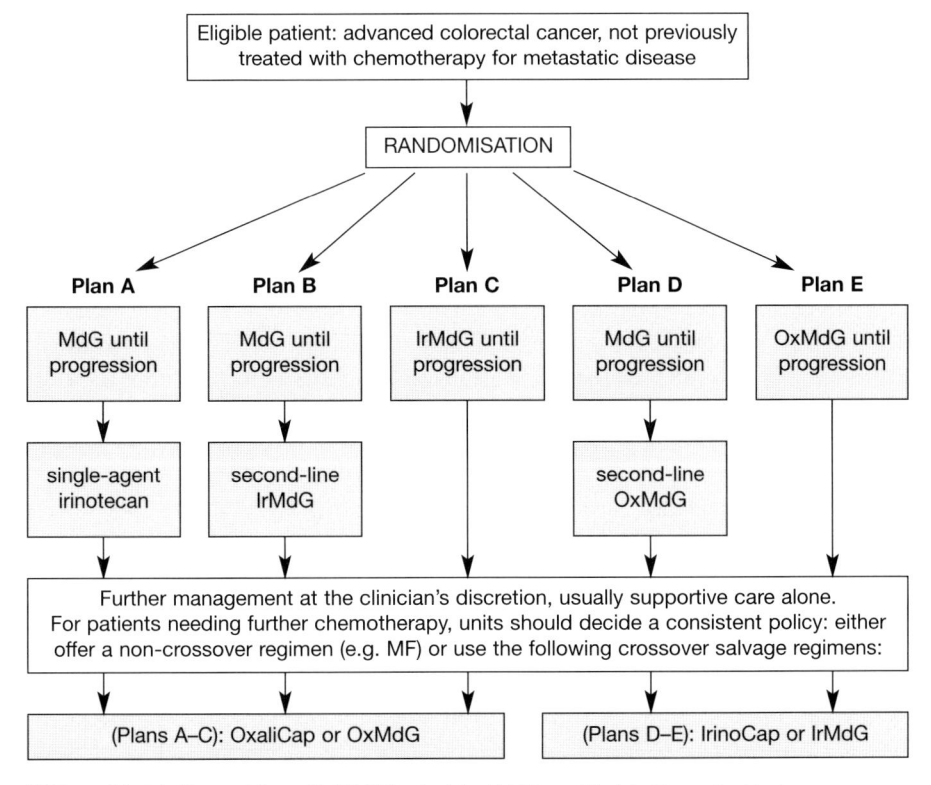

Evidence and opinion for combination therapy **141**

```
┌─────────────────────────────────────────────────────────┐
│ Eligible patient: advanced colorectal cancer, not       │
│ previously treated with chemotherapy for metastatic disease │
└─────────────────────────────────────────────────────────┘
                            │
                            ▼
                   ┌──────────────────┐
                   │  RANDOMISATION   │
                   └──────────────────┘
```

Plan A	Plan B	Plan C	Plan D	Plan E
MdG until progression	MdG until progression	IrMdG until progression	MdG until progression	OxMdG until progression
↓	↓		↓	
single-agent irinotecan	second-line IrMdG		second-line OxMdG	

Further management at the clinician's discretion, usually supportive care alone. For patients needing further chemotherapy, units should decide a consistent policy: either offer a non-crossover regimen (e.g. MF) or use the following crossover salvage regimens:

(Plans A–C): OxaliCap or OxMdG   (Plans D–E): IrinoCap or IrMdG

MdG: modified de Gramont 2-weekly 5FU/FA schedule. IrMdG: modified de Gramont + irinotecan. IrinoCap: 2-weekly irinotecan/capecitabine. OxMdG: modified de Gramont + oxaliplatin. OxaliCap: 2-weekly oxaliplatin/capecitabine. MF: PVI 5FU + mitomycin.

Figure 11.1 Trial design for the FOCUS study. 2100 patients will be randomised. Selection criteria include: evaluable advanced colorectal cancer: PS 0-2 and fit for any of the treatments; not previously treated with chemotherapy for metastatic disease; at least 6 months from last cycle of adjuvant chemotherapy; no previous oxaliplatin or irinotecan. Randomisation will be as shown in the flow diagram, with 1/3rd of patients in the control arm A and 1/6th in each of the experimental arms B–E. Principal endpoint is overall survival, with secondary endpoints PFS, response rate, quality of life and economic evaluation.

Combination with capecitabine

Capecitabine has also been integrated into combinations, the XELOX Phase II trial of 96 ACRC patients treated with 1000mg/m^2 bd Days 1–14 oral capecitabine and 130mg/m^2 day 1 oxaliplatin in a 3 weekly cycle, has recently been published (Cassidy *et al.* 2004). This showed response rates of 55%, PFS of 7.6 months and OS of 19.5 months, which is similar to the FOLFOX 4 regimen used in the MOSAIC trial. The toxicity profile was similar to FOLFOX 4 with slightly more diarrhoea and hand foot syndrome. There is now a Phase III trial comparing FOLFOX 4 to XELOX. There has also been a Phase II trial comparing capecitabine (1000mg/m² bd days 1–14) and oxaliplatin (70mg/m² day 1) to capecitabine and irinotecan 3-weekly with the dose of irinotecan given initially at 100mg/m² day 1 but then reduced to 80mg/m² at the interim analysis (Jordan *et al.* 2002). There was a high 60-day mortality with 6.37% (5/79) patients in the capecitabine/irinotecan group dying while one of the capecitabine/oxaliplatin patients died within 60 days. The grade 3/4 toxicities were similar in both treatments except for the hand and foot syndrome and neurotoxicity seen mainly in patients receiving the oxaliplatin containing regimen. There was no significant difference in the RR, PFS and OS. The results of capecitabine combined with either irinotecan or oxaliplatin show similar RR, PFS and OS to the combinations with 5FU instead of capecitabine (see Table 11.4). However, these are retrospective and based on historical data so we will have to await the Phase III trials being conducted at the moment comparing FOLFOX with XELOX to see if this is born out.

Table 11.4 Capecitabine and oxaliplatin efficacy as first line therapy.

Study	XELOX (n = 96)	CAPOX (n = 80)	FOLFOX4 (n = 267)	FOLFOX4 N = 210
PR + CR	55	51	45	50
PFS months	7.7	7.2	8.7	8.2
OS months	19.5	>17	19.5	16.2

Targeted Therapies
Bevacizumab (Avastin)

A number of studies have examined the prognostic biomarkers that influence outcome in colon cancer. VEGFR was found to be an independent prognostic indicator of OS or time to recurrence in 4 of 5 studies (Amaya *et al.* 1997; Ishigami *et al.* 1998; Maeda *et al.* 2000; Takahashi *et al.* 1997; Zheng *et al.* 2003). VEGF has been implicated in tumour angiogenesis and blocking VEGFR in preclinical studies has prevented new vessel formation limiting the size of tumours and acting as a cytostatic agent (Connolly *et al.* 1989). A monoclonal antibody targeted to VEGFR known as bevacizumab has now been tested in a Phase III randomised trial in conjunction with bolus IFL. Patients were randomised to bolus IFL (bolus 5FU 500mg/m², leucovorin 20mg/m², irinotecan 125mg/m² given 4/6 weeks) with or without bevacizumab or bolus 5FU (500mg/m² and 500mg/m² leucovorin) with bevacizumab (Hurwitz *et al.* 2004). The bevacizumab was given at a dose of 5mg/m² every 2 weeks. The overall response rate was 34.8 % in the IFL group and 44.85% with the addition of bevacizumab. The PFS was 6.2 versus 10.6 months and the survival in months was 15.6 in the IFL alone group and 20.3 in the IFL and bevacizumab group. Clearly this shows a significant improvement with the addition of this biological therapy. There are now a number of Phase III trials that have been undertaken examining the addition of bevacizumab to the FOLFOX and XELOX regimens. Recently, the results of TREE2 and E3200 were presented at ASCO 2005 and these data and their clinical significance will be discussed in considerable detail in the Fifth Edition of this volume (currently 'in press': publication anticipated late 2005).

Cetuximab

Another successful biological agent used in the treatment of colorectal cancer is a monoclonal antibody which targets the EGFR (epidermal growth factor receptor). This is a transmembrane protein with an intracellular tyrosine kinase domain. The ligand for EGFR is either TGFa (transmembrane growth factor) or EGF. On binding to the ligand the tyrosine kinase causes phosphorylation of tyrosine residues which leads to induction of a signalling cascade that can induce a number of genes involved in cell proliferation, metastasis and angiogenesis. Cetuximab is a chimeric IgG1 monoclonal antibody, which has greater affinity for the EGFR than its natural ligands. On binding to the receptor it induces internalisation and degradation of EGFR (Huang & Harari, 1999). Colon cancer overexpresses EGFR and treatment with cetuximab has a cytostatic effect on the tumours. Furthermore, cetuximab is synergistic with chemotherapeutic agents and this has been shown in the clinic setting. A Phase II study of 138 patients treated with a loading dose of cetuximab at 400mg/m^2 then 250mg/m^2 weekly in combination with irinotecan showed a median survival of 8.4 months with a one year survival of 32% (Cunningham *et al.* 2004). Interestingly, in patients who had developed irinotecan-resistant disease, the addition of cetuximab led to sensitivity to further irinotecan. Cunningham *et al.* randomised patients whose disease had progressed within 3 months of being treated with irinotecan-containing regimens to either cetuximab alone or the combination of cetuximab and irinotecan – the cetuximab alone group could on progression cross over to the combination. They found a response rate of 22.9% versus 10.8%, a time to progression of 4.1 versus 1.5 months with a median survival of 8.9 versus 6.9 months in favour of the combination arm. All patients had tumours that were EGFR-positive although there was no correlation between the EGFR positivity and the degree of response. However, the numbers of responders were greater in those with more severe skin reaction, a known toxicity from cetuximab treatment, which has previously correlated with response in other clinical trials. Importantly, this is the first biological therapy which has changed a specific chemotherapy resistant tumour to a more sensitive phenotype. Cetuximab has also been combined with the FOLFOX regimen in a small study of 20 people giving impressive results. 7 patients proceeded to curative liver surgery, there were 5% complete responses and 76% partial responses. An updated abstract published in ASCO involved 43 patients treated with cetuximab and FOLFOX, 14 patients (48.3%) had a partial response and 12 patients (41.3%) had stable disease with only 2 patients (5.9%) had progressed (Tabernero *et al.* 2004).

Clearly, we have moved forward from the 1980s when the outlook for patients with metastatic colon cancer was grim with most people given supportive care and with median survivals of about 6 months. The advent of newer combination chemotherapy agents have increased the OS for patients to around 20 months and it is hoped with the addition of biological agents we may push survival to greater than 2 years.

Management of liver metastases

In colorectal cancer the presence of liver metastases is the most accurate predictor of survival. Liver metastases are found in about 50% of patients at some time during follow up. The liver is the only site of tumour recurrence in 30% of patients with metastatic disease. Synchronous liver metastases are found in 15–30% of patients at the time of surgery for their primary tumour and metachronous tumours develop in 15–30% of patients usually within 3 years of diagnosis. The only chance of cure for these patients is surgical resection. However, only 10% are amenable to resection. The 5 year survival for patients with curative liver resection varies between 20–50% whereas it is only 5% for those with unresectable tumours (Adam *et al.* 2001; Adson *et al.* 1984; Fong *et al.* 1997; Jaeck *et al.* 1997; Scheele *et al.* 1995). Using the newer combination chemotherapy agents more people are down staging their metastases to enable them to undergo surgical resections. Using chronomodulated combination chemotherapy with oxaliplatin and 5FU there was a 13.6% conversion from non resectable to resectable liver metastases. The 5 year survival for these patients was 35% which is in a similar range to resectable disease at outset not requiring down staging chemotherapy (Adam *et al.* 2004). Similarly, Giachetti et al reported in a group of 151 patients a 50% conversion to resectable tumours using FOLFOX with 58 patients (38%) achieving complete resections and of these an impressive 50% five year survival (Giacchetti *et al.* 2000). These appear to be long term cures as the survival curves continue out at 9 years. The other trials wait maturing of their data but the conversion rates and complete resections remain within this range of 13.6–50%.

Experimental therapies

With the success of bevacizumab and cetuximab there are now a number of other experimental therapies being developed. Some of these are alternative approaches to blocking EGFR and associated pathways. Erlotinib (Tarceva) is an EGFR tyrosine kinase inhibitor that has been used in a Phase II study of metastatic colorectal patients in combination with capecitabine and oxaliplatin. It was well tolerated with the commonest toxicity being rash and diarrhoea. Of the 25 patients evaluable 24% had partial response and 40% had stable disease indicating activity of this regimen. (Meyerhardt *et al.* 2004). A Phase II study of 148 patients treated with the monoclonal antibody pantumumab (ABX-EGF) directed at EGFR was also presented at ASCO and showed encouraging results with 15 (10.1%) partial responses and 54 (36.5%)

stable disease after 8 weeks this was an interim analysis and the final data are awaited (Hecht *et al.* 2004). More novel approaches have also been examined such as using immunotherapy with autologous dendritic cells transfected with carcinoembryonic antigen mRNA. The use of dendritic cells has given limited results. Last year, however, Morse *et al.* published a Phase II trial demonstrating an immunological response with little toxicity although the responses remained small with 1 compete response by tumour marker, 2 minor responses and 3 stable diseases (Morse *et al.* 2003). More recently, the role of Cox II inhibitors in colon cancer has also been examined as both preclinical and clinical data have shown an over expression of cyclooxygenase-2 in primary and metastatic colon cancer. Furthermore, data has shown synergy with 5FU chemotherapy. This has led to studies of combination 5FU and rofecoxib in metastatic colon cancer. However the toxicity was found to be high and in a study of 10 patients 4 developed upper GI bleeds with no responses seen so the study was terminated (Becerra *et al.* 2003). Rofecoxib has recently been withdrawn from the market due to cardiovascular toxicity and therefore although the use of non NSAIDs in colon cancer remains interesting it may not be beneficial at this stage and may be used more in a preventative role (ASCO 2004).

Current state of the art

The development of the affymetrix gene chip and the use of proteomics have resulted in a profile of different tumours being gradually built up in all cancer fields. In a crude sense the presence of EGFR staining of tumours is a forerunner of this. In the same way that we can now target cancer that are positive for EGFR with cetuximab we may be able to do this on a more refined scale. Using the present technology of gene chips and proteomics thousands of genes involved in the tumour process are being identified. As we develop targets for them we may be able to treat selected tumours with a combination of biological therapies, which are known to be involved in that particular patient's tumour development. Furthermore, these genes may possibly be able to tell us whether tumours are likely to develop resistance to chemotherapeutic agents. This is, of course, simply speculation at the time of writing and we will continue to use a combination of chemotherapies and biological agents for sometime. This field remains a rapidly expanding area with the combinations of chemotherapy agents such as irinotecan and oxaliplatin with 5FU or oral fluoropyrimidines being used to treat colon cancer and the incorporation of biological therapies. Furthermore, with the adjuvant trials showing a disease free advantage with some combination therapies such as FOLFOX 4, they maybe used up front to prevent relapse which may then alter the choice of treatments to be used in the metastatic setting. There are a number of trials awaited to answer this question which means that the treatments will continue to alter rapidly and as newer therapies emerge from the laboratory they too may come to have a significant impact.

References

Meta-analysis Group in Cancer. (1998a). Efficacy of intravenous continuous infusion of fluorouracil compared with bolus administration in advanced colorectal cancer. *Journal of Clinical Oncology* **16**, 301–308.

Meta-Analysis Group In Cancer (1998b). Toxicity of fluorouracil in patients with advanced colorectal cancer: effect of administration schedule and prognostic factors. *Journal of Clinical Oncology* **16**, 3537–3541.

Adam, R., Avisar, E., Ariche, A., Giachetti, S., Azoulay, D., Castaing, D., Kunstlinger, F., Levi, F. & Bismuth, F. (2001). Five-year survival following hepatic resection after neoadjuvant therapy for nonresectable colorectal cancer. *Annals of Surgical Oncology* **8**, 347–353.

Adam, R., Delvart, V., Pascal, G., Valeanu, A., Castaing, D., Azoulay, D., Giacchetti, S., Paule, B., Kunstlinger, F., Ghemard, O., Levi, F. & Bismuth, H. (2004). Rescue surgery for unresectable colorectal liver metastases downstaged by chemotherapy: a model to predict long-term survival. *Annals of Surgery* **240**, 644–657; discussion 657–658.

Adson, M. A., van Heerden, J. A., Adson, M. H., Wagner, J. S. & Ilstrup, D. M. (1984). Resection of hepatic metastases from colorectal cancer. *Archives of Surgery* **119**, 647–651.

Amaya, H., Tanigawa, N., Lu, C., Matsumura, M., Shimomatsuya, T., Horiuchi, T. & Muraoka, R. (1997). Association of vascular endothelial growth factor expression with tumor angiogenesis, survival and thymidine phosphorylase/platelet-derived endothelial cell growth factor expression in human colorectal cancer. *Cancer Letters* **119**, 227–235.

Becerra, C. R., Frenkel, E. P., Ashfaq, R. & Gaynor, R. B. (2003). Increased toxicity and lack of efficacy of rofecoxib in combination with chemotherapy for treatment of metastatic colorectal cancer: A phase II study. *International Journal of Cancer* **105**, 868–872.

Beretta, G., Bollina, R., Cozzi, C., Beretta, G., Moriabito, A. (1997). Should we consider the weekly 5-fluorouracil plus folinic acid a standard treatment for advanced/metastatic carcinoma of the digestive tract in elderly patients? *Proceedings of the American Society of Clinical Oncology* **16**: A920.

Cassidy, J., Tabernero, J., Twelves, C., Brunet, R., Butts, C., Conroy, T., Debraud, F., Figer, A., Grossmann, J., Sawada, N., Schoffski, P., Sobrero, A., Van Cutsem, E. & Diaz-Rubio, E. (2004). XELOX (capecitabine plus oxaliplatin): active first-line therapy for patients with metastatic colorectal cancer. *Journal of Clinical Oncology* **22**, 2084–2091.

Connolly, D. T., Heuvelman, D. M., Nelson, R., Olander, J. V., Eppley, B. L., Delfino, J. J., Siegel, N. R., Leimgruber, R. M. & Feder, J. (1989). Tumor vascular permeability factor stimulates endothelial cell growth and angiogenesis. *Journal of Clinical Investigation* **84**, 1470–1478.

Cunningham, D., Pyrhonen, S., James, R. D., Punt, C. J., Hickish, T. F., Heikkila, R., Johannesen, T. B., Starkhammar, H., Topham, C. A., Awad, L., Jacques, C. & Herait, P. (1998). Randomised trial of irinotecan plus supportive care versus supportive care alone after fluorouracil failure for patients with metastatic colorectal cancer. *The Lancet* **352**, 1413–1418.

Cunningham, D., Humblet, Y., Siena, S., Khayat, D., Bleiberg, H., Santoro, A., Bets, D., Mueser, M., Harstrick, A., Verslype, C., Chau, I., Van Cutsem, E. (2004). Cetuximab monotherapy and cetuximab plus irinotecan in irinotecan-refractory metastatic colorectal cancer. *New England Journal of Medicine* **351**, 337–345.

de Gramont, A., Bosset, J. F., Milan, C., Rougier, P., Bouche, O., Etienne, P. L., Morvan, F., Louvet, C., Guillot, T., Francois, E. & Bedenne, L. (1997). Randomized trial comparing monthly low-dose leucovorin and fluorouracil bolus with bimonthly high-dose leucovorin and fluorouracil bolus plus continuous infusion for advanced colorectal cancer: a French intergroup study. *Journal of Clinical Oncology* **15**, 808–815.

de Gramont, A., Figer, A., Seymour, M., Homerin, M., Hmissi, A., Cassidy, J., Boni, C., Cortes-Funes, H., Cervantes, A., Freyer, G., Papamichael, D., Le Bail, N., Louvet, C., Hendler, D., de Braud, F., Wilson, C., Morvan, F. & Bonetti, A. (2000). Leucovorin and fluorouracil with or without oxaliplatin as first-line treatment in advanced colorectal cancer. *Journal of Clinical Oncology* **18**, 2938–2947.

de Gramont, A., Cervantes, A., Andre, T., Figer, A., Lledo, G., Flesch, M., Mineur, L., Russ, G., Quinaux, E., Etienne, P.-L (2004). OPTIMOX study: FOLFOX 7/LV5FU2 compared to FOLFOX 4 in patients with advanced colorectal cancer. ?????**22**, 3525.

Douillard, J. Y., Cunningham, D., Roth, A. D., Navarro, M., James, R. D., Karasek, P., Jandik, P., Iveson, T., Carmichael, J., Alakl, M., Gruia, G., Awad, L. & Rougier, P. (2000). Irinotecan combined with fluorouracil compared with fluorouracil alone as first-line treatment for metastatic colorectal cancer: a multicentre randomised trial. *The Lancet* **355**, 1041–1047.

Fong, Y., Cohen, A. M., Fortner, J. G., Enker, W. E., Turnbull, A. D., Coit, D. G., Marrero, A. M., Prasad, M., Blumgart, L. H. & Brennan, M. F. (1997). Liver resection for colorectal metastases. *Journal of Clinical Oncology* **15**, 938–946.

Giacchetti, S., Perpoint, B., Zidani, R., Le Bail, N., Faggiuolo, R., Focan, C., Chollet, P., Llory, J.F., Letourneau, Y., Coudert, B., Bertheaut-Cvitkovic, F., Larregain-Fournier, D., Le Rol, A., Walter, S., Adam, R., Misset, J.L. & Levi, F. (2000). Phase III multicenter randomized trial of oxaliplatin added to chronomodulated fluorouracil-leucovorin as first-line treatment of metastatic colorectal cancer. *Journal of Clinical Oncology* **18**, 136–147.

Giacchetti, S., Bjarnason, G., Garufi, C., Tubiana-Mathieu, N., Iacobelli, S., Dogliotti, L., Smaaland, R., Focan, C., Coudert, B., Lévi, F. (2004). First line infusion of 5-fluorouracil, leucovorin and oxaliplatin for metastatic colorectal cancer : 4-day chronomodulated (FFL4-10) versus 2-day FOLFOX2. A multicenter randomized Phase III trial of the Chronotherapy Group of the European Organization for Research and Treatment of Cancer (EORTC 05963). *Proceedings of the American Society of Clinical Oncology* **22**, 3526.

Glimelius, B., Hoffman, K., Graf, W., Haglund, U., Nyren, O., Pahlman, L. & Sjoden, P. O. (1995). Cost-effectiveness of palliative chemotherapy in advanced gastrointestinal cancer. *Annals of Oncology* **6**, 267–274.

Goldberg, R. M., Sargent, D. J., Morton, R. F., Fuchs, C. S., Ramanathan, R. K., Williamson, S. K., Findlay, B. P., Pitot, H. C. & Alberts, S. R. (2004). A randomized controlled trial of fluorouracil plus leucovorin, irinotecan, and oxaliplatin combinations in patients with previously untreated metastatic colorectal cancer. *Journal of Clinical Oncology* **22**, 23–30. Epub 2003 Dec 09.

Grothey, A., Deschler, B., Kroening, H., Ridwelski, K., Reichardt, P., Kretzschmar, A., Clemens, M., Hirschmann, W., Lorenz, M., Asperger, W., Buechele, T., Schmoll, H.-J. (2002). Phase III study of bolus 5-fluorouracil (5-FU)/folinic acid (FA) (Mayo) vs weekly high-dose 24h 5-FU infusion/FA + oxaliplatin (OXA) (FUFOX) in advanced colorectal cancer (ACRC). *Proceedings of the American Society of Clinical Oncology* **22**, 512.

Grothey, A., Sargent, D., Goldberg, R. M. & Schmoll, H. J. (2004). Survival of patients with advanced colorectal cancer improves with the availability of fluorouracil-leucovorin, irinotecan, and oxaliplatin in the course of treatment. *Journal of Clinical Oncology* **22**, 1209–1214.

Hoff, P. M., Ansari, R., Batist, G., Cox, J., Kocha, W., Kuperminc, M., Maroun, J., Walde, D., Weaver, C., Harrison, E., Burger, H. U., Osterwalder, B., Wong, A. O. & Wong, R. (2001). Comparison of oral capecitabine versus intravenous fluorouracil plus leucovorin as first-line treatment in 605 patients with metastatic colorectal cancer: results of a randomized phase III study. *Journal of Clinical Oncology* **19**, 2282–2292.

Hecht, J. R., Patnaik, A., Malik, I., Venook, A., Berlin, J., Croghan, G., Wiens, B. L, Visonneau, S., Jerian, S., Meropol, N. J. (2004). ABX-EGF monotherapy in patients (pts) with metastatic colorectal cancer (mCRC): An updated analysis. *Proceedings of the American Society of Clinical Oncology* **22**, 3511.

Huang, S. M. & Harari, P. M. (1999). Epidermal growth factor receptor inhibition in cancer therapy: biology, rationale and preliminary clinical results. *Invest New Drugs* **17**, 259–269.

Hurwitz, H., Fehrenbacher, L., Novotny, W., Cartwright, T., Hainsworth, J., Heim, W., Berlin, J., Baron, A., Griffing, S., Holmgren, E., Ferrara, N., Fyfe, G., Rogers, B., Ross, R. & Kabbinavar, F. (2004). Bevacizumab plus irinotecan, fluorouracil, and leucovorin for metastatic colorectal cancer. *New England Journal of Medicine* **350**, 2335–2342.

Ishigami, S. I., Arii, S., Furutani, M., Niwano, M., Harada, T., Mizumoto, M., Mori, A., Onodera, H. & Imamura, M. (1998). Predictive value of vascular endothelial growth factor (VEGF) in metastasis and prognosis of human colorectal cancer. *British Journal of Cancer* **78**, 1379–1384.

Jaeck, D., Bachellier, P., Guiguet, M., Boudjema, K., Vaillant, J. C., Balladur, P. & Nordlinger, B. (1997). Long-term survival following resection of colorectal hepatic metastases. Association Francaise de Chirurgie. *British Journal of Surgery* **84**, 977–980.

Jordan, K., Kellner, O., Mueller, P. L, Thomas, K., Schmoll, H.-J., Grothey, A. (2002). Capecitabine plus irinotecan or oxaliplatin in patients with advanced gastrointestinal tumours – Results of a pilot study. *Annals of Oncology* **19**(5), 79.

Kawato, Y., Aonuma, M., Hirota, Y., Kuga, H. & Sato, K. (1991). Intracellular roles of SN-38, a metabolite of the camptothecin derivative CPT-11, in the antitumor effect of CPT-11. *Cancer Research* **51**, 4187–4191.

Köhne, C.-H., Van Cutsem, E., Wils, J., Bokemeyer, C., El-Serafi, M., Lutz, M., Lorenz, M., Anak, O., Genicot, B., Nordinger, B. (2003). Irinotecan improves the activity of the AIO regimen in metastatic colorectal cancer: Results of EORTC GI group study 40986. *Proceedings of the 12th European Cancer Conference European. Journal of Cancer Suppl* **1**(5), 1088.

Maeda, K., Nishiguchi, Y., Yashiro, M., Yamada, S., Onoda, N., Sawada, T., Kang, S. M. & Hirakawa, K. (2000). Expression of vascular endothelial growth factor and thrombospondin-1 in colorectal carcinoma. *International Journal of Molecular Medicine* **5**, 373–378.

Maughan, T. S., James, R. D., Kerr, D. J., Ledermann, J. A., Seymour, M. T., Topham, C., McArdle, C., Cain, D. & Stephens, R. J. (2003). Comparison of intermittent and continuous palliative chemotherapy for advanced colorectal cancer: a multicentre randomised trial. *The Lancet* **361**, 457–464.

Meyerhardt, J. A, Xhu, A., Enzinger, P. C., Ryan, D. P., Clarke, J. W., Kulke, M. J., Michelini, A., Vincitore, M., Thomas, A., Fuchs, C. S. (2004). Phase II study of capecitabine, oxaliplatin and erlotinib in previously treated patients with metastatic colorectal cancer (MCRC). *Proceedings of the American Society of Clinical Oncology* **22**, 3580.

Morse, M. A., Nair, S. K., Mosca, P. J., Hobeika, A. C., Clay, T. M., Deng, Y, Boczkowski, D., Proia, A., Neidzwiecki, D., Clavien, P.-A., Hurwitz, H. I., Schlom, J., Gilboa, E., Lyerly, H. K. (2003). Immunotherapy with autologous, human dendritic cells transfected with carcinoembryonic antigen mRNA. *Cancer Invest* **21**, 341–349.

Nordic Gastrointestinal Tumour Adjuvant Therapy Group (1992). Expectancy or primary chemotherapy in patients with advanced asymptomatic colorectal cancer: a randomized trial. *Journal of Clinical Oncology* **10**, 904–911.

Pluzanska, A., Mainwaring, P., Cassidy, J. *et al.* (2005). Final results of a randomised phase III study evaluating the addition of oxaliplatin in first line to 5-FU followed by irinotecan at progression in advanced colorectal cancer. (LIFE study). *Proceedings of the American Society of Clinical Oncology* **23**, Abstract 3517.

Rothenberg, M.L., Meropol, N.J., Poplin, E.A., Van Cutsem, E. & Wadler, S. (2001). Mortality associated with irinotecan plus bolus fluorouracil/leucovorin: summary findings of an independent panel. *Journal of Clinical Oncology* **19**, 3801–7.

Rougier, P., Van Cutsem, E., Bajetta, E., Niederle, N., Possinger, K., Labianca, R., Navarro, M., Morant, R., Bleiberg, H., Wils, J., Awad, L., Herait, P. & Jacques, C. (1998). Randomised trial of irinotecan versus fluorouracil by continuous infusion after fluorouracil failure in patients with metastatic colorectal cancer. *The Lancet* **352**, 1407–1412.

Saltz, L. B., Cox, J. V., Blanke, C., Rosen, L. S., Fehrenbacher, L., Moore, M. J., Maroun, J. A., Ackland, S. P., Locker, P. K., Pirotta, N., Elfring, G. L. & Miller, L. L. (2000). Irinotecan plus fluorouracil and leucovorin for metastatic colorectal cancer. Irinotecan Study Group. *New England Journal of Medicine* **343**, 905–914.

Scheele, J., Stang, R., Altendorf-Hofmann, A. & Paul, M. (1995). Resection of colorectal liver metastases. *World Journal of Surgery* **19**, 59–71.

Scheithauer, W., Rosen, H., Kornek, G.V., Sebesta, C. & Depisch, D. (1993). Randomised comparison of combination chemotherapy plus supportive care with supportive care alone in patients with metastatic colorectal cancer. *British Medical Journal* **306**, 752–755.

Slatter, J. G., Schaaf, L. J., Sams, J. P., Feenstra, K. L., Johnson, M. G., Bombardt, P. A., Cathcart, K. S., Verburg, M. T., Pearson, L. K., Compton, L. D., Miller, L. L., Baker, D. S., Pesheck, C. V. & Lord, R. S., 3rd. (2000). Pharmacokinetics, metabolism, and excretion of irinotecan (CPT-11) following I.V. infusion of [(14)C]CPT-11 in cancer patients. *Drug Metab Dispos* **28**, 423–433.

Tabernero, J. M., Van Cutsem, E., Sastre, J., Cervantes, A., Van Laethem, J.-L., Humblet, Y., Soulié, P., Corretgé, S., Mueser, M., de Gramont, A. (2004). An international phase II study of cetuximab in combination with oxaliplatin/5-fluorouracil (5-FU)/folinic acid (FA) (FOLFOX-4) in the first-line treatment of patients with metastatic colorectal cancer (CRC) expressing Epidermal Growth Factor Receptor (EGFR). Preliminary results. *Proceedings of the American Society of Clinical Oncology* **22**, 3512.

Takahashi, Y., Tucker, S. L., Kitadai, Y., Koura, A. N., Bucana, C. D., Cleary, K. R. & Ellis, L. M. (1997). Vessel counts and expression of vascular endothelial growth factor as prognostic factors in node-negative colon cancer. *Archives of Surgery* **132**, 541–546.

Tournigand, C., Andre, T., Achille, E., Lledo, G., Flesh, M., Mery-Mignard, D., Quinaux, E., Couteau, C., Buyse, M., Ganem, G., Landi, B., Colin, P., Louvet, C. & de Gramont, A. (2004). FOLFIRI followed by FOLFOX6 or the reverse sequence in advanced colorectal cancer: a randomized GERCOR study. *Journal of Clinical Oncology* **22**, 229–237. Epub 2003 Dec 02.

Van Cutsem, E., Twelves, C., Cassidy, J., Allman, D., Bajetta, E., Boyer, M., Bugat, R., Findlay, M., Frings, S., Jahn, M., McKendrick, J., Osterwalder, B., Perez-Manga, G., Rosso, R., Rougier, P., Schmiegel, W. H., Seitz, J. F., Thompson, P., Vieitez, J. M., Weitzel, C. & Harper, P. (2001). Oral capecitabine compared with intravenous fluorouracil plus leucovorin in patients with metastatic colorectal cancer: results of a large phase III study. *Journal of Clinical Oncology* **19**, 4097–4106.

Zheng, S., Han, M. Y., Xiao, Z. X., Peng, J. P. & Dong, Q. (2003). Clinical significance of vascular endothelial growth factor expression and neovascularization in colorectal carcinoma. *World Journal of Gastroenterology* **9**, 1227–1230.

Chapter 12

Evidence and opinion for the use of combined modality treatment in rectal cancer

Rob Glynne-Jones and Suzy Mawdsley

Introduction

The optimal management of stage II and III rectal cancer remains a challenge for oncologists. Although surgery is the mainstay of treatment, historically a high risk of local recurrence and poor survival has been reported. Because only 40–55% of patients survive five years after a curative resection, a combined modality approach is increasingly being explored. There is, therefore. an increasing enthusiasm for the use of chemoradiation in rectal cancer, and more than 50 papers have been published on this theme in the past year.

The current evidence base suggests that the standard of care for stage II and III rectal cancer is surgery followed by post-operative adjuvant chemoradiation to doses of 45–54 Gy. The most convincing results have been achieved with infusional 5-fluorouracil (5-FU) in a study where post-operative chemoradiation has been shown to reduce distant metastases (O'Connell 1996).

The Swedish Rectal Cancer Trial results (The Swedish Rectal Cancer Trial Group 1997) represented the 'blanket' approach, which offered a quick, effective, practical and cheap schedule that dramatically reduced the risk of local recurrence from 27% to 11% and even improved overall five-year survival from 48% to 58%. For this reason, this strategy with a five-fraction schedule has been widely adopted in parts of Europe. In the UK, COG guidelines recommend the use of pre-operative radiotherapy if a surgeon has rates of local recurrence in excess of 10%.

The efficacy of pre-operative radiotherapy has been explored in two recent meta-analyses (Camma *et al.* 2000; Colorectal Cancer Collaborative Group 2001). Although both appear to show a significant reduction in local recurrence, the latter study using individualised data failed to confirm a significant survival advantage from pre-operative radiotherapy.

In addition to chemotherapy and radiotherapy, there have been significant recent improvements in surgical technique. A major reduction in the risk of local recurrence has been observed when the surgeon performs an R0 resection (defined as a circumferential margin of greater than 1 mm) and patients now have a higher expectation of undergoing sphincter-sparing surgery.

Recent randomised studies in rectal cancer have confirmed that total mesorectal excision (TME) can significantly contribute to reducing the risk of local recurrence.

In the Dutch TME study, local recurrence following pre-operative radiotherapy and surgery was 2.4% at two years compared with 8.4% after surgery alone (Kapiteijn 2001). The current CRUK study CR07 is addressing the question as to whether a blanket approach of short-course radiotherapy is better than post-operative chemoradiation selected on the basis of high-risk pathological factors.

The challenge remains that although surgeons appear to achieve near optimal local control for early resectable cancers, very low local recurrence rates do not appear to impact on overall survival. In addition a further 20–25% of patients present with locally advanced cancers that can be predicted to have a higher than average risk of a positive circumferential margin and hence local recurrence and metastatic disease.

The incidence of distant metastases does not appear to be reduced by improved local surgical control (Kockerling *et al.* 1998). In the Erlangen series, the risk of metastatic disease remained at 25% between 1974 and 1991 despite major improvements in surgical technique during the period. Also, the Dutch TME study confirms that metastases were present at two years in 16% of patients. Data from the Norwegian rectal cancer project show that with a median follow-up of 29 months, 40% of patients who had a positive circumferential margin (CRM) developed metastatic disease compared with 12% where the margin was more than 1 mm (Wibe *et al.* 2002).

Therefore, TME alone appears insufficient for more locally advanced rectal cancers in the lower third of the rectum requiring APER, and those with positive lymph nodes (T4 N0–N2, T3N1). Further improvements in survival are likely only to be gained with the more strategic use of more effective chemotherapy.

Pre-operative chemoradiation allows systemic chemotherapy to be integrated early on in the disease. It has a theoretical advantages of potentially reducing tumour seeding at operation and the promise of greater radio-sensitivity than radiotherapy delivered in the post-operative setting where many of the potentially active cells will be in scar tissue and hence relatively hypoxic. In addition, pre-operative chemoradiation offers a potential method of defining high- and low-risk groups. It is increasingly recognised that patients who still have positive involved lymph nodes after chemoradiation have a very poor prognosis, with an overall five-year survival in the region of 25%. In contrast, some of the few studies which have presented five-year survival have documented that downstaging after chemoradiation (yPT0, PT1, PT2, N0) confers a very high chance of five-year survival in the region of 90% (Ruo *et al.* 2002; Valentini *et al.* 2002). The aims of the pre-operative approach are therefore to facilitate the surgeon achieving a curative (R0) resection, to enhance the opportunity for performing sphincter-sparing surgery, and to reduce the incidence of metastases – and hence impact on both survival and quality of life.

The weakness in the evidence base lies in the fact that reported clinical trials are mainly in the phase II setting. There are no published meta-analyses examining chemoradiation in rectal cancer. The benefits observed are usually small, not always conclusively reproducible and often balanced by an increased risk of non-cancer-related death in the chemoradiation arm.

Major questions remain as to the ideal schedule, and whether the concomitant or sequential use of chemotherapy drugs is best. Would any beneficial effects still persist if the radiotherapy component were to be optimised (e.g. with IMRT)? Can the beneficial effects be generalisable to more adventurous strategies of delivering radiotherapy—i.e. accelerated/hyperfractionated radiotherapy? In addition, a major disadvantage to the chemoradiation approach is that so little is known of the late effects.

So what we have learnt about chemoradiation from recent studies?

Data from recent studies of radiotherapy/chemoradiation
Post-operative chemoradiation

Although the standard of care remains post-operative adjuvant chemoradiation, we have not yet defined the optimal combination of chemotherapy and radiotherapy; the optimal drugs and the optimal sequencing of chemotherapy and radiotherapy. Evidence from the final results of the Intergroup 0144 study using a bolus 5-FU regimen, suggests there is no advantage with either the addition of levamisole or modulation with folinic acid in this context (Tepper *et al.* 2002).

A study from Korea (Lee *et al.* 2002) enrolled patients with stage II and stage III rectal cancer following TME surgery. This study aimed to investigate whether early postoperative radiotherapy with chemotherapy was the optimal sequence, ie early radiotherapy versus late radiotherapy in combination with chemotherapy.

Radiotherapy started on day 1 on the *first* cycle of chemotherapy in the early RT group and day 1 of the *third* cycle of chemotherapy in the late RT arm. With a median follow up of 37 months, 61 (22%) of the 274 eligible patients had experienced a recurrence of their rectal cancer, 23 in the early radiotherapy group and 38 in the late radiotherapy group. The four-year rate of disease-free survival was 81% for early radiotherapy and 71% for late radiotherapy. Both distant metastases and local regional recurrence appeared to show a trend towards being less frequent for early radiotherapy (15% versus 22%) and (2% versus 6%) respectively. However, the four-year overall survival was similar in both groups (84% versus 82%).

This study seems to confirm the hypothesis that early radiotherapy may be an advantage and mirrors data from studies of early radiotherapy in small cell lung cancer and nasopharyngeal cancer. This is a thought-provoking study, not least because starting post-operative chemoradiation within four–six weeks of surgical resection would not be feasible in the UK because of inappropriately long waiting times for radiotherapy.

Pre-operative chemoradiation

There is no published evidence from phase III studies that neoadjuvant chemoradiation in the preoperative setting improves survival over surgery alone or surgery followed by post-operative chemoradiation. However, with the increasing emphasis on pre-operative imaging, meticulous surgical technique and accurate pathological reporting of the circumferential or radial margin, and the favourable results of the Swedish rectal cancer trial – pre-operative radiotherapy and pre-operative chemoradiation are being used widely throughout Europe. At a recent international meeting in Barcelona, 75% of the audience were routinely using 5-FU-based chemoradiation pre-operatively in locally advanced rectal cancers.

Neoadjuvant chemotherapy using continuous infusion 5-FU in combination with mitomycin C prior to chemoradiation has also been explored (Chau *et al*. 2002) and appears safe without compromising compliance.

Molecular predictive indicators in patients with locally advanced rectal cancer

The main prognostic factors in rectal cancer following surgery remain the extent of the primary tumour (T stage), regional lymph node status (N stage), the histological grade, the presence of vascular invasion and whether there is a sufficient circumferential resection margin. These factors are not easy to predict pre-operatively. Thus, there have been considerable efforts to define accurate pre-operative histological, pathological and molecular information, which has a bearing on proliferation, apoptosis and other molecular targets and can hence predict future outcome.

In addition, with the exciting drive to develop drugs with new mechanisms of action based on signal transduction inhibitors, cyclo-oxygense inhibitors and angiogenesis, new possibilities for treatment are opening up. Interesting interactions have been reported at a cellular level between these drugs and radiation, and many are currently in phase I/phaseII development.

There has been enormous thrust to develop laboratory techniques to study these potentially useful prognostic markers both at the gene and protein level. Many of these marker proteins can be assayed using standard immunohistochemical techniques, from formalin-fixed, paraffin-embedded tissue or by Western blot or flow cytometric analysis. Other laboratory techniques have been developed to identify specific genetic alterations using the reverse-transcriptase polymerase chain reaction and DNA sequencing.

The p53 tumour suppressor gene plays a critical role in cell cycle progression, DNA repair and apoptosis. Mutation of this gene is found in many tumours and loss of its function has been reported to increase radioresistance. Numerous studies have been reported in colorectal cancer with conflicting results. In rectal cancer non-functional p53 can be found in up to 84% of cases (Marijnen. Kapiteijn & van de

Velde 2002) but its prognostic significance is controversial. A study by Schwandner et al. (2000) suggests p53 had an independent effect on recurrence and disease-free survival and Diez et al. (2000) found that in colorectal cancer the presence of p53 overexpression was an indicator of a high risk of recurrence only after the first year of follow-up. More recently a study with mature follow-up from Lyon (Rebischung et al. 2002) showed that the prevalence of mutated p53 was significantly higher in patients who failed to respond to pre-operative radiotherapy. In a multivariate analysis, p53 mutation status remained a prognostic factor, which was associated with a shorter overall survival, independent of stage.

Ki67 is a marker of proliferation and is expressed in all phases of the cell cycle except G0. High levels of ki67 expression have been associated with a decreased survival in several tumour types. In rectal cancer, however, fast-proliferating tumours have been shown to demonstrate a high immediate response to high-dose radiation therapy and an improved response to chemoradiation (Kim et al. 2001). Interestingly, in a study by Adell (2001) using short-course preoperative radiotherapy, a high ki67 predicted for an increased risk of treatment failure suggesting that those patients whose tumours demonstrate a higher proliferation rate should be offered the longer-course chemoradiation schedules. A similar marker to ki67 is the apoptotic index. In rectal cancer, a reduced local recurrence is observed following both surgery alone and pre-operative chemoradiation, in tumours demonstrating a higher apoptotic index (Adell et al. 2001; Rodel et al. 2002). In cancers with a lower apoptotic index, recurrence rates were improved with the addition of pre-operative radiotherapy.

Bcl2 is an intra-cellular membrane protein capable of inhibiting programmed cell death; this potentially could promote resistance to chemotherapy and radiotherapy. Spitz et al. (1996) found a better response to pre-operative chemoradiotherapy in bcl2 negative tumours; however, other studies have failed to confirm this finding (Qui et al. 2000; Okonkwo et al. 2001; Rodel et al. 2002).

$P27^{kip1}$ inhibits cell cycle progression from G1 into S phase by binding to and inhibiting cyclin E/CDK2. Studies in rectal cancer have shown that a higher $P27^{kip1}$ expression is associated with a poorer response to pre-operative radiation and chemoradiation (Esposito et al. 2001).

There is currently considerable interest in angiogenesis and its role in the growth of solid tumours. Microvessel density within tumours has been suggested as an indirect way of looking at angiogenesis, which may act as a prognostic factor. High microvessel density has been shown to be associated with an increased risk of tumour recurrence and metastases in breast cancer, non small cell lung cancer and melanomas. Some investigators have shown a relationship between high microvessel density and lymph node and distant metastases in colorectal cancer. Galindo-Gallego (2000), in a study of rectal cancers, showed that the presence of microvessels was prognostic for overall survival but not progression-free survival.

A study from the University of Florence (*Cianchi et al.* 2002) aimed to analyse retrospectively the value of microvessel density in 170 patients with T2, T3 N0, M0 (i.e. node negative patients) with rectal cancer. The aim was to compare the standard prognostic factors such as differentiation and vascular involvement and the Jass staging, and see whether microvessel density offered any additional prognostic promotion.

The authors used the median microvessel density of all patients as a cut-off to define low and high levels. The presence of a conspicuous lymphocytic infiltration appeared significantly associated with increased microvessel density but no significant association could be determined between microvessel density and survival. It does not, therefore, appear that microvessel density offers any additional prognostic information as compared with standard histopathological details in rectal cancer with negative lymph nodes. However, microvessel counts may yield conflicting results because they involve selection of areas near or at the edge of a tumour to identify the highest areas of activity, thereby introducing selection bias.

A study from the Royal Marsden Hospital (George *et al.* 2001) aimed to assess whether indirect measures of angiogenesis could be used to predict and assess response to treatment in 57 patients with rectal cancer. The relationship between circulating VEGF levels and tumour VEGF levels was investigated. They compared DCE-MRI estimates of tumour vascular permeability with circulating VEGF levels and changes in serum VEGF and DCE-MRI tumour permeability during chemoradiotherapy in patients with T3/T4 rectal cancer. This relationship may prove useful in monitoring response and downstaging of locally advanced rectal cancers treated with pre-operative chemoradiotherapy, and in the follow-up of resected tumours – but no longitudinal studies have been reported so far.

A recent paper (Giralt *et al.* 2002) examined tumour specimens of patients with rectal cancer treated by pre-operative chemoradiation; 64% demonstrated EGFR + tumours. EGFR positivity was not associated with either the primary stage or the nodal stage of the tumour. EGFR status appeared the only factor associated with response to chemoradiation, and there was a significant association between EGFR expression recurrence of disease. This study strongly suggests that high tumour EGFR expression predicts poor response to chemoradiation and a lower disease-free survival. If the hypothesis in this study can be validated, then EGFR expression could identify patients at high risk of failure who might benefit from novel therapeutic modalities that target this receptor.

Locally advanced rectal cancer offers a unique model for defining histological and genetic changes because access to histological material is relatively easy without the requirements of an anaesthetic. Rectal cancers develop along a variety of molecular pathways. Each tumour involves multiple, sequential genetic alterations different from the next. Many markers have been studied; however, their specific prognostic and predictive value in rectal cancer has yet to be definitively validated. This is in part due to the use of polyclonal and monoclonal antibodies, different scoring systems and stage of disease, and differing treatments. The majority of studies are also small and have combined colon with rectal cancers so that the effect of these markers in rectal cancer, which is often biologically more aggressive, is unclear. What is needed is the study of tumours in large prospective randomised trials using similar staining and scoring systems so that results can be compared between institutions. At present it is too early to incorporate these predictive markers into the routine diagnostic workup to give information to the clinician and help with decisions regarding treatment.

The importance of the CRM

Traditionally, histopathologists have reported only the proximal and distal bowel margins in rectal cancer and the majority of American studies do not accurately report the circumferential or radial margin status. There is also a lack of clarity about the definitions, which makes the literature difficult to interpret. The current American Joint Committee on Cancer manual (6th edition) defines an R0 resection as 'complete resection, margins histologically negative, no residual tumour left after resection' (AJCC 2002).

The work of Phil Quirke has shown that circumferential margin of 1 mm or less is associated with a very high risk of local recurrence *and* metastatic disease The Dutch TME study also showed particularly high risks of a positive CRM and local recurrence after TME alone for cancers in the low rectum and those where an AP excision of the rectum was performed. Other groups have confirmed that involvement of the CRM predicts a higher risk of both local and metastatic disease (Ng *et al*. 1993; de Haas-Kock *et al*. 1996; Wibe *et al*. 2002). In recent data from Leeds, the risk of a positive CRM has not reduced for tumours in the low rectum despite the introduction of TME techniques (Birbeck *et al*. 2001). A distance of < 1 mm has been prospectively defined as CRM involvement in several studies (MRC CR07 and Dutch TME study). In the Dutch TME study, despite optimised surgery and impressive rates of local pelvic control, 18% of patients overall demonstrated a positive resection margin (<1 mm). The Dutch TME study suggests that <2 mm may be a more appropriate definition (Nagtegaal *et al*. 2002). The cut-off of 2 mm is also supported by data from the Norwegian rectal cancer project. Data show that with a median follow-up of 29 months, 40% percent of patients who had a positive circumferential margin (CRM) developed metastatic disease compared with 12% where the margin was more than 2 mm (Wibe *et al*. 2002).

So, rather than local recurrence, a positive CRM is probably at the present time the most appropriate surrogate endpoint for survival. And of all the risk factors for local recurrence and metastatic disease, the circumferential margin is the one that could potentially be influenced by to the greatest extent treatment.

Residual cell density

The histopathological appearances following preoperative chemoradiation for rectal cancer have been poorly documented. There remains a marked lack of any standardised approach to characterising and quantifying these changes. The tumour regression scale described by Mandard *et al*. (1994) in oesophageal cancers after chemoradiation used a five-point scale basing the grades on the amount of residual tumour cells and the extent of fibrosis achieved.

Others have tried to grade tumour necrosis as a percentage of the tumour mass. A recent paper (Bouzourene *et al*. 2002) found a strong correlation between different levels of post-chemoradiation tumour regression and necrosis and demonstrated that patients who exhibited large amounts of tumour necrosis appeared to survive longer but with a non-significant difference. In this study, although tumour downstaging did not appear to correlate with survival, the tumour regression grade 2–4, i.e. responders, compared favourably with those not exhibiting any regression, i.e. tumour regression grade 5. On multivariate analysis, tumour regression grade remained an independent prognostic indicator for long-term local tumour control.

An interesting paper from Oxford (Wheeler *et al*. 2002) retrospectively reviewed patients treated with pre-operative chemoradiation and recommended a modified staging system with only three grades of response. Grade 1 demonstrated either complete pathological response or only microscopic residual foci of adenocarcinoma; grade 2 represented marked fibrosis with the presence of macroscopic residual tumour. According to this system rectal cancer regression grades 1 and 2 were demonstrated in 13/26 (50 %).

In contrast a relatively recent study (Vecchio *et al*. 2002) used the pathological response score system with five grades after pre-operative combined modality therapy. The five-year cumulative incidence rates of metastases for TRG 1 was 7.6%, 5.6% for TRG 2, 10% for TRG 3, and 44% for TRG 4. This study strongly suggests tumour regression grade can be used to predict metastases-free survival in rectal cancer. However, it is not yet clear how reproducible residual cell density (RCD) is as an endpoint as many pathologists consider the system to be too subjective.

Clinical significance of the pathologist in quality control

Further data from the Dutch TME study (Nagtegaal *et al*. 2002) examined 180 patients about whom full information as to the quality of the mesorectum was available. In this study, 102 specimens (56.6%) were classified as complete, 35 (19%) nearly complete and 43 (24%) incomplete. The distance of the tumour from the anal verge is strongly associated with the quality of the mesorectal excision. Only 39% of tumours within 5 cm of the anal verge were classified as complete excision compared with 67% in those tumours located more 10 cm from the anal verge, i.e. upper rectum. AP excision of the rectum showed only a complete mesorectum in 34% compared with 73% in those patients who underwent low anterior resection. Otherwise, there was no association between age or sex of the patient and the scoring of the resection specimen.

Incomplete resections were associated with a higher recurrence rate at two years of follow-up (35%) compared with 21% with a nearly complete mesorectum. There was no difference in survival rates.

Even in patients who had a negative resection margin, an incomplete mesorectum seemed to confer a higher overall recurrence rate (26.6% versus 14.9%) so it is clear that defining the quality of the mesorectal excision is clinically important in addition to the specific comments about a positive circumferential margin. Overall, the survival for patients with a complete mesorectum was 90.5% versus 76.9% with an incomplete mesorectum. This study quite clearly confirms that the pathologist has a major role to play in evaluating the quality of surgery and will be a strong requirement in the future in any rectal cancer study.

Downstaging/lack of downstaging

We know that many of the same factors that predict for a higher risk of local failure in rectal cancer following chemoradiation also predict for distant metastases – that is to say, higher T stages, undifferentiated tumours and positive lymph nodes. Outcome appears better for patients who had significant downstaging /downsizing, i.e. path CR and pT1 pT2 N0 as compared with those patients who had persistent T3 cancers or persistent N1 / N2 positive lymphadenopathy within the pelvis.

Retrospective studies in anal cancer showed the response to chemoradiation in terms of the local tumour control was highly important for overall outcome. Anal cancers that failed to respond to chemoradiation and persisted were usually associated with a very high risk of metastatic disease. Why is local failure associated with an increased risk of metastatic disease? Some tumours may have an inherently more aggressive behaviour. Hypoxic tumours are more resistant to treatment and may also be more likely to metastasise at an early stage. In contrast, it is possible that local failure/persistence of the tumour with the accumulated changes induced by the radiotherapy may somehow be more likely to switch on angiogenic pathways and metastasise. Whatever view one accepts, it is important to aggressively pursue local control of the tumour with high doses of radiotherapy and the most effective concomitant chemotherapy available.

Lymph node assessment

Even after short-term pre-operative radiotherapy there is a significant reduction in the number of lymph nodes retrieved from irradiated specimens. Data from the large Dutch TME study includes 1,306 patients randomised to preoperative radiotherapy or immediate surgery (Nagtegaal *et al*. 2002). Significantly fewer nodes were obtained from irradiated specimens (7.7 versus 9.7). This reduction in the number of nodes found was noted in the MRC 2 rectal cancer study after 40 Gy and an interval of 45 days (MRC 2).

Data suggest the overall number of lymph nodes retrieved by the pathologist is of prognostic significance in both colon cancer (Le Voyer *et al.* 2000) and rectal cancer (Tepper *et al.* 2001) whether involved or not. Results from the Intergroup 0114 study demonstrated a 34% five-year relapse rate and a 73% five-year survival for node negative patients with five to eight nodes identified, compared with 19% and 82 %, respectively, if 14 or more nodes were identified (Tepper *et al.* 2001). It has been suggested that the higher the number of lymph nodes examined, the more accurate the staging.

Many authors have observed that lymph nodes in the surgical specimen appear to be effaced by pre-operative radiotherapy and chemotherapy (Wheeler 2002). Pathologists often are unable to find sufficient lymph nodes to confidently pronounce on stage. Retrospective studies have shown that these lymph nodes are often smaller and are less likely to contain malignant cells (Wichmann *et al.* 2002). This retrospective study showed that in patients who received surgery alone, there were 19.1 lymph nodes available for pathological examination compared with 13.6 in those receiving pre-operative radiotherapy. A mean of 3.1 lymph nodes in surgery alone patients compared with 1.4 in the pre-operative radiotherapy were observed to be infiltrated by cancer cells. Pathologists retrieved an inadequate number of lymph nodes for accurately defining nodal status in 13 patients (13.1%) in those treated by surgery alone versus 11 in the pre-operative radiotherapy group (11.9%).

Rinkus *et al.* (2002) also identified 292 patients with rectal cancer between 1984 and 1998, and examined the effect of pre-operative chemoradiation on the lymph node status and resected specimens of rectal cancer particularly in view of the fact that positive lymph nodes, i.e. Dukes' C status has usually been the best predictor of future outcome and has in general led clinicians to offer post-operative adjuvant chemotherapy. For the 251 evaluable patients, pre-operative radiotherapy does not appear to appreciably alter the nodal status of the population under study. Both groups had a rate of node positivity of approximately 45% and this continues to reflect future outcome quite strongly. What the study does not show is whether there is any additional advantage using post-operative adjuvant chemotherapy for those patients who still have residual positive lymph nodes following pre-operative chemoradiation.

Acute toxicity and complications

The Dutch TME study comprised 1,861 patients randomised to surgery alone, or pre-operative radiotherapy followed by surgery. A further report examined the acute side effects and complications after short-term pre-operative radiotherapy combined with total mesorectal excision in primary rectal cancer in 1,530 Dutch patients. (Marijnen *et al.* 2002). Patients received radiotherapy to a dose of 25 Gy in five fractions over 5–7 days. The radiotherapy fields encompassed the pelvis from the level of the sacral promontory but the perineum was only included if an AP excision of the rectum was planned and 3 cm from the anal verge if an anterior resection was intended.

In patients undergoing pelvic radiotherapy, transient neurological symptoms were documented in 53 patients, the majority of whom (35) experienced only grade 1 toxicity. However, 13 patients had their treatment interrupted because of pain in the buttocks or legs. Only 4 patients had documented other grade 3 toxicities (less than 1%).

Radiotherapy did not appear to complicate surgery as there was no significance difference as regards operation time or hospital stay between the treatment arms. Although a higher total blood loss was noted in the radiotherapy group, it was mainly confined to those patients undergoing a low anterior resection.

Post-operative complication rate was 48% for the radiotherapy arm and 41% for the surgery alone arm. This difference was mainly attributable to slow perineum wound healing after radiotherapy (29% versus 18%)—although there is no difference in abdominal wound complications. Interestingly, the percentage of patients who demonstrated a clinical leak post-operatively was no different whether they received radiotherapy or not (11% versus 12%). Although leakage was less commonly observed in patients who had a diverting stoma (8% versus 16%).

Mortality was 4% for the radiotherapy arm and 3.3% for the TME alone group. In the radiotherapy group, 10 patients had cardiac problems from which they died in contrast to only 3 in the surgery alone group. It is of note that 23% of all in hospital mortalities was due an anastomotic leak.

The Dutch TME study shows quite convincingly that short fractionation pre-operative radiotherapy does not appear to complicate TME surgery although there is some delay in perineal wound healing.

Finally, findings from a prospective database of 187 patients treated with neoadjuvant preoperative chemoradiation at Mount Vernon Cancer Centre (R. Glynne-Jones, unpublished data 2003) for locally advanced rectal cancer (T3/T4) suggest the following conclusions can be drawn. Patients downstaged to path CR pT1 T2 N0 have a *low* risk of either local relapse or systemic relapse. In contrast, patients who have residual positive lymph nodes have very high risk of systemic relapse and very poor overall survival.

Discussion

It seems reasonable to assume that by reducing distant failure we would improve both survival and quality of life, which supports the view that an aggressive approach to gaining local control by pre-operative chemoradiation may be warranted since surgical resection does not appear to alter the risk of subsequent metastatic disease.

Currently, there is a major European study in T3/T4 resectable rectal cancer supported by the EORTC which is a 2 × 2 factorial design randomising pre-operative radiotherapy alone versus chemoradiation to a dose of 45 Gy with or without chemotherapy, with 5-FU and leucovorin according to the above regimen, and further randomising post-operatively to adjuvant chemotherapy, with 5-FU and low-dose leucovorin or control. This trial has been completed, having accrued 992 patients. The EORTC trial is unique in that it should help to clarify the role of combined modality treatment compared with radiotherapy alone in the pre-operative setting and the role of adjuvant chemotherapy in the post-operative setting.

However, this trial was designed in 1991 and the only endpoints are overall and disease-free survival. Sadly, this trial will not provide accurate and robust information on the R0 resection rate after radiotherapy or chemoradiotherapy because of the lack of quality assurance of pathological reporting and the fact that TME surgery was not mandated.

The German CAO/ARO/AIO–94 protocol was initiated in 1995 to compare preoperative 5-FU based chemoradiation with standard conventionally fractionated radiotherapy versus postoperative combined modality treatment for stage II/III resectable rectal cancer. The primary endpoints of the study were overall and relapse free survival; local regional distant control with the secondary endpoints including the rate of curative (R0) resections, sphincter-saving procedures, toxicity, and surgical complications. Owing to premature closure of the Intergroup and the NSABP pre- versus post-operative chemoradiation studies, the 800 patients recruited in the German study offer crucial information.

Conclusion

The evidence base remains scanty. Very few studies of neoadjuvant chemoradiotherapy report long-term survival or late morbidity. Commonly, the median follow-up is only 24–32 months. The debate continues regarding pathological reporting and the optimal endpoints. It also seems unlikely that the intensity of chemoradiotherapy currently delivered in the neoadjuvant setting in rectal cancer is sufficient to prevent the development of metastatic disease in a significant number of patients. Patients who still have positive lymph nodes in the definitive surgical specimen following neoadjuvant chemoradiation have a very high risk of metastatic disease and a poor overall survival. Metastatic disease in lung and liver remains the cause of death in the vast majority of patients with rectal cancer who get TME surgery. It seems likely that further improvements in overall survival are only going to be achieved by reducing metastatic disease. Thus, is better/stronger/more chemoradiotherapy the key?

The best approach for the future would appear to lie in better and more intensive chemotherapy in the neoadjuvant setting and *different* (non-5-FU-based?) post-operative chemotherapy for those patients for whom the pathologist finds significant residual local disease and/or positive lymph nodes, rather than increasing the radiation dose.

We need the results of the current trials, mostly planned more than a decade ago, to refine and to design the next generation of trials incorporating the new drugs and all the achievements in surgery and pathology. We also need clear information on late effects. Future improvements in overall survival will almost certainly depend on the integration of all modalities, especially the new chemotherapy drugs irinotecan, oxaliplatin and capecitabine, and possibly the newer molecular targets.

References

Adell, G., Zhang, H., Jansson, A. et al. (2001). Decreased tumour cell proliferation as an indication of the effect of preoperative radiotherapy of rectal cancer. *International Journal of Radiation Oncology, Biology, Physics* **50**(3), 659–663.

Adell, G. C. E., Zhang, H., Evertsson, S. et al. (2001). Apoptosis in rectal carcinoma: prognosis and recurrence after preoperative radiotherapy. *Cancer* **91**(10), 1870–1875.

AJCC (2002). *American Joint Committee on Cancer Manual*. Philadelphia PA, Lipincott Raven.

Birbeck, K. F., Macklin, C. P., Tiffin, N. et al. (2001). Rates of circumferential resection margin involvement vary between surgeons and predict outcomes in rectal cancer surgery. *Annals of Surgery* **235**, 449–457.

Bouzourene, H., Bosman, F. T., Seelenta, G. W. et al. (2002). Importance in tumour regression assessment in predicting the outcome in patients with locally advanced rectal carcinoma who are treated with preoperative radiotherapy. *Cancer* **94**, 1121–1130.

Camma, C., Giunta, M., Fiorica, F., Pagliaro, L., Craxi, A., Cottone, M. (2000). Preoperative radiotherapy for resectable rectal cancer: A meta-analysis. *Journal of the American Medical Association* **284**, 1008–1015.

Chau, I., Allen, M., Cunningham, D. et al. (2002). Neoadjuvant systemic 5FU and mitomycin C (MMC) prior to synchronous chemoradiation is an effective strategy in locally advanced rectal cancer. *Proceedings of the American Society of Clinical Oncology* **21**, 637 (abstract).

Cianchi, F., Palomba, A., Masserini, L. et al. (2002). Tumor angiogenesis in lymph node negative rectal cancer: correlation with clinicopathological parameters and prognosis. *Annals of Surgical Oncology* **9**, 20–26.

Colorectal Cancer Collaborative Group (2001). Adjuvant radiotherapy for rectal cancer: a systematic overview of 8507 patients from 22 randomised trials. *Lancet* **358**, 1291–1304.

De Haas-Kock, D. F. N., Baeten, C. G. M. I., Jager, J. J. et al. (1996). Prognostic significance of radial margins of clearance in rectal cancer. *British Journal of Surgery* **83**, 781–785.

Diez, M., Pollan, M., Mugerza, J. M. et al. (2000). Time-dependency of the prognostic effect of carcinoembryonic antigen and p53 protein in colorectal adenocarcinoma. *Cancer* **88**, 35–41.

Edler, D., Hallstrom, M., Johnston, P. et al. (2000). Thymidylate synthase expression: an independent prognostic factor for local recurrence, distant metastasis, disease free and overall survival in rectal cancer. *Clinical Cancer Research* **6**, 1378–1384.

Elsaleh, H., Soontrapornchai, P. A., Grieu, F. et al. (1999). p53 alterations have no prognostic or predictive significance in Dukes' C rectal carcinomas. *International Journal of Oncology* **15**, 1239–1243.

Esposito, G., Pucciarelli, S., Alaggio, R. et al. (2001). $p27^{kip1}$ expression is associated with tumour response to preoperative chemoradiotherapy in rectal cancer. *Annals of Surgical Oncology* **8**, 311–318.

Galindo-Gallego, M., Fernandez-Acenero, M. J., Sanz-Ortega, J. et al. (2000). Prognostic significance of microvascular counts in rectal carcinoma. *Pathology, Research and Practice* **196**, 607–612.

George, M. L., Dzik-Jurasz, A. S. K., Padhani, A R. et al. (2001). Non-invasive methods of assessing angiogenesis and their value in predicting response to treatment in colorectal cancer. *British Journal of Surgery* **88**, 1628–1636.

Giralt, J., Eraso, A., Armengol, A. et al. (2002). Epidermal growth factor receptor is a predictor of tumour response in locally advanced rectal cancer patients treated with preoperative radiotherapy. *International Journal of Radiation Oncology, Biology, Physics* **54**, 1460–1465.

Kapiteijn, E., Marijnen, C. A. M., Nagtegaal, I. D. *et al.* (2001). Preoperative radiotherapy combined with total mesorectal excision for resectable rectal cancer. *New England Journal of Medicine* **345**, 638–646.

Kim, N. K., Park, J. K., Lee, K. Y. *et al.* (2001). p53, bcl2, and ki67 expression according to tumour response after concurrent chemoradiotherapy for advanced rectal cancer. *Annals of Surgical Oncology* **8**, 418–424.

Kockerling, F., Reymond, N. A., Altendorf Hoffmann, A. *et al.* (1998). Influence of surgery on metachronous distant metastases and survival in rectal cancer. *Journal of Clinical Oncology* **16**, 324–329.

Le Voyer, T. E., Sigurdson, E. R., Hanlon, A. L. *et al.* (2000). Colon cancer survival is associated with increasing number of lymph nodes removed. A secondary analysis of INT-0089. *Journal of Clinical Oncology* **19**, 925 (abstract).

Lee, J. H., Lee, J. H., Ah, J. H. *et al.* (2002). Randomized trial of postoperative adjuvant therapy in stage II and III rectal cancer to define the optimal sequence of chemotherapy and radiotherapy: a preliminary report. *Journal of Clinical Oncology* **20**, 1751–1758.

Marijnen, C. A., Kapiteijn, E. & van de Velde, C. J. H. *et al.* (2002). Acute side effects and complications after short-term preoperative radiotherapy combined with total mesorectal excision in primary rectal cancer: report of a multicenter randomised trial. *Journal of Clinical Oncology* **20**, 817–825.

Marijnen, C. A., Kapiteijn, E., Nagtelgaal, I. D. *et al.* (2002). p53 expression in human rectal tissues after radiotherapy: upregulation in normal mucosa versus functional loss in rectal carcinomas. *International Journal of Radiation Oncology, Biology, Physics* **52**, 720–728.

Medical Research Council Rectal Cancer Working Party (MRC 2) (1996). Randomized trial of surgery versus radiotherapy followed by surgery for potentially operable locally advanced rectal cancer. *The Lancet* **348**,1605–1610.

Nagtegaal, I. D., van der Velde, C. J. H., van de Worp, E. *et al.* (2001). Macroscopic evaluation of rectal cancer resection specimen: clinical significance of the pathologist in quality control. *Journal of Clinical Oncology* **20**, 1729–1734.

Nagtegaal, I. D., Marijnen, C. A. M., Kranenberg, E. *et al.* (2002). Short-term preoperative radiotherapy interferes with the determination of pathological parameters in rectal cancer. *Journal of Pathology*, 1729–1734.

Nehls, O, Klump, B., Holzmann, K. *et al.* (1999). Influence of p53 status on prognosis in preoperatively irradiated rectal carcinoma. *Cancer* **85**, 2541–2548.

Ng, I. O., Luk, I. S., Yuen, S. T. *et al.* (1993). Surgical lateral clearance in resected rectal carcinomas. A multivariate analysis of clinicopathologic features. *Cancer* **71**, 1972–1976.

O'Connell, M. J., Martenson, J. A., Wieand, H. S. *et al.* (1994). Improving adjuvant therapy of rectal cancer by combining protracted infusional fluorouracil with radiation therapy after curative surgery. *New England Journal of Medicine* **331**, 502–507.

Okonkwo, A., Musunuri, S., Talamonti, M. *et al.* (2001). Molecular markers and prediction of response to chemoradiation in rectal cancer. *Oncology Reports* **8**, 497–500.

Qui, H., Sirivongs, P., Rothenberger, M. *et al.* (2000). Molecular prognostic factors in rectal cancer treated by radiation and surgery. *Diseases of Colon and Rectum* **43**, 451–459.

Rinkus, K. M., Russell, G. B., Levine E. A. (2002). Prognostic significance of nodal disease following preoperative radiation for rectal adenocarcinoma. *American Surgeon*, **68**, 482–87.

Rodel, C., Grabenbauer, G. G., Papadopoulos, T. *et al.* (2002). Apoptosis as a cellular predictor for histopathologic response to neoadjuvant radiochemotherapy in patients with rectal cancer. *International Journal of Radiation Oncology, Biology, Physics* **52**(2), 294–303.

Rebischung, C., Gerard, J. P., Gayet, J. *et al.* (2002). Prognostic value of p53 mutations in rectal carcinoma. *International Journal of Cancer* **100**, 131–135.

Ruo, L., Tickoo, S., Klimstra, D. *et al.* (2002). Long-term prognostic significance of extent of rectal cancer response to preoperative radiation and chemotherapy. *Annals of Surgery* **236**, 75–81.

Schwandner, O., Schiedeck, T. H. K., Bruch, H. P. *et al.* (2000). p53 and bcl2 as significant predictors of recurrence and survival in rectal cancer. *European Journal of Oncology* **36**, 348–356.

Spitz, F. R., Giacco, G. G., Hess, K. *et al.* (1995). p53 immunohistochemical staining predicts residual disease after chemoradiation in patients with high-risk rectal cancer. *British Journal of Cancer* **72**, 435–441.

Swedish Rectal Cancer Trial (1997). Improved survival with preoperative radiotherapy in resectable rectal cancer. *New England Journal of Medicine* **336**, 980–987.

Tepper, J. E., O'Conell, M. J., Niedzwiecki, D. *et al.* (2001). Impact of number of nodes retrieved on outcome in patients with rectal cancer. *Journal of Clinical Oncology* **19**, 157–163.

Tepper, J. E., O'Connell, M., Niedzwiecki, D. *et al.* (2002). Adjuvant therapy in rectal cancer analysis of stage, sex and local control: final report of Intergroup 0114J. *Clinical Oncology* **20**, 1744–1750.

Valentini, V., Coco, C., Picchiocci, A. *et al.* (2002). Does downstaging predict improved outcome after preoperative chemoradiation for extraperitoneal locally-advanced rectal cancer? A long-term analysis of 165 patients. *International Journal of Radiation Oncology, Biology, Physics* **53**, 664–674.

Wheeler, J. M. D., Warren, B. F., Mortensen, N. J. M. *et al.* (2002). Quantification of histologic regression of rectal cancer after irradiation: a proposal for a modified staging system. *Diseases of Colon and Rectum* **45**, 1051–1056.

Wibe, A., Rendedal, P. R., Svensson, E. *et al.* (2002). Prognostic significance of the circumferential resection margin following total mesorectal excision for rectal cancer. *British Journal of Surgery* **20**, 327–334.

Wichmann, M. W., Muller, C., Meyer, G. *et al.* (2002). Effect of preoperative radiochemotherapy on lymph node retrieval after resection of rectal cancer. *Archives of Surgery* **137**, 206–210.

Chapter 13

Intermittent or continuous palliative chemotherapy in metastatic colorectal cancer

Tim Maughan and Richard Stephens

Introduction

Over most of the past 40 years oncologists treating metastatic colorectal cancer have only had one option for treatment: 5-fluorouracil (5-FU). This drug has modest activity but practically no cumulative toxicity. In the absence of any second-line therapy, it became common practice to treat with chemotherapy until progression on the unproven assumption that this maximised the benefits from the palliative chemotherapy. The question arose as to whether this is the optimal way to use palliative chemotherapy in this disease. Much evidence had been established in other cancers that shorter courses of chemotherapy were equally effective in terms of survival, but no data existed in the literature with respect to palliative treatment of colorectal cancer. In recent years, with the advent of oxaliplatin and irinotecan, this historical pattern of therapy has been adapted, as two or three lines of therapy are now available to the oncologist: single agent 5-FU-based therapy, oxaliplatin plus 5-FU and irinotecan, alone or in combination. The pattern continues in many countries and is perpetuated in most clinical trial protocols of treatment with first-line chemotherapy to progression. This chapter presents data from the recent Medical Research Council trial (MRC CR06B), which has compared intermittent and continuous palliative chemotherapy for patients with metastatic colorectal cancer (Maughan *et al.* 2003). We are grateful to the many patients, research nurses and clinicians across the UK who have enabled us to obtain these data, which challenge the accepted norms of treatment in this disease setting.

In 1995, a survey conducted by our group indicated that policies regarding duration of treatment varied across the UK. While all agreed that patients with progressive disease should stop chemotherapy, for patients who were responding, approximately 30% of clinicians stopped chemotherapy after three months, 50% after six months, and the remaining 20% gave 'open-ended' chemotherapy (Seymour *et al.* 1997).

No previous trials had addressed this issue in advanced colorectal cancer, although previous randomised trials in adjuvant colon cancer (O'Connell *et al.* 1996; Ito *et al.* 2000) and other cancer sites[*] have generally shown that short-course treatment is as

---

[*]See the following references: Smalley *et al.* 1976; Coates *et al.* 1987; The Ludwig Breast Cancer Study Group 1988; Buccheri *et al.* 1989; Einhoen *et al.* 1989; Harris *et al.* 1990; Muss *et al.* 1991; Early Breast Cancer Trialists' Collaborative Group 1992; Hakes *et al.* 1992; Bertelsen *et al.* 1993; Ejlertsen *et al.* 1993; The Medical Research Council Lung Cancer Working Party 1993; The Childhood ALL Collaborative Group 1996; The International Breast Cancer Study Group. 1996; Gregory *et al.*1997; Pavlovsky *et al.* 1997; Beith *et al.* 1998; Elonen *et al.* 1998; Sculier *et al.* 1998; Sauerbrei *et al.* 2000; Smith *et al.* 2001; The French Epirubicin Study Group 2000.

effective as long-course. One consistent finding is that patients receiving short-course therapy may experience a shorter time to disease progression, but several papers (Smalley *et al.* 1976; Fisher *et al.* 1979; Paccagnella et al. 1983; Coates *et al.* 1987; Harris *et al.* 1990; The French Epirubicin Study Group 2000; Muss *et al.* 1991; Ejlertsen *et al.* 1993) have reported that at the time of progression patients may be successfully re-challenged with the same regimen.

The MRC CR06B trial

This trial was designed to compare the outcomes in patients who had received 12 weeks of palliative chemotherapy and had stable or responding disease and who at that point either stopped chemotherapy (with the plan to restart the same chemotherapy on progression) or who continued on chemotherapy until progression (Maughan *et al.* 2003). Initially the trial was open only to patients who were participating in the MRC CR06 trial (Maughan *et al.* 2002). This was a randomised comparison of the following three chemotherapy regimens: De Gramont (De Gramont *et al.* 1997) – 2-weekly cycles of i.v. folinic acid 200 mg/m^2 (max 350 mg) over 2 hours, followed by 5-FU 400 mg/m^2 bolus over 5 minutes and 5-FU infusion 600 mg/m^2 over 22 hours, repeated on day 2; Lokich (Lokich *et al.* 1991) – continuous i.v. infusion 5-FU 300 mg/m^2/day given via an ambulatory pump; and raltitrexed (Cunningham *et al.* 1996) – 3 mg/m^2 given intravenously over 15 minutes every 3 weeks. This trial had shown equivalence in response rate and survival between these three regimens, though an increase in toxicity with raltitrexed (Maughan *et al.* 2002). After the closure of the CR06 trial, the current trial remained open to patients who fulfilled the same criteria, i.e. had satisfied the same entry criteria and received one of the three 'CR06' chemotherapy regimens, with stable or responding disease after 12 weeks (87 patients).

Results

Three hundred and fifty-four patients were entered into the study. The key patient characteristics are easily memorable: 64% were male, 64% had carcinoma of the colon (the remainder having rectal cancer) and the median age was 64 years; 80% were World Health Organization performance status 0 or 1, 41% had either complete or partial response, and the remainder stable disease, after the initial 12 weeks of chemotherapy.

Treatment

The 'intermittent' policy

After a median of 130 days (SD 129 days), 66 patients (37%) on the 'intermittent' policy re-started their first-line chemotherapy, because of disease progression (85%), patient choice (11%) or clinical decision (3%), and on average received a further course of 12 weeks of chemotherapy. Overall, on average, patients received a total of

18 weeks' treatment on their original regimen. Of the 66 patients, 24 subsequently received second-line chemotherapy (different drugs or a different schedule of drugs). A further 38 patients (21% of the whole group) did not restart their original chemotherapy but moved straight onto second-line treatment (Figure 13.1).

Further chemotherapy	INTERMITTENT	CONTINUE
Number of patients	62	53
5FU-based regimens	26	18
Raltitrexed	5	1
Irinotecan	20	17
Oxaliplatin	0	6
5-FU + mitomycin	7	8
Other	4	3

Figure 13.1 Chemotherapy administered

The 'continue' policy

Patients allocated to 'continue' remained on the same chemotherapy regimen as they had received for the first 12 weeks of treatment. On average, patients received chemotherapy for a further 92 days (SD 86 days); 46% then stopped because of disease progression, although toxicity (18%), clinical decision (16%), patient choice (14%), and other treatment indicated (3%) were also recorded as reasons for stopping. In addition, a further 3% of patients died during chemotherapy. Overall, on average, patients received a total of 28 weeks' treatment on their original regimen; 53 patients (30%) subsequently received second-line chemotherapy (Figure 13.1).

Response

At randomisation, 41% of patients had a complete or partial response and the remainder had stable disease. Of the 66 patients on the 'intermittent' policy who progressed while off treatment and were then re-started on the same chemotherapy, 14 (21%) responded and a further 17 were reported as having stable disease during this phase. There did not appear to be a relationship between time off treatment and subsequent response. Nineteen per cent of patients who re-started within three months had a response, compared to 24% who re-started after more than three months. Only 14 (8%) of the 176 patients on the 'continue' policy improved their response status while on the continuing phase of treatment (9 improved from stable disease to a response, 5 from partial to complete response).

When patients moved onto a different (second-line) therapy (Figure 13.1), 6 (10%) of the 62 'intermittent' patients responded and a further 14 (23%) were reported as having stable disease, compared with 5 (9%) and 6 (11%), respectively, of the 53 patients in the 'continue' group.

Toxicity

The policy of continuing chemotherapy resulted in a total of 17 treatment-related serious adverse events (SAEs), compared to 6 on the 'stop' policy. The only patient reported as having a fatal SAE was admitted as an emergency 11 days after their 10th cycle of raltitrexed with neutropenic sepsis and died two days later. Clinician-reported symptoms differed only in the frequency of a rash, which was greater in those continuing chemotherapy ($p = 0.002$).

Patient-reported quality of life

Before randomisation and at six-weekly intervals thereafter, patients completed the Hospital Anxiety and Depression Scale (HADS) (Zigmond & Snaith 1983) and the EORTC Quality of Life core questionnaire (QLQ-C30) (Aaronson et al. 1993) plus six similarly structured questions covering trial-specific symptoms and how acceptable and worthwhile patients considered their treatment to be. Patients on the 'continue' policy reported more specific chemotherapy-related side effects (dry or sore mouth, discomfort with hand and feet (see Figure 13.2a,b). This did not have a statistically significantly impact on functioning or overall health (see Figure 13.2c,d), although throughout patients on 'continue' reported consistently slightly poorer functioning. There was no evidence of a difference in terms of general symptoms or psychological distress, and most patients in both groups considered their treatment to have been very worthwhile (see Figure 13.2e,f).

Progression-free survival

There was a strong indication that a policy of continuing chemotherapy delayed the time to progression although this difference was non-significant and the benefit was only about a month (median 3.7 months for 'intermittent', 4.9 months for 'continue') (see Figure 13.3). The overall hazard ratio was 1.20 (favouring 'continue'), 95% confidence intervals (CIs) 0.96–1.49, $p = 0.10$.

Survival

Overall survival was the primary endpoint of the trial. Median survival from randomisation (after the initial 12 weeks of treatment) was 10.8 months for the 'intermittent' group, 11.3 months for the 'continue' group, with the one- and two-year survival figures being 46% and 19% for 'intermittent', and 45% and 13% for 'continue'. Overall, there was no evidence of a benefit in survival to either group (see Figure 13.4) (hazard ratio = 0.87 (favouring 'intermittent'), 95% CIs 0.69–1.09, $p = 0.23$). There was no indication that any subgroup of patients benefited more or less from either of the policies, though the hazard ratios consistently (though non-

A. Dry and/or sore mouth

B. Discomfort with hands/feet

C. Physical functioning

Based on the following numbers of patients:

week	intermittent	continue
0	125–147	132–147
6	85–102	104–112
12	62–76	69–77
18	43–55	58–64
24	38–52	44–49
30	31–42	38–39

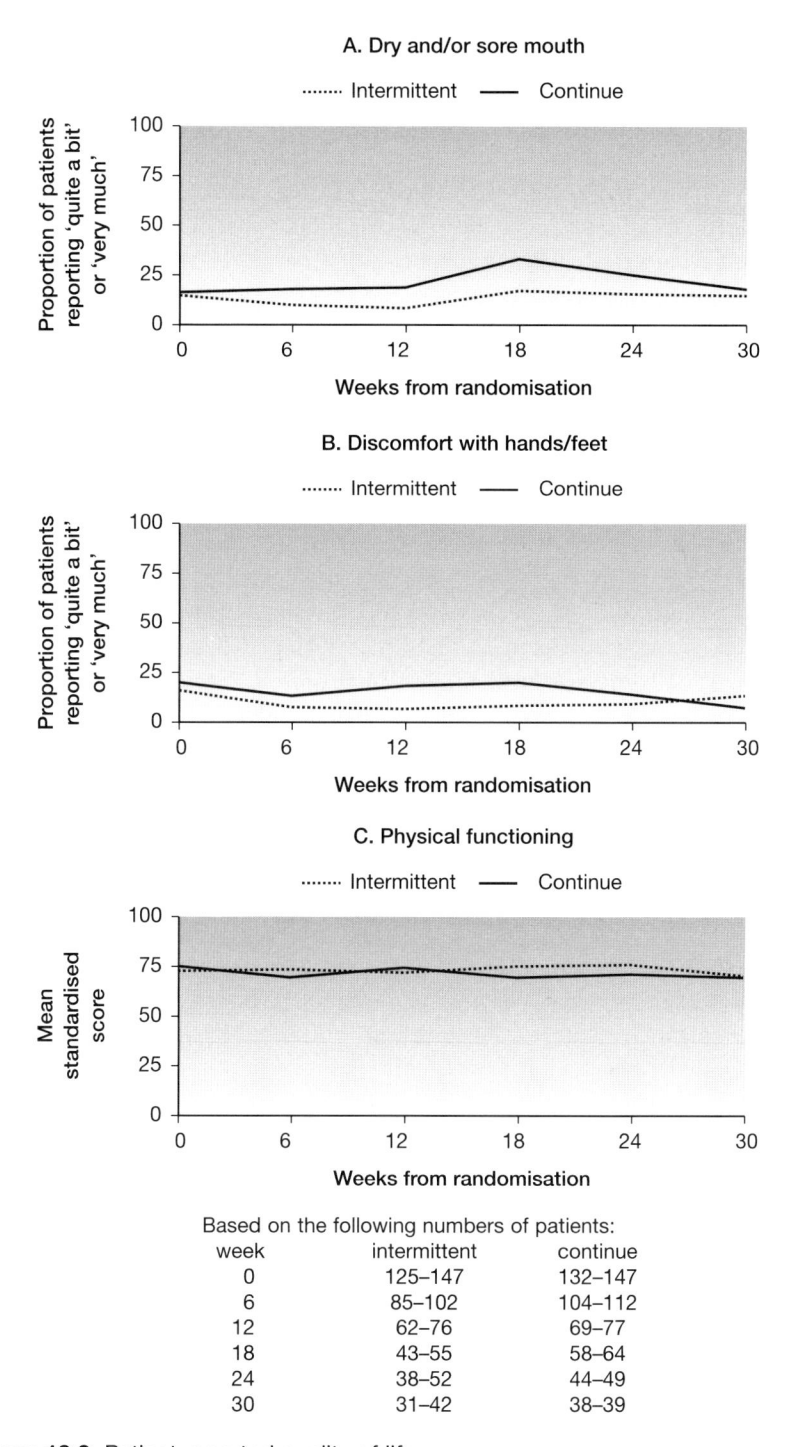

Figure 13.2 Patient-reported quality of life.

D. Global health status

······ Intermittent — Continue

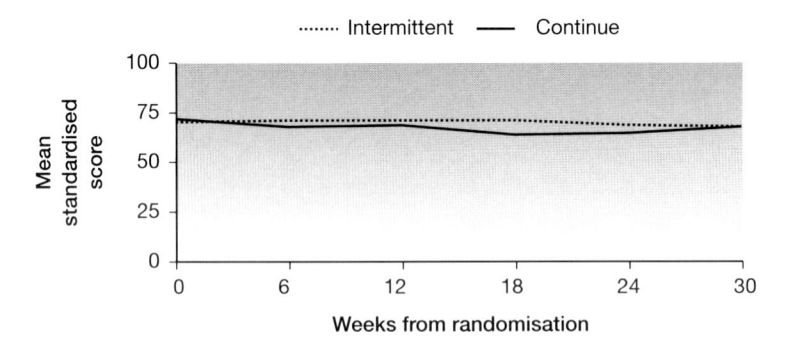

E. Treatment intefered with normal activities

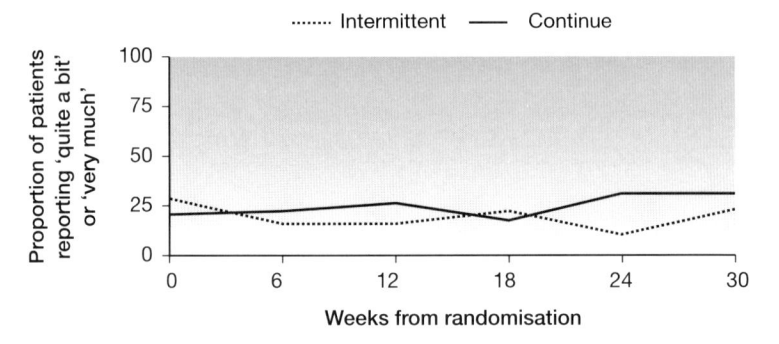

······ Intermittent — Continue

F. How worthwhile has treatment been?

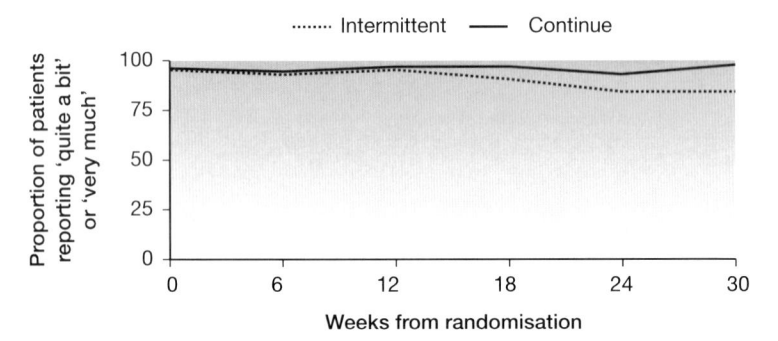

······ Intermittent — Continue

Based on the following numbers of patients:

week	intermittent	continue
0	125–147	132–147
6	85–102	104–112
12	62–76	69–77
18	43–55	58–64
24	38–52	44–49
30	31–42	38–39

Figure 13.2 contd.

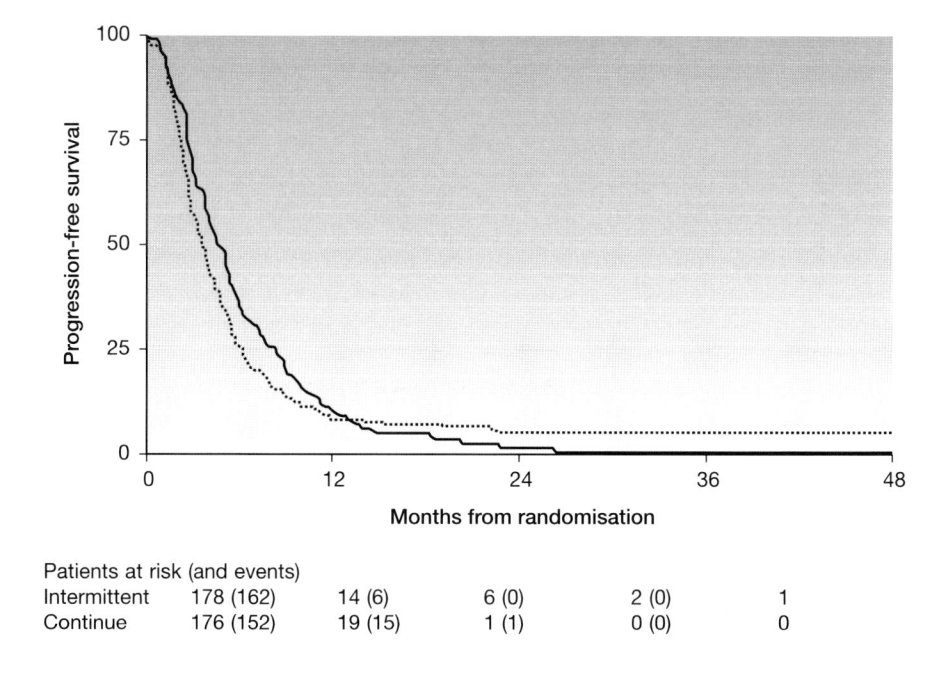

Palliative chemotherapy in metastatic colorectal cancer 173

Patients at risk (and events)					
Intermittent	178 (162)	14 (6)	6 (0)	2 (0)	1
Continue	176 (152)	19 (15)	1 (1)	0 (0)	0

Figure 13.3 Progression-free survival.

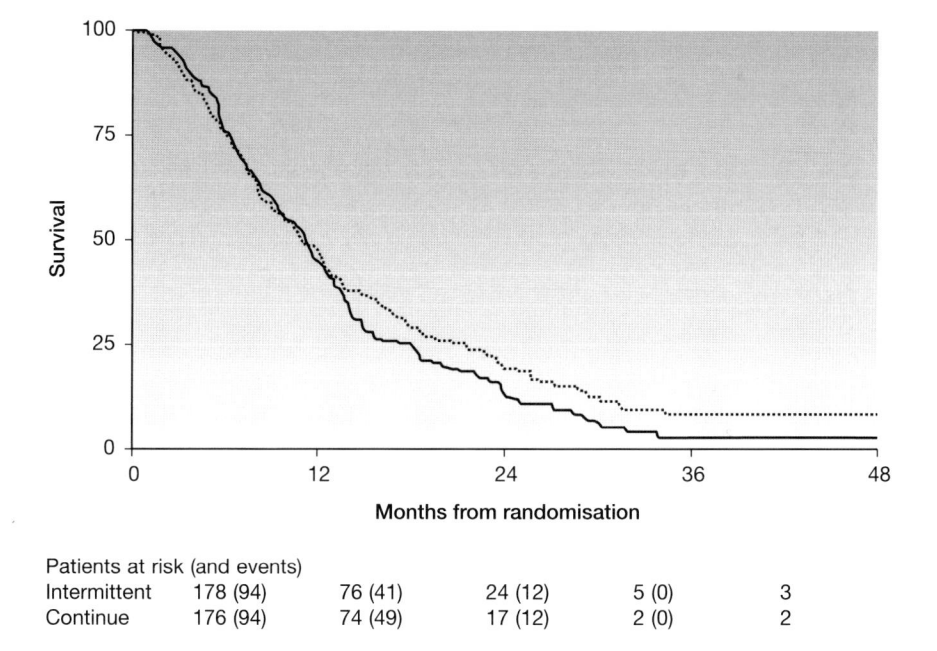

Patients at risk (and events)					
Intermittent	178 (94)	76 (41)	24 (12)	5 (0)	3
Continue	176 (94)	74 (49)	17 (12)	2 (0)	2

Figure 13.4 Overall survival.

significantly) favour those patients given intermittent therapy. The only exception to this was that there was a suggestion of a trend towards younger patients doing slightly better on continuous therapy.

Generalisability

Most of the patients in this trial were also participating in MRC CR06 (Maughan *et al.* 2002). We have therefore been able to analyse the outcome of all the other patients in that trial who were eligible for the current trial but, because of their own or their clinicians' choice, were not randomised into the comparison of 'pause' versus 'continue'.

In all, 461 of the 905 CR06 patients had responding or stable disease after the initial 12 weeks of treatment; 267 were randomised (131 to stop, 136 to continue). Of the 194 patients not randomised, 99 stopped treatment (55% because of patient choice) and 95 continued (72% because of patient choice). The characteristics of these three groups were very similar.

The survival of the four groups of patients – randomised to 'pause'; randomised to 'continue'; chose to stop; and chose to continue – from the time of initial randomisation to CR06 (the only common timepoint for all these patients), is shown in Figure 13.5. There is no evidence of any difference, suggesting that the randomised group were representative of the whole population. Note that the top line on the survival curve was from those patients who chose to stop.

Conclusion

These provocative results challenge the accepted orthodoxy that for optimal outcomes patients should be treated with cytotoxic chemotherapy until progression. In practice, many oncologists give a six-month course of chemotherapy and give patients a rest at that time. However, clinical experience informs us that those second 12 weeks of therapy are increasingly exhausting for the patients. These data give an evidence base for discontinuing therapy after 12 weeks, which is much appreciated by patients if they are previously informed that this is the planned scheme of chemotherapy. There are several practical points that need to be considered when implementing this policy:

- The induction chemotherapy must be of sufficient duration and efficacy to ensure that most responses are achieved during the induction period. In the current trial only 8% of patients on the 'continue' arm improved their response status during the 'continue' phase of chemotherapy. However, a long induction treatment may induce drug resistance and subsequent re-challenging may be less effective.
- There must be a good response to the re-use of the same chemotherapy. In the current trial 47% of patients re-challenged had responding or stable disease on re-exposure to their initial chemotherapy.
- There may need to be a reasonable gap between stopping induction treatment and

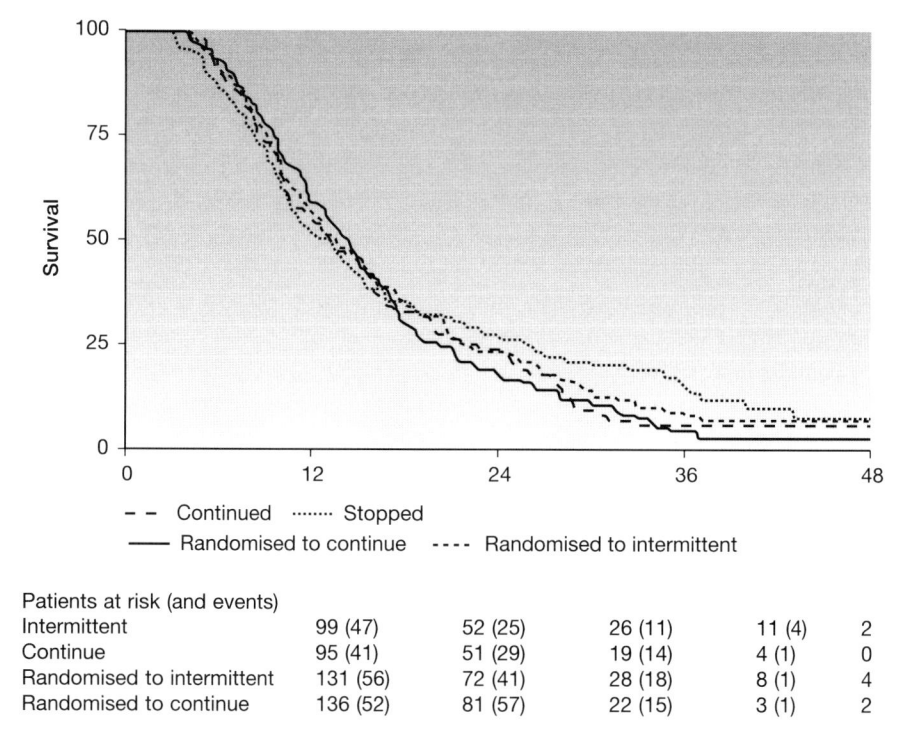

Figure 13.5 Overall survival of randomised and non-randomised patients in MRC CR06 trial.

Patients at risk (and events)

Intermittent	99 (47)	52 (25)	26 (11)	11 (4)	2
Continue	95 (41)	51 (29)	19 (14)	4 (1)	0
Randomised to intermittent	131 (56)	72 (41)	28 (18)	8 (1)	4
Randomised to continue	136 (52)	81 (57)	22 (15)	3 (1)	2

progression. Fisher et al. (1979) and Harris et al. (1990) both reported that patients who had a longer gap between stopping and re-starting were more likely to respond, although this pattern was not observed in the current trial.

- Observation of patients off chemotherapy must be diligent. Coates et al. (1987) argue that patients on continuous chemotherapy are less anxious because they are reassured by regular hospital contact and maintained symptom control. Spiro and Souhami (1990) suggest that patients may prefer to continue, feeling that more of what was doing them good would be better. Patients off treatment must be regularly followed up to ensure that treatment can be re-introduced at the first sign of progression and to provide reassurance and optimal symptom control during the interval off therapy.

These shortened exposures to chemotherapy also have a beneficial economic effect. The health economic evaluation shows that 10 less weeks of chemotherapy were administered to those on the intermittent schedule (Hale et al. 2002).

These data are not directly transferable to combination chemotherapy regimens and this may be addressed in future trials. However, the data do point towards an altered paradigm for treatment of patients with metastatic colorectal cancer in the more modern era of effective combination chemotherapy and novel cytostatic agents. With combination regimens a disease control rate, combining responding and stable disease approaching 90% has been reported (Cassidy *et al.* 2004). After a short period of induction chemotherapy, patients with controlled disease would be suitable for trials of cytostatic agents such as anti-angiogenic agents, epidermal growth factor receptor targeted therapy, cox-2 inhibitors, or immunotherapy in an attempt to prolong this time interval off cytotoxic chemotherapy. Recent experience with the epidermal growth factor receptor tyrosine kinase (Iressa) trials in non small cell lung cancer has shown that the combination of these novel agents with chemotherapy can have unpredictable outcomes (Herbst *et al.* 2004). This approach would allow clear demonstration of the benefits of such agents against a placebo in a group of patients relatively early in their metastatic disease course.

Acknowledgements

This chapter gives data from a trial of the British Medical Research Council Colorectal Cancer Group. Clinicians and research nurses from 45 hospital contributed and are listed in *The Lancet*. The trial was funded by an MRC grant, and AstraZeneca provided raltitrexed at no cost and a financial grant to support research costs of the participating centres.

References

Aaronson, N. K., Ahmedzai, S., Bergman, B. *et al.* (1993). The European Organization for Research and Treatment of Cancer Quality of LifeQ-C30: a quality of life instrument for use in international clinical trials in oncology. *Journal of the National Cancer Institute* **85**, 365–376.

Beith, J. M., Clarke, S. J., Woods, R. L. *et al.* (1996). Long-term follow-up of a randomised trial of combined chemoradiotherapy induction treatment, with and without maintenance chemotherapy in patients with small cell carcinoma of the lung. *European Journal of Cancer* **32A**, 438–443.

Bertelsen, K., Jakobsen, A., Stroyer, I. *et al.* (1993). A prospective randomized comparison of 6 and 12 cycles of cyclophosphamide, adriamycin, and cisplatin in advanced epithelial ovarian cancer: a Danish Ovarian Study Group trial (DACOVA). *Gynaecologic Oncology* **49**, 30–36.

Buccheri, G. F., Ferrigno, D., Curcio, A. *et al.* (1998). Continuation of chemotherapy versus supportive care alone in patients with inoperable non-small cell lung cancer and stable disease after two or three cycles of MACC. *Cancer* **63**, 428–432.

Cassidy, J., Tabernero, J., Twelves, C., Brunet, R., Butts, C., Conroy, T., Debraud, F., Figer, A., Grossmann, J., Sawada, N., Schoffski, P., Sobero, A., Van Cutsem, E. & Diaz-Rubio, E. (2004). XELOX (capecitabine plus oxaliplatin): active first-line therapy for patients with metastatic colorectal cancer. *Journal of Clinical Oncology* **22**, 2084–2091.

Childhood ALL Collaborative Group (1996). Duration and intensity of maintenance chemotherapy in acute lymphoblastic leukaemia: overview of 42 trials involving 12000 randomised children. *The Lancet* **347**, 1783–1788.

Coates, A., Gebski, V., Bishop, J. F. *et al.* (1987). Improving the quality of life during chemotherapy for advanced breast cancer. *New England Journal of Medicine* **317**, 1490–1495.

Cunningham, D., Zalcberg, J. R., Rath, U. et al. (1996). Final results of a randomised trial comparing 'Tomudex' (raltitrexed) with 5-fluourouracil plus leucovorin in advanced colorectal cancer. 'Tomudex' Colorectal Cancer Study Group. *Annals of Oncology* **7**, 961–965.

De Gramont, A., Bosset, J. F., Milan, C. et al. (1997). Randomized trial comparing monthly low-dose leucovorin and fluorouracil bolus with bimonthly high-dose leucovorin and fluorouracil bolus plus continuous infusion for advanced colorectal cancer: a French Intergroup trial. *Journal of Clinical Oncology* **15**, 808–815.

Early Breast Cancer Trialists' Collaborative Group (1992). Systemic treatment of early breast cancer by hormonal, cytotoxic, or immune therapy. *The Lancet* **339**, 71–85.

Einhorn, L. H., Williams, S. D., Loehrer, P.J. et al. (1989). Evaluation of optimal duration of chemotherapy in favorable-prognosis disseminated germ cell tumors: a Southeastern Cancer Study Group protocol. *Journal of Clinical Oncology* **7**, 387–391.

Ejlertsen, B., Pfeiffe,r P., Pedersen, D. et al. (1993). Decreased efficacy of cyclophosphamide, epirubicin and 5-fluorouracil in metastatic breast cancer when reducing treatment duration from 18 to 6 months. *European Journal of Cancer* **29A**, 527–531.

Elonen, E., Almqvist, A., Hanninen, A. et al. (1998). Comparison between four and eight cycles of intensive chemotherapy in adult acute myeloid leukemia: a randomized trial of the Finnish Leukemia Group. *Leukemia* **12**, 1941–1048.

Fisher, R. I., DeVita, V. T., Hubbard, S. P. et al. (1979). Prolonged disease-free survival in Hodgkin's disease with MOPP reinduction after first relapse. *Annals of International Medicine* **90**, 761–763.

French Epirubicin Study Group (2000). Epirubicin-based chemotherapy in metastatic breast cancer patients: role of dose-intensity and duration of treatment. *Journal of Clinical Oncology* **18**, 3115–3124.

Gregory, R. K., Powles, T. J., Chang, J. C. & Ashley S. (1997). A randomised trial of six versus twelve courses of chemotherapy in metastatic carcinoma of the breast. *European Journal of Cancer* **33**, 2194–2197.

Hakes, T. B., Chalas, E., Hoskins, W J. et al. (1992). Randomized prospective trial fo 5 versus 10 cycles of cyclophosphamide, doxorubicin, and cisplatin in advanced ovarian carcinoma. *Gynaecologic Oncology* **45**, 284–289.

Hale, J. P., Cohen, D. R., Maughan. T. S. & Stephens R. J. (2002). Costs and consequences of different chemotherapy regimens in metastatic colorectal cancer. *British Journal of Cancer* **86**, 1684–1690.

Harris, A. L., Cantwell, B. M. J., Carmichael, J. et al. (1990). Comparison of short-term and continuous chemotherapy (mitozantrone) for advanced breast cancer. *The Lancet* **335**, 186–190.

Herbst, R., Giaccone, G., Schiller, J. H. et al. (2004). Gefitinib in combination with paclitaxel and carboplatin in chemotherapy in advanced non-small–cell lung cancer: a phase III trial INTACT 2. *Journal of Clinical Oncology* **22**, 785–794.

International Breast Cancer Study Group (1996). Duration and reintroduction of adjuvant chemotherapy for node-positive premenopausal breast cancer patients. *Journal of Clinical Oncology* **14**, 1885–1894.

Ito, K., Kato, T., Koike, A. et al. (2000). Optimum duration of oral adjuvant chemotherapy of HCFU for colorectal cancer: review of 5-year follow-up. *Anticancer Research* **20**, 4681–4686.

Lokich, J. J., Ahlgren, J. D., Cantrell, J. et al. (1991). A prospective randomized comparison of protracted infusional 5-fluorouracil with or without weekly bolus cisplatin in metastatic colorectal carcinoma. A Mid-Atlantic Oncology Program study. *Cancer* **67**, 14–19.

Ludwig Breast Cancer Study Group (1988). Combination adjuvant chemotherapy for node-positive breast cancer. *New England Journal of Medicine* **319**, 677–683.

Maughan, T. S., James, R. D., Kerr, D. *et al.* (2002). Comparison of survival, palliation and quality of life with three chemotherapy regimens in metastatic colorectal cancer: a multicentre randomised trial. *The Lancet* **359**, 1555–1563.

Maughan, T. S., James, R. D., Kerr, D. J., Ledermann, J. A., Seymour, M. T. *et al.* (2003). Comparison of intermittent and continuous palliative chemotherapy for advanced colorectal cancer: a multicentre randomised trial. *The Lancet* **361**, 457–464.

Medical Research Council Lung Cancer Working Party. (1993). A randomised trial of three or six courses of etoposide cyclophosphamide methotrexate and vincristine or six courses of etoposide and ifosfamide in small cell lung cancer (SCLC) I: survival and prognostic factors. *British Journal of Cancer* **68**, 1150–1156.

Muss, H. B., Case, L. D., Richards, F. II *et al.* (1991). Interrupted versus continuous chemotherapy in patients with metastatic breast cancer. *New England Journal of Medicine* **325**, 1342–1348.

O'Connell, M. J., Laurie, J. A., Shepherd, L. *et al.* (1996). A prospective evaluation of chemotherapy duration and regimen as surgical adjuvant treatment for high-risk colon cancer: a collaborative trial of the North Central Cancer Treatment Group and the National Cancer Institute of Canada Clinical Trials Group. *Proceedings of American Society of Clinical Oncology* **15**, 209, 478 (abstract).

Paccagnella, A., Cartei, G., Fosser, V. *et al.* (1983). Treatment of multiple myeloma with M-2 protocol and without maintenance therapy. *European Journal of Cancer* **19**, 1345–1351.

Pavlovsky, S., Schvartzman, E., Lastiri, F. *et al.* (1997). Randomized trial of CVPP for three versus six cycles in favorable-prognosis and CVPP versus AOPE plus radiotherapy in intermediate-prognosis untreated Hodgkin's disease. *Journal of Clinical Oncology* **15**, 2652–2658.

Sauerbrei, W., Bastert, G., Bojar, H. *et al.* (2000). Randomized 2x2 trial evaluating hormonal treatment and the duration of chemotherapy in node-positive breast cancer patients: an update based on 10 years' follow-up. *Journal of Clinical Oncology* **18**, 94–101.

Sculier, J. P., Berghmans, T., Castaigne, C. *et al.* (1998). Maintenance chemotherapy for small cell lung cancer: a critical review of the literature. *Lung Cancer* **19**, 141–151.

Seymour, M. T., Stenning, S. P. & Cassidy, J. (1997). Attitudes and practice in the management of metastatic colorectal cancer in Britain. Colorectal Cancer Working Party of the UK Medical Research Council. *Clinical Oncology* **9**, 248–251.

Smalley, R. V., Murphy, S., Huguley, C. M. Jr & Bartolucci, A. A. (1976). Combination versus sequential five-drug chemotherapy in metastatic carcinoma of the breast. *Cancer Research* **36**, 3911–3916.

Smith, I. E., O'Brien, M. E. R., Talbot, D. C. *et al.* (2001). Duration of chemotherapy in advanced non-small cell lung cancer: a randomized trial of three versus six courses of mitomycin, vinblastine, and cisplatin. *Journal of Clinical Oncology* **19**, 1336–1343.

Spiro, S. G. & Souhami, R. L. (1990). Duration of chemotherapy in small cell lung cancer. *Thorax* **45**, 1–2.

Zigmond, A. S. & Snaith, R. P. (1983). The Hospital Anxiety and Depression Scale. *Acta Psychologica Scandinavica* **67**, 361–370.

Chapter 14

Novel approaches in the management of colorectal cancer

Anjana Kulkarni and Daniel Hochhauser

Introduction

Colorectal cancer (CRC) remains a leading cause of cancer mortality in the Western world. Despite significant advances in the treatment of CRC with surgery, radiotherapy and chemotherapy, there remains a need to improve upon current therapies, with increased cure rates in early cases and better survival in advanced disease.

Over the past decade, there have been major advances in our understanding of the molecular factors involved in the development and progression of CRC (Vogelstein *et al.* 1996). This knowledge is already being translated into novel strategies using agents directed against various intracellular targets.

The advent of microarray and proteomic technologies has had major implications for oncological practice. The principle of microarray expression is transcriptional profiling. It has numerous applications:

(a) as a screening test to identify potential novel drug targets, prognostic and predictive markers;
(b) as a method of analysing cell behaviour and the response of genes to specific therapies;
(c) as a classification tool, allowing identification of patients with differing clinical outcomes, such as good responders to a given treatment or long-term survivors (Pusztai *et al.* 2003).

Microarrays have already been used to improve classification of tumours, such as non-Hodgkin's lymphoma, and have demonstrated that they can predict important clinical outcomes in breast cancer (van de Vijver *et al.* 2002). This has enabled the identification of intracellular targets that play a role in the response to anti-cancer agents.

Research has focused on genetic abnormalities that contribute to the development of malignancy. These alterations result in altered protein expression (Liotta *et al.* 2001). De-regulation of cellular proteins activates aberrant signal transduction pathways that contribute to oncogenesis. Proteins are, thus, potential diagnostic and prognostic markers. The field of proteomics has experienced rapid growth, with advances in techniques and improvements upon current methods, such as mass spectrometry coupled with protein microarrays. Only small amounts of tissue or samples of body fluid are necessary for proteomic pattern analysis (Rosenblatt *et al.* 2004).

Studies have shown that this method can be used for the diagnosis of ovarian (Petricoin *et al.* 2002), breast (Li *et al.* 2002), prostate (Adam *et al.* 2002) and liver cancer (Poon *et al.* 2003). It was first described in the detection of early-stage ovarian cancer (Petricoin *et al.* 2002). Using a few microlitres of serum in the assay, this study found that 18 patients with stage 1 disease were correctly identified, as well as those with more advanced disease; 63 of 66 non-cancer cases were correctly identified, demonstrating that the technique has high sensitivity and specificity. Other clinical applications include measurement of response and toxicity to drugs and the identification of new drug targets.

This article gives a brief overview of some of the new and promising agents, directed against molecular targets. There is no attempt to comprehensively cover the strategies being evaluated.

Epidermal growth factor receptor

Studies have shown that many epithelial cancers over-express the receptor for epidermal growth factor (EGFR), including breast, colon, lung, prostate, ovary, pancreas and bladder (Kim *et al.* 2001). Also, over-expression of EGFR has been associated with a poorer prognosis in patients with cancer (Modjahedi *et al.* 1998). Approximately 25–77% of CRCs have abnormalities in the EGFR pathway (Nicum *et al.* 2003). This has stimulated interest in developing agents designed to block or downregulate EGFR, including monoclonal antibodies, tyrosine kinase inhibitors, ligand-linked toxins and antisense approaches (Kim *et al.* 2001).

EGFR (HER-1) is a member of the erb-B family of receptor tyrosine kinases (Carpenter *et al.* 1990). It is a transmembrane protein comprising three domains, including an intracellular tyrosine kinase region (Harari *et al.* 2000). Binding of specific ligands to the receptor induces internalisation of the complex and activates the protein kinase by autophosphorylation. This leads to further activation of downstream signal transduction pathways, which, in turn, result in cell proliferation, tumour growth, progression of invasion and metastasis (Kim *et al.* 2000). These signal transduction pathways also play a key part in processes such as inhibition of apoptosis, angiogenesis, tumour cell motility and cell cycle progression, all of which are contributory factors in the development of malignancies (DeJong *et al.* 1998, Radinsky *et al.* 1995, Nagane *et al.* 1996).

Novel agents targeting EGFR are being evaluated in combination with chemotherapy and radiotherapy. There is preclinical evidence that this may result in synergistic activity against tumours (Sartor *et al.* 2000):

Monoclonal antibodies: cetuximab (Erbitux)

Cetuximab is a chimerized IgG monoclonal antibody, which binds to the EGFR with high affinity, stimulating internalisation of the complex without activation of the tyrosine kinase. This blocks EGFR-mediated signal transduction resulting in cellular apoptosis.

Cetuximab has shown synergistic anti-tumour activity with chemotherapy drugs and radiotherapy, in both *in vitro* and *in vivo* models (Kim *et al.* 2001). In colorectal cancer xenograft models, the combination of cetuximab and irinotecan significantly inhibited tumour growth, resulting in regression rates of 100% and 60% respectively for the two models used. In an irinotecan-refractory tumour model, combined treatment with irinotecan and cetuximab significantly inhibited growth (Prewett *et al.* 2002)

Cetuximab was well tolerated in early trials. The main toxicities are nausea, vomiting, diarrhoea and skin rashes. Previously, it was studied in combination with irinotecan in 121 CRC patients who were EGFR-positive and refractory to both 5-fluorouracil (5-FU) and irinotecan. Seventeen per cent showed a partial response for a median duration of 84 days. 31% had stable disease or a minor response (Saltz *et al.* 2004). These encouraging results led to further phase II studies.

The recent 'BOND' (Bowel Oncology with Cetuximab Antibody) study evaluated the use of cetuximab, in combination with irinotecan or as a single agent, in patients with EGFR-expressing irinotecan-refractory metastatic CRC (Cunningham *et al.* 2004). Five hundred and seventy-seven patients with CRC, who had progressed within three months of irinotecan-based chemotherapy, were initially screened for EGFR expression. Of these, 82% (474 patients) expressed the EGFR on tumour cells; 329 patients were randomised, in a 2:1 ratio, to an infusion of cetuximab followed by weekly cetuximab, with or without irinotecan at the same dose and schedule on which they had been progressing. Those who received cetuximab alone had the option to switch to the combination after progression.

The primary endpoint of the study was objective response rate with secondary endpoints of time to progression, survival time and safety. Of patients receiving the combination of cetuximab and chemotherapy, 22.9% had a measurable response, whereas cetuximab alone demonstrated a response rate of 10.8%. Disease control (complete response + partial response + stable disease) was seen in 55.5% of the combination arm compared with 32.4% of the monotherapy arm. Tumour progression was delayed by a median of 4.1 months in the combination group compared with 1.5 months in the group receiving cetuximab alone. Survival time was 8.6 months compared with 6.9 months. There was no statistically significant difference between the two groups. However, some authors argue that this was probably due to the high level of cross-over from the cetuximab monotherapy arm to combination treatment (56 of 111 patients). For the safety profile of cetuximab in combination with irinotecan, the grade 3/4 toxicities were diarrhoea (21.2%), asthenia (13.7%), acneiform rash (9.4%) and neutropenia (9.5%). Single-agent cetuximab had less toxicity. Importantly, a significant proportion of patients randomised in the study had been heavily pre-treated with conventional irinotecan- and oxaliplatin-based regimens.

The results of this impressive study show that the addition of cetuximab has significant and important activity in patients resistant to chemotherapy, a sub-group for whom there are limited options. Cetuximab may re-sensitise resistant cells to conventional chemotherapy but the mechanisms by which this may occur remain unclear. This study has, thus, raised further issues about the optimal use of cetuximab in chemotherapy regimens for CRC and its potential role in first-line treatment. Larger phase III trials of cetuximab in advanced CRC are now underway.

Tyrosine kinase inhibitors: gefitinib (Iressa)

Small molecules that compete for the ATP-binding site of the EGFR tyrosine kinase have also been investigated as potential therapeutic agents. One of these is gefitinib, which is currently undergoing extensive preclinical and clinical investigation and has shown promising results in several solid tumour types.

One study examined the effects of ZD1839 alone and in combination with cytotoxic drugs in four human cancer cell lines that express EGFR, including GEO colon cancer cells. ZD1839 showed a cytostatic effect on tumour growth and this was associated with a dose-dependent increase in cell apoptosis. Also of particular importance was the finding that, although the effect was cytostatic rather than cytotoxic, the animals treated with ZD1839 showed improved survival (Ciardiello *et al.* 2000).

Gefitinib has been studied in phase II and III studies in non-small-cell lung cancer, and has shown some promising results (Miller *et al.* 2001, Fukuoka *et al.* 2002, Kris *et al.* 2002). This has stimulated interest in further evaluating its use in other solid tumour types, including CRC. There is no current evidence for efficacy of gefitinib in colon cancer. This is of interest in that it suggests that the agents targeting EGFR may have important differences in mechanism of action that translate into variable clinical outcomes.

Studies have shown that ZD1839 may reverse resistance to the active metabolite of irinotecan in human colon tumour cells, through its inhibition of EGFR-tyrosine kinase activity (Braun *et al.* 2002). Ongoing trials are further investigating gefitinib in combination with different regimens and doses of 5-FU and leucovorin. One phase III trial, currently open to recruitment, is the INFORM study which is investigating the safety and efficacy of gefitinib, in conjunction with 5-FU, in irinotecan and 5-FU-refractory CRC patients.

Vascular endothelial growth factor

Tumour-related neovascularisation plays a crucial role in the progression of CRC, with angiogenesis being an essential requirement for tumour growth, invasion and metastasis. Not surprisingly, increased angiogenesis in the primary tumour in CRC has been associated with poor prognosis and relapse of disease (Takebayashi et al. 1996). Factors that play an important role include integrins, fibroblast growth factor and vascular endothelial growth factor (VEGF) (Stoeltzing et al. 2003). This has stimulated interest in the development of anti-angiogenic therapies that target these molecules.

VEGF induces endothelial cell migration, proliferation and invasion and increases vascular permeability in preclinical studies. It mediates angiogenesis via one or more of three tyrosine kinase receptors, which are mainly expressed on endothelial cells. Each receptor plays a role in different signal transduction pathways (Stoeltzing et al. 2003).

Overexpression of VEGF and its receptors correlates with the development of metastases in CRC (Takahashi et al. 1995) Novel agents targeting the VEGFR/ligand system are currently under investigation and include antibodies to VEGF and its receptors and tyrosine kinase inhibitors that block downstream signalling.

Bevacizumab (Avastin)

One of the more extensively investigated agents targeting this system is bevacizumab, a recombinant humanized monoclonal antibody to VEGF. Currently, there are several phase II and III clinical trials studying the efficacy of this agent in metastatic CRC, focusing in particular on its use in combination with standard chemotherapy regimens.

A recent landmark phase III trial evaluated bevacizumab in combination with bolus irinotecan/5-FU/leucovorin (IFL) as first-line treatment in patients with metastatic CRC (Hurwitz et al. 2004). The prospective study randomised 800 patients with metastatic CRC to receive standard chemotherapy with IFL or the same regimen plus bevacizumab.

The primary endpoint was survival, with secondary endpoints of response rate (partial response + complete response), progression-free survival, response duration, quality of life and safety. Results showed a significant improvement in several endpoints in the arm randomised to receive bevacizumab. Median survival was 20.3 months in the bevacizumab arm, compared with 15.6 months with the IFL and placebo regimen. Progression-free survival was also significantly improved by the addition of bevacizumab, 10.6 months compared with 6.2 months. IFL and bevacizumab showed an overall response rate of 45% compared with 35% in the placebo arm.

Importantly, the addition of bevacizumab to standard chemotherapy appears to be well tolerated. Phase II trials had identified bleeding, thrombosis, proteinuria and hypertension as possible safety issues. However, the main adverse effect that appeared to be clearly increased in the bevacizumab plus chemotherapy regimen, in this phase III trial, was hypertension easily managed by oral medications. There was a 1.5% incidence of bowel perforation, although these events are uncommon. The study concluded that bevacizumab in combination with IFL had an acceptable side-effect profile and significantly increased survival, progression-free survival, response rate and duration of response in patients with previously untreated metastatic CRC.

This trial is the first phase III validation of an anti-angiogenesis strategy to treat CRC. It raises important issues with regards to the future use of bevacizumab, in combination with conventional cytotoxic agents and in conjunction with other new agents directed at intracellular targets. These promising results in metastatic CRC have stimulated interest in the potential benefits of bevacizumab in the adjuvant setting. Further trials are necessary to clarify the appropriate scheduling and length of treatment with bevacizumab. Other studies evaluating bevacizumab, in combination with other cytotoxic drugs in CRC and other tumour types, including metastatic renal carcinoma and locally recurrent/metastatic breast cancer, are currently underway.

Cyclooxygenase-2 inhibitors

Cyclooxygenase (COX) is a key enzyme involved in prostaglandin synthesis (DuBois *et al.* 1998). Prostaglandins regulate numerous physiological processes and are produced in a diverse range of tissues throughout the body. Two isoforms of the COX enzyme have been identified. Studies show COX-1 is expressed in most tissues in the body constitutively, whereas COX-2 is not normally present in most tissues. Instead its production is induced in sites of inflammation by specific growth factors and cytokines (Smith *et al.* 2000). Conventional non-steroidal anti-inflammatory drugs (NSAIDs) are known to inhibit both COX-1 and COX-2. Studies have suggested that the analgesic and anti-inflammatory properties of these drugs are based on their inhibition of COX-2, whereas the gastrointestinal side effects are due to lack of COX-1-mediated prostaglandin production in gastric epithelium (Masferrer *et al.* 1994). This stimulated the search for specific inhibitors of COX-2.

COX-2 expression and colorectal cancer

The major prostaglandin produced by the COX pathway in epithelial cells is prostaglandin E2, raised levels of which have been demonstrated in human colonic tumours (Rigas *et al.* 1993). Studies have shown an association between COX-2 protein expression and the development of tumours; moreover this expression seems to occur early in the disease process. Also, importantly, these studies showed that the degree of protein expression correlates with tumour size and depth of invasion, which has implications for its use as a prognostic indicator (Church *et al.* 2003).

Various mechanisms of action have been proposed, including induction of tumour cell apoptosis, inhibition of angiogenesis and inhibition of other enzymes, such as matrix metalloproteinases, which may play a role in the invasion of malignant tumours (Church *et al.* 2003). The inhibition of COX and the resulting fall in prostaglandin levels has been established (Fitzgerald *et al.* 2001), though how this translates into downstream cellular events remains unclear.

Non-steroidal anti-inflammatory drugs

Past epidemiological studies have suggested that conventional non-steroidal anti-inflammatory drugs (NSAIDs) such as aspirin, may reduce the incidence of or the risk of death from CRC by 50% in regular users (Thun *et al.* 1991). There is a significant body of evidence supporting the anti-cancer effect of NSAIDs *in vivo*. Studies looking at the effect of indomethacin on intestinal tumours in rats showed that tumour development was significantly reduced or even prevented compared with growth in control animals (Pollard *et al.* 1980; Narisawa *et al.* 1981). Studies have shown similar anti-tumour benefits of other conventional NSAIDs, for example aspirin, piroxicam, sulindac and ibuprofen. Also, studies in patients with familial adenomatous polyposis (FAP) have shown reductions in the number and size of colonic polyps in patients taking NSAIDs (Cruz-Correa *et al.* 2002).

As mentioned previously, the main drawback of conventional NSAIDs is their side-effect profile. However, the newer COX-2 inhibitors have fewer in the way of gastrointestinal risks. These drugs have potential therapeutic applications in both prevention and treatment of CRC and are currently being assessed in phase II and III settings.

Clinical applications of COX-2 inhibitors

Chemoprevention

A recent multi-centre trial in the USA studied the use of oral celecoxib, a COX-2 selective inhibitor, in patients with FAP. Patients received celecoxib or placebo for six months. Results showed a decrease in polyp numbers from the baseline by a mean of 28% compared with 4.5% in the control group. The overall size of polyps and polyp burden was also reduced in those taking celecoxib (Steinbach *et al.* 2000). This trial has prompted the recent approval of the use of celecoxib as a chemoprevention agent in patients with FAP.

It has been noted that drugs such as celecoxib and rofecoxib may cause renal impairment in the elderly and increase the risk of cardiovascular events in some users (Ahmad *et al.* 2002; Mukherjee *et al.* 2001). Furthermore, it is not yet clear whether the results above translate into benefits for patients with sporadic colonic tumours. Studies have demonstrated that COX-2 expression may be higher in sporadic tumours compared with hereditary non-polyposis colonic cancer (Sinicrope *et al.* 1999).

Adjuvant therapy

The use of COX-2 inhibitors in the adjuvant setting is an attractive concept, especially in view of the significant rate of relapse in patients with Duke's B and C disease after potentially curative surgery. The rationale for their use is based on their anti-angiogenic and pro-apoptotic properties discussed previously.

Trials were planned to evaluate the role of these agents in the prevention of recurrence after potentially curative surgery. The VICTOR study is a phase III randomised, double-blind, placebo-controlled trial evaluating rofecoxib, a COX-2–selective inhibitor, in CRC patients after curative therapy. It is currently open to recruitment and is an international multicentre trial aiming to recruit 7,000 patients over five years. Patients are randomised to receive either rofecoxib or placebo once daily, for either two or five years.

The primary hypothesis is that rofecoxib administered for two years will result in greater overall survival compared with placebo. The secondary hypotheses are that rofecoxib administered for two years will result in greater relapse-free survival compared with placebo, and that rofecoxib administered for five years will result in greater overall and relapse-free survival than rofecoxib administered for two years.

Importantly, rofecoxib appears to be reasonably well-tolerated and has been evaluated for safety in approximately 12,000 individuals, including 1,000 patients treated for one year or longer.

Advanced disease

The use of COX-2 inhibitors in conjunction with chemotherapy has already shown benefit in some *in vitro* and *in vivo* studies. For example, one study used celecoxib and irinotecan to treat colonic cancer xenograft tumours in nude mice. Combined treatment resulted in 91.4% reduction in tumour growth compared with 28.7% for irinotecan alone and 72.3% for celecoxib alone. There was also a reduction in the incidence of irinotecan-induced diarrhoea when used in association with celecoxib (Trifan *et al.* 2002).

Phase II trials have also shown promising results with the use of COX-2 inhibitors as an adjunct to standard chemotherapy regimens (Blanke *et al.* 2002). Several clinical trials were designed to evaluate these agents further in the setting of advanced CRC and to test their efficacy and safety when used in conjunction with standard cytotoxic drugs. However, because of the observed high incidence of cardiovascular toxicities (including myocardial infarction and cerebrovascular events) observed with rofecoxib (Vioxx), the drug was withdrawn in October of last year (2004) and the VICTOR study was terminated. It remains unclear as to whether all COX-2 inhibitors will prove to have a similar toxicity profile (Fitzgerald 2004; Topol 2004).

Other strategies

Other strategies, currently under relatively earlier investigation, involve other targets:

Proteasome inhibitors

The ubiquitin–proteasome pathway has been shown to play an important role in cell cycle regulation (Hilt & Wolf 1996). This occurs by programmed intracellular protein breakdown, which in turn leads to downstream changes in specific signal transduction pathways. Lactacystin, peptide aldehydes and dipeptide boronate derivatives are a few of the inhibitors of this pathway that have been identified.

One specific inhibitor, PS-341 (Velcade, bortezomib), has shown anti-tumour activity in various human tumour cells *in vitro* (Adams *et al.* 1999). It has also shown a synergistic effect in combination with radiation, cyclophosphamide, cisplatin, fluorouracil, gemcitabine, irinotecan and adriamycin (Teicher *et al.* 1999). In phase I studies, partial responses and stable disease have been observed in non-small-cell lung cancer, melanoma and sarcoma (Aghajanian *et al.* 2001, Hamilton *et al.* 2001). Ongoing phase II trials of PS-341, as a single-agent and in combination with conventional cytotoxics, are currently underway in breast, brain and other solid tumours (Wright *et al.* 2000).

Histone deacetylase inhibitors

The action of several transcription factors, involved in cell cycle regulation, is dependent on histone acetylation by histone acetyltransferases (Struhl 1998). The process of carcinogenesis in several tumour types has been associated with disruption of acetylation. In contrast, histone deacetylases (HDACs) suppress this transcriptional activity and thereby potentially promote the development of cancer (Wolffe *et al.* 1996). Thus, drugs that inhibit HDAC activity are currently under development. Examples of HDAC inhibitors that have been identified include butyrate, trichostatin A, suberoylanilide hydroxamic acid (SAHA), desipeptide and benzamide compounds.

MS-275 is a benzamide derivative that has already shown promise in preclinical studies and is currently being assessed in phase I and II trials. It induces cell cycle arrest and has shown significant anti-tumour activity on a variety of human tumour cell lines, including myeloma, colon, lung and ovarian tumours. In colon cancer xenograft models, it has demonstrated comparable or superior antitumour effects to fluorouracil (Saito *et al.* 1999). A phase I trial of MS-275 in lymphomas and other solid tumours is now underway.

SAHA is one of the more extensively tested HDAC inhibitors. One study of the effect of SAHA on mammary tumours in rats showed a reduction in the incidence of tumours by 40% and a mean reduction in tumour volume of 78% without toxic side effects (Marks *et al.* 2001). Also, this agent suppressed growth of androgen-dependent prostate tumours in nude mice, with a reduction in the mean tumour volume of up to 97% (Butler *et al.* 2000). Phase I clinical trials have shown that SAHA is well tolerated at doses that cause accumulation of acetylated histones in tumour cells. It also resulted in significant anti-tumour activity in these studies (Kelly *et al.* 2001).

Conclusion

Many novel agents are under investigation in the prevention and management of early and advanced CRC. This brief overview highlights several promising approaches that target pathways involved in angiogenesis, invasion and metastasis. There have been significant advances in our understanding of these mechanisms and their translation into therapeutic applications, with the treatment of CRC entering a new era. However, there needs to be further investigation into the cost–benefit issues that have been highlighted, because of the fact, for example, that cetuximab with irinotecan may cost up to £12,000 per full course of treatment (and bevacizumab *possibly* up to £20,000 per course of treatment). It is likely that the other novel therapies may well also incur similar levels of costs.

These new agents, in combination with conventional cytotoxic regimens, are already showing promise in phase II and III settings, in terms of increased remission rates, prolonged progression-free and overall survival, and positive effects on time free of symptoms and quality of life. The continuing challenge is to use these more complex treatment strategies as effectively as possible, thus ensuring the maximal benefit for individual patients.

References

Adam, B. L., Qu, Y., Davis, J. W. *et al.* (2002). Serum protein fingerprinting coupled with a pattern-matching algorithm distinguishes prostate cancer from benign prostate hyperplasia and healthy men. *Cancer Research* **62**, 3609–3614.

Adams, J., Palombella, V. J., Sausville, E. A. *et al.* (1999). Proteasome inhibitors: a novel class of potent and effective antitumor agents. *Cancer Research* **59**, 2615–2622.

Aghajanian, C., Soignet, S., Dizon, D. S. *et al.* (2001). A phase I trial of the novel proteasome inhibitor PS341 in advanced solid tumor malignancies. *Proceedings of the American Society of Clinical Oncology* **20**, 338a (abstract).

Ahmad, S. R., Kortepeter, C., Brinker, A., Chen, M. & Beitz, J. (2002). Renal failure associated with the use of celecoxib and rofecoxib. *Drug Safety* **25**, 537–544.

Blanke, C. D., Benson III, A. B., Dragovich, T., Lenz, H. J., Haller, D., Robles, C. *et al.* (2002). A phase II trial of celecoxib (CX), irinotecan (I), 5-fluorouracil (5FU), and leucovorin (LCV) in patients (pts) with unresectable or metastatic colorectal cancer (CRC). *Proceedings of the American Society of Clinical Oncology* **21**, 127a (abstract).

Braun, A., Dirsch, O., Lindtner, B. *et al.* (2002). Inhibition of the epidermal growth factor receptor by ZD1839 ('Iressa') reverses resistance to the active metabolite irinotecan (SN-38) in human colon tumor cells. *Proceedings of the American Association for Cancer Research* **43**, 952 (abstract A4713).

Butler, L. M., Agus, D. B., Scher, H. I. *et al.* (2000). Suberoylanilide hydroxamic acid, an inhibitor of histone deacetylase, suppresses the growth of prostate cancer cells in vitro and in vivo. *Cancer Research* **60**, 5165–5170.

Carpenter, G. & Cohen, S. (1990). Epidermal growth factor. *Journal of Biological Chemistry* **265**, 7709–7712.

Church, R. D., Fleshman, J. W. & McLeod, H. L. (2003). Cyclo-oxygenase inhibition in colorectal cancer therapy. *British Journal of Surgery* **90**, 1055–1067.

Ciardiello, F., Caputo, R., Bianco, R. et al. (2000). Antitumor effect and potentiation of cytotoxic drugs activity in human cancer cells by ZD-1839 (Iressa), an epidermal growth factor receptor-selective tyrosine kinase inhibitor. *Clinical Cancer Research* **6**, 2053–2063.

Cruz-Correa, M., Hylind, L. M., Romans, K. E., Booker, S. V., Giardiello, F. M. (2002). Long-term treatment with sulindac in familial adenomatous polyposis: a prospective cohort study. *Gastroenterology* **122**, 641–645.

Cunningham, D., Humblet, Y., Siena, S., Khayat, D., Bleiberg, H., Santoro, A., Bets, D., Mueser, M., Harstrick, A., Verslype, C., Chau, I. & Van Cutsem, E. (2004). Cetuximab monotherapy and cetuximab plus irinotecan in irinotecan-refractory metastatic colorectal cancer. *New England Journal of Medicine* **351**, 337–345.

DeJong, J. S., van Diest, P. J., van der Valk P. et al. (1998). Expression of growth factors, growth-inhibiting factors, and their receptors in invasive breast cancer. II: correlations with proliferation and angiogenesis. *Journal of Pathology* **184**, 53–57.

DuBois, R. N. et al. (1998). Cyclooxygenase in biology and disease. *FASEB Journal* **12**, 1063–1073.

FitzGerald, G. A. (2004). Coxibs and cardiovascular disease. *New England Journal of Medicine* **351**, 1709–1711.

FitzGerald, G. A. & Patrono, C. (2001). The coxibs, selective inhibitors of cyclooxygenase-2. *New England Journal of Medicine* **345**, 433–442.

Fukuoka, M. & Yano, S., Giaccone G et al. (2002). Final results from a Phase II trial of ZD1839 ('Iressa') for patients with advanced non-small-cell lung cancer (IDEAL 1). *Proceedings of the American Society of Clinical Oncology* **21**, 298a.

Hamilton, A. L., Eder, J. P., Pavlick, A. C. et al. (2001). PS-341: phase I study of a novel proteasome inhibitor with pharmacodynamic endpoints. *Proceedings of the American Society of Clinical Oncology* **20**, 336a (abstract).

Harari, P. M. & Huang, S. M. (2000). Modulation of molecular targets to enhance radiation. *Clinical Cancer Research* **6**, 323–325.

Hilt, W. & Wolf, D. H. (1996). Proteasomes: destruction as a programme. *Trends in Biochemical Sciences* **21**, 96–102.

Hurwitz, H., Fehrenbacher, L., Novotny, W., Cartwright, T., Hainsworth, J., Heim, W., Berlin, J., Baron, A., Griffing, S., Holmgren, E., Ferrara, N., Fyfe, G., Rogers, B., Ross, R. & Kabbinavar, F. (2004). Bevacizumab plus irinotecan, fluorouracil, and leucovorin for metastatic colorectal cancer *New England Journal of Medicine* **350**, 2335–2342.

Kelly, W. K., Richon, V. M., Troso-Sandoval, T. et al. (2001). Suberoylanilide hydroxamic acid (SAHA), a histone deacetylase inhibitor: biologic activity without toxicity. *Proceedings of the American Society of Clinical Oncology* **20**, 87a (abstract).

Kim, E.S., Khuri, F.R., Herbst, R.S. (2001). Epidermal growth factor receptor biology (IMC-C225). *Current Opinion in Oncology* **13**, 506–513.

Kris, M. G., Natale, R. B., Herbst, R. S. et al. (2002). A Phase II trial of ZD1839 ('Iressa') in advanced non-small-cell lung cancer (NSCLC) patients who had failed platinum- and docetaxel-based regimens (IDEAL 2). *Proceedings of the American Society of Clinical Oncology* **21**, 292a.

Li, J., Zhang, Z., Rosenzweig, J. et al. (2002) Proteomics and bioinformatics approaches for identification of serum biomarkers to detect breast cancer. *Clinical Chemistry* **48**, 1296–1304.

Liotta, L., Kohn, E. C. & Petricoin, E. F. (2001). Clinical proteomics: personalized molecular medicine. *Journal of the American Medical Association* **286**, 2211–2214.

Malcolm, R. (2002). ZD1839 (Iressa™): For more than just non-small cell lung cancer. *Oncologist* **7**(4), 16–24.

Marks, P. A., Richon, V. M., Breslow, R. & Rifkind, R. A. (2001). Histone deacetylase inhibitors as new cancer drugs. *Current Opinion in Oncology* **13**, 477–483.

Masferrer, J. L. et al. (1994). Selective inhibition of inducible cyclooxygenase-2 in vivo is anti-inflammatory and nonulcerogenic. *Proceedings of the National Academy of Sciences of the United States of America* **91**, 3228–3232.

Miller, V. A., Johnson, D. H., Heelan, R. T. et al. (2001). A pilot trial demonstrates the safety of ZD1839 (Iressa), an oral epidermal growth factor receptor tyrosine kinase inhibitor (EGFR-TKI), in combination with carboplatin (C) and paclitaxel (P) in previously untreated advanced non-small cell lung cancer. *Proceedings of the American Society of Clinical Oncology* **20**, 326a (abstract).

Modjahedi, H., Affleck, K., Stubberfield, C. et al. (1998). EGFR blockade by tyrosine kinase inhibitor or monoclonal antibody inhibits growth, directs terminal differentiation and induces apoptosis in human squamous cell carcinoma HN5. *International Journal of Oncology* **13**, 335–342.

Mukherjee, D., Nissen, S. E. & Topol, E. J. (2001). Risk of cardiovascular events associated with selective COX-2 inhibitors. *Journal of the American Medical Association* **286**, 954–959.

Nagane, M., Coufal, F., Lin, H., et al. (1996). A common mutant epidermal growth factor receptor confers enhanced tumorigenicity on human glioblastoma cells by increasing proliferation and reducing apoptosis. *Cancer Research* **56**, 5079–5086.

Narisawa, T., Sato, M., Tani, M., Kudo, T., Takahashi, T. & Goto, A. (1981). Inhibition of development of methylnitrosourea-induced rat colon tumors by indomethacin treatment. *Cancer Research* **41**, 1954–1957.

Nicum, S., Midgley, R., Kerr, D. J. (2003). Colorectal cancer. *Acta Oncologica* **42**, 263–275.

Petricoin, E. F., Ardekani, A. M., Hitt, B. A. et al. (2002). Use of proteomic patterns in serum to identify ovarian cancer. *The Lancet* **359**, 572–577.

Pollard, M. & Luckert, P. H. (1980). Indomethacin treatment of rats with dimethylhydrazine-induced intestinal tumors. *Cancer Treatment Reports* **64**, 1323–1327.

Poon, T. C., Yip, T. T., Chan, A. T. et al. (2003). Comprehensive proteomic profiling identifies serum proteomic signatures for detection of hepatocellular carcinoma and its subtypes. *Clinical Chemistry* **49**, 752–760.

Prewett, M. C., Hooper, A. T., Bassi, R., Ellis, L. M., Waksal, H. W., Hicklin, D. J. (2002). Enhanced antitumor activity of anti-epidermal growth factor receptor monoclonal antibody IMC-C225 in combination with irinotecan (CPT-11) against human colorectal tumor xenografts. *Clinical Cancer Research* **8**, 994–1003.

Pusztai, L., Ayers, M., Stec, J., Hortobágyi, G. N. (2003). Clinical application of cDNA microarrays in oncology. *Oncologist* **8**, 252–258.

Radinsky, R., Risin, S., Fan, Z. et al. (1995). Level and function of epidermal growth factor receptor predict the metastatic potential of human colon carcinoma cells. *Clinical Cancer Research* **1**, 19–31.

Rigas, B., Goldman, I. S. & Levine, L. (1993). Altered eicosanoid levels in human colon cancer. *Journal of Laboratory and Clinical Medicine* **122**, 518–523.

Rosenblatt, K. P., Bryant-Greenwood, P., Killian, J. K., Mehta, A., Geho, D., Espina, V., Petricoin, E. F. & Liotta, L. A. (2004). Serum proteomics in cancer diagnosis and management. *Annual Review of Medicine* **55**, 97–112.

Saito, A., Yamashita, T., Mariko, Y. et al. (1999). A synthetic inhibitor of histone deacetylase, MS-27-275, with marked in vivo antitumor activity against human tumors. *Proceedings of the National Academy of Sciences of the United States of America* **96**, 4592–4597.

Saltz, L. B., Meropol, N. J., Loehrer Sr, P. J., Needle, M. N., Kopit, J. & Mayer, R. J. (2004). Phase II trial of cetuximab in patients with refractory colorectal cancer that expresses the epidermal growth factor receptor. *Journal of Clinical Oncology* **22**, 1201–1208.

Sartor, C. (2000). Biological modifiers as potential radiosensitizers: targeting the epidermal growth factor receptor family. *Seminars in Oncology* **27** (Suppl. 11), 15–20.

Sinicrope, F. A., Lemoine, M., Xi, L., Lynch, P. M., Cleary, K. R., Shen, Y. et al. (1999). Reduced expression of cyclooxygenas 2 proteins in hereditary nonpolyposis colorectal cancers relative to sporadic cancers. *Gastroenterology* **117**, 350–358.

Smith, W. L., DeWitt, D. L. & Garavito, R. M. (2000). Cyclooxygenases: structural, cellular and molecular biology. *Annual Review of Biochemistry* **69**, 145–182.

Steinbach, G., Lynch, P. M., Phillips, R. K., Wallace, M. H., Hawk, E., Gordon, G. B. et al. (2000). The effect of celecoxib, a cyclooxygenase-2 inhibitor, in familial adenomatous polyposis. *New England Journal of Medicine* **342**, 1946–1952.

Stoeltzing, O., Liu, W., Reinmuth, N., Parikh, A., Ahmad, S., Jung, Y. D., Fan, B. S. & Ellis, L. M. (2003). Angiogenesis and antiangiogenic therapy of colon cancer liver metastasis. *Annals of Surgical Oncology* **10**, 722–733.

Struhl, K. (1998). Histone acetylation and transcriptional regulatory mechanisms. *Genes and Development* **12**, 599–606.

Takahashi, Y., Kitadai, Y., Bucana, C. D., Cleary, K. R. & Ellis, L. M. (1995). Expression of vascular endothelial growth factor and its receptor, KDR, correlates with vascularity, metastasis, and proliferation of human colon cancer. *Cancer Research* **55**, 3964–3968.

Takebayashi, Y., Aklyama, S., Yamada, K., Akiba, S., Aikou, T. (1996). Angiogenesis as an unfavorable prognostic factor in human colorectal carcinoma. *Cancer* **78**, 226–231.

Teicher, B. A., Ara, G., Herbst, R. et al. (1999). The proteasome inhibitor PS-341 in cancer therapy. *Clinical Cancer Research* **5**, 2638–2645.

Thun, M. J., Namboodiri, M. M. & Heath Jr, C. W. (1991). Aspirin use and reduced risk of fatal colon cancer. *New England Journal of Medicine* **325**, 1593–1596.

Topol, E. J. (2004). Failing the public health—rofecoxib, Merck, and the FDA. *New England Journal of Medicine* **351**, 1707–1709.

Trifan, O. C., Durham, W. F., Salazar, V. S., Horton, J., Levine, B. D., Zweifel, B. S. et al. (2002). Cyclooxygenase-2 inhibition with celecoxib enhances antitumor efficacy and reduces diarrhoea side effect of CPT-11. *Cancer Research* **62**, 5778–5784.

van de Vijver, M. J., He, Y. D., van't Veer, L. J., Dai, H., Hart, A. A., Voskuil D. W. et al. (2002). A gene-expression signature as a predictor of survival in breast cancer. *New England Journal of Medicine* **347**, 1999–2009.

Vogelstein, B. & Kinzler, K. W. (1996). Lessons from hereditary colorectal cancer. *Cell* **87**, 159–170.

Wolffe, A. P. (1996). Histone deacetylase: a regulator of transcription. *Science* **272**, 371–372.

Wright, J., Hillsamer, V. L., Gore-Langton, R. E. et al. (2000). Clinical trials referral resource. Current clinical trials for the proteasome inhibitor PS-341. *Oncology (Huntington NY)* **14**, 1589–1590, 1593–1594, 1597.

PART 4

Clinical governance of colorectal cancer services

Chapter 15

Recent judgements of the National Institute for Clinical Excellence: their scientific basis, clinical credibility and moral implications

Catherine A. McBain and Mark P. Saunders

Introduction

Around half of the 35,390 patients diagnosed with colorectal cancer each year in the UK will go on to develop metastases and will die of their disease (Office for National Statistics 2000). Without treatment, the median survival of these patients with advanced colorectal cancer (ACRC) is around six months, with few surviving beyond one year. Until relatively recently, treatment options were limited; 5-fluorouracil (5-FU) has been the mainstay of treatment for 40 years, its use about doubling median survival.

The development of new agents active in the treatment of ACRC has greatly altered the management of this disease. Combinations of irinotecan and oxaliplatin with 5-FU have brought new opportunities to prolong survival and improve quality of life. New oral fluoropyrimidines such as capecitabine offer convenient oral alternatives to intravenous treatments and the development of surgical resection of hepatic and pulmonary metastases offers the hope of cure.

The cost of these new agents for the many patients with ACRC, and the ensuing funding implications for the NHS, have made the treatment of this malignancy the subject of detailed scrutiny and the issuance of guidelines by the National Institute for Clinical Excellence (NICE). The aim of this chapter is to discuss the guidelines, to review their scientific basis and to discuss their implications in terms of financial cost and impact on patient care and on UK oncology practice.

The National Institute for Clinical Excellence

On 1 April 1999, the National Institute of Clinical Excellence (NICE) was established to evaluate the clinical and cost-effectiveness of various medical technologies, including pharmaceuticals. Its remit includes providing patients, health professionals and the public with authoritative, robust and reliable guidance on current 'best practice' and encouraging improvement in the quality of healthcare delivered nationally. Initially, Appraisal Committee considers a technology the using evidence from commissioned independent assessments and submissions from professional and patient groups and industry. The form of evidence is specified as clinical outcomes, cost per quality adjusted life year (QALY) and the impact on the cost of NHS and social services. Particular attention is paid to high quality, adequately powered randomised controlled trials. A provisional advisory document (PAD) is produced and comments invited from all interested parties before release of the final advisory document (FAD). Appeals may be lodged after this final guidance is produced, but if an appeal is unsuccessful, the process stops and the *Technology Appraisal Guidance* (TAG) is published on the NICE website and as a booklet.

NICE guidelines relating to advanced colorectal cancer

The guidance on the use of irinotecan, oxaliplatin and raltitrexed for the treatment of advanced colorectal cancer (ACRC) was published in March 2002 (NICE 2002). The process began in August 2000 with reports submitted by the pharmaceutical industry, UKCCCR, CancerBACUP, Macmillan Cancer Relief and ScHARR (the School of Health and Related Research, University of Sheffield). Advice was also sought from the MRC Trials Unit and from the Royal College of General Practitioners. The appraisal committee included a single external expert and a patient advocate (NICE TAG33, 2002). A FAD was published in April 2001 but interested parties successfully appealed and after further consideration of the evidence, a revised FAD was produced in December 2001. Following a second appeal, NICE guidance was finally published on 7 March 2002.

The guidance issued to date is as follows:

- *5-fluorouracil and folinic acid (5-FU/FA)* are advocated as first line treatment. On the balance of clinical and cost-effectiveness, neither irinotecan nor oxaliplatin in combination with 5-FU/FA are recommended for routine first-line therapy for advanced colorectal cancer.
- *Irinotecan* monotherapy is recommended in patients who have failed an established 5-FU containing treatment regime.
- *Oxaliplatin* should be considered for use as first-line therapy, in combination with 5-FU/FA, in advanced colorectal cancer in patients with metastases confined solely to the liver *and* may become resectable ('downstaged') following treatment.
- *Raltitrexed* is not recommended for use outside appropriately designed clinical studies.
- Enrolment of patients into the MRC CR08 FOCUS trial, which is evaluating the first- and second-line use and sequencing of irinotecan and oxaliplatin, is encouraged.

Chemotherapy in advanced colorectal cancer

Before discussing the clinical credibility of these NICE guidelines and their impact on the management of advanced colorectal cancer in the UK, it is necessary to review and discuss the evidence for the use of these agents to date.

5-fluorouracil

5-FU has been in use for approximately 40 years and various different administration regimes have been developed and investigated. Bolus injection of 5-FU results in a response rate of only around 10% with no survival benefit, largely due to the very short half-life of the parent compound and its metabolites. When given as a continuous infusion, response rates are increased (22% versus 14%) and a small survival benefit results (Meta-analysis Group in Cancer 1998). Modulation with folinic acid (FA) essentially prolongs the effect of 5-FU, conferring benefit similar to that seen with a continuous infusion. Many combinations of 5-FU and FA exist and two of the most common have been directly compared (de Gramont et al. 1997). The European infusional 5-FU/FA approach pioneered by Professor de Gramont was found to be better than the North American bolus 5-FU/FA strategy developed at the Mayo clinic. The response rate for the de Gramont regimen was significantly higher at 32.6% compared with 14.4% with the Mayo regimen ($p = 0.0004$). Progression-free survival (PFS) was increased, although median overall survival was similar (Mayo 56.8 weeks; de Gramont 62 weeks, $p = 0.067$).

The de Gramont regimen was also much better tolerated, with significantly less mucositis. Nonetheless, there is still an Atlantic divide in the chosen way of administering 5-FU and FA. Overall, when either of these regimens is used, the response rate is generally about 20–25% and the median overall survival is increased to approximately 12 months.

When should chemotherapy be instigated?: evidence for early intervention

Treatment early in the disease process, when the patient is fit and well, is preferable. An important paper by the Nordic GI Tumour Adjuvant Therapy Group (Nordic GI Group, 1992) randomised 183 asymptomatic patients with ACRC to early treatment with 5-FU/FA chemotherapy, or no treatment until symptoms appeared. The patients treated early had a longer median survival (14 versus 9 months) and an increased median symptom-free period (10 versus 2 months). This emphasised the need to treat patients soon after they present with metastatic disease, rather than wait until they are symptomatic and may well not be fit enough to receive chemotherapy at all.

Irinotecan

Irinotecan is a topoisomerase 1 inhibitor that does not exhibit cross-resistance with 5-FU. There are now four published randomised controlled trials with irinotecan, which show a survival benefit over 5-FU/FA combinations. Two initial trials used irinotecan monotherapy given 'second-line' to patients who had failed 5-FU/FA chemotherapy. Cunningham et al (1998) randomised patients whose disease had progressed after receiving 5-FU/FA to either irinotecan or best supportive care (BSC); Rougier et al. (1998) randomised patients who had failed bolus 5-FU/FA to receive either irinotecan or an infusional 5-FU regimen. Both studies showed a significant survival benefit (median survivals of 9.2 versus 6.5 months, $p = 0.0001$, Cunningham, Pyrhonen & James 1998; and 10.8 versus 8.5 months, $p = 0.035$, Rougier *et al*. 2000), with an improved quality of life (QoL).

The evidence for the use of irinotecan and 5-FU/FA together as first-line treatment of patients with ACRC is also compelling. Two large randomised trials involving more than 1,000 patients have been published from Europe and North America. Both showed improved response rates, increased median times to progression and treatment failure and significant survival benefits when patients received an Ir.5-FU/FA combination compared with 5-FU/FA alone (median survival 17.4 versus 14.1 months, Douillard *et al*. 2000; median survival 14.8 versus 12.6 months, Saltz *et al*. 2000). These overall survival (OS) benefits were achieved despite a significant number of the control patients 'crossing over' to the irinotecan containing arm on disease progression (31% and 56% in the two studies, respectively), suggesting that the survival benefit would probably be even greater if 'crossover' were not allowed. It also suggests that giving irinotecan 'up-front' is advantageous, since patients in the irinotecan first-line arms of both studies still fared better, despite the considerable number of patients in the control arms who crossed over to receive irinotecan 'second line' on 5-FU/FA failure. Irinotecan is now licensed in the UK for the treatment of patients with ACRC either 'up-front' in combination with 5-FU/FA, or as a single agent after they have failed 5-FU. When it is combined with 5-FU/FA and given as first-line treatment to patients with metastatic disease, the response rate is 40–50% and the median overall survival is approximately 15–17 months.

Oxaliplatin

Oxaliplatin is a new platinum derivative that has been found to be active in colorectal cancer. Approximately, a 40–50% response rate is achieved when it is given in combination with 5-FU/FA (Ox.5-FU/FA) to patients with ACRC. There have been two large randomised studies comparing first-line 5-FU/FA to a similar regimen but also containing oxaliplatin (de Gramont *et al*. 2000; Giacchetti *et al*. 2000). In the de Gramont study the response rate was increased from under 23% to more than 50%. PFS was increased from approximately 6 to 9 months but an OS benefit was not achieved by the addition of oxaliplatin (16.2 versus 14.7 months, $p = 0.12$). In the Giacchetti paper, the OS for *both* the control and treatment arms was in the order of 19 months. This length of survival in the control arm was much longer than would be expected for a simple 5-FU/FA regimen, where a median OS of about one year would be predicted. This probably reflects the crossover effect from the control arm to oxaliplatin-based therapy on disease progression. If crossover was not allowed, a significant survival benefit may well have been achieved.

Oxaliplatin before liver resection

Patients with metastatic colorectal cancer have a five-year survival of less than 5% whatever chemotherapy regimen is chosen. However, a small proportion of patients develop liver or lung metastases that can be removed (1–2% of all patients with colorectal cancer). In such instances, the five-year survival is increased to around 30–40%. A few patients present with inoperable liver metastases that can be downstaged with chemotherapy to make them operable. Bismuth *et al.* (1996, updated by Adam *et al.* 2001) showed that, from a group of more than 700 patients with inoperable liver disease, 13.5% were downstaged enough to have a curative resection. The survival of these patients was improved considerably (35% five-year survival). Giacchetti *et al.* (1999) also retrospectively showed that 38% of patients with inoperable liver disease could be downstaged with oxaliplatin-based chemotherapy to allow a curative resection and improved survival (50% five-year survival). Therefore, the advent of oxaliplatin has provided some hope for this small group of patients with inoperable liver disease.

Combined irinotecan and oxaliplatin

Since irinotecan and oxaliplatin have been shown to be extremely active in patients with ACRC, the obvious step forward would be to give patients both of these new drugs. The FOLFOX/FOLFIRI study by Tournigand *et al.* (2004) randomised patients to receive either Ox.5-FU/FA (FOLFOX) or Ir.5-FU/FA (FOLFIRI) initially, crossing over to receive the other arm when the disease progressed. The first-line response rate to FOLFIRI was 56% and to FOLFOX6 was 54%, while the median PFS was 8.5 and 8.0 months, respectively. The second-line response rate to both regimens was low, being 4% for FOFIRI and 15% for FOLFOX6. The median survival exceeded that seen in any previous advanced CRC studies (*ca.* 21 months in both treatment arms: data presented later at the American Society of Clinical Oncology (ASCO), San Francisco, 2001). A GI intergroup study (N9741) was initially presented by Goldberg at ASCO 2002 and later at the colorectal perspectives meeting in Barcelona (Goldberg *et al.* 2004). Just under 800 patients were randomised into three arms (1: Ir + bolus 5-FU/FA; 2: FOLFOX; 3: Ir.Ox). The response rate of the irinotecan arms (arms 1 and 3) was 31% and 35%, respectively, whereas it was 45% for the FOLFOX arm (arm 2). The median overall survival was also significantly increased in this arm compared with the others (arm 1: 15.0 months, arm 2: 19.5 months, arm 3: 17.4 months). However, two main concerns arise. The patients in arm 2 (who had the highest response rate and longest overall survival) received infusional 5-FU, rather than none or bolus, and also had the opportunity to receive irinotecan on disease progression. Very few patients treated in the irinotecan arms were able to receive second-line oxaliplatin since it was generally unavailable in North America at that time. Overall, however, the evidence for both drugs is rapidly emerging and as Dr Leonard Saltz (Memorial Sloan-Kettering) stated at ASCO in May 2002: 'We need all three drugs. We have conflicting data about how to best use them, but, clearly, we need to have them all available to our patients.'

Table 15.1 Summary of approximate response rates and survival advantages for chemotherapy regimes used in ACRC (see text for definitions of abbreviations)

Treatment	Response rate (%)	Median survival (months)
Best supportive care (BSC)	–	5–8
5-FU/FA	20–25	12
Ox.5-FU/FA	40–50	16–19
Ir.5-FU/FA	40–50	15–17
Ir.5FU/FA / Ox.5FU/FA	50–60	18–21

Oral fluoropyrimidines

The oral fluoropyrimidines such as capecitabine and tegafur/uracil are more convenient and acceptable forms of chemotherapy compared with the intravenous fluoropyrimidine, 5-FU. Both are prodrugs of 5-FU. Two randomised studies with capecitabine (Van Cutsem *et al.* 2001; Hoff *et al.* 2001) and two with tegafur/uracil (Douillard *et al.* 2002; Carmichael *et al.* 2002) have shown equivalence to bolus i.v . 5-FU/FA. They have not been compared with an infusional 5-FU regimen and therefore a conclusion about their comparative efficacy in this situation cannot be made. Capecitabine can result in hand foot syndrome, troublesome in approximately 15% of patients, but overall, both appear at least as good as 5-FU with acceptable toxicity profiles. Although both drugs cost more than 5-FU/FA, there will be savings in terms of central venous catheters, infusion pumps, hospital visits and staff time. NICE produced guidance in May 2003 and stated 'oral therapy with either capecitabine or tegafur with uracil (in combination with folinic acid) is recommended as an option for the first-line treatment of metastatic colorectal cancer'. In terms of patient preference, oral fluoropyrimidines have been shown to be more acceptable than intravenous 5-FU (Borner et al, 2002) and NICE also stated that the individual and clinician should make the choice of regimen jointly.

Raltitrexed

Raltitrexed, a direct thymidylate synthetase inhibitor, was launched in 1996, its major advantages being ease of administration and lack of cardiac toxicity. Its inclusion as one of three arms in the MRC CR06 trial (comparing it with infusional 5-FU administered by either the Lokich or de Gramont regimens) showed comparable response rates and median overall survival times, but increased toxicity and a very much higher rate of treatment related deaths (Maughan *et al.* 2002). While indications for its use are not widespread, it remains a useful option to be considered in patients with problematic cardiac arrhythmias or ischaemic heart disease.

NICE guidelines and trial evidence: areas of conflict

The NICE guidelines issued in relation to advanced colorectal cancer have been controversial, eliciting dispute from clinicians and patient groups and generating letters to the national and medical press (*Daily Telegraph* June 2002; Cassidy *et al.* 2002; Benjamin *et al.* 2002; Saunders and Valle. 2002). The Health Technology Board for Scotland (HTBS), the Scottish equivalent of NICE, have 'rubber-stamped' the NICE decision or, as Dorothy-Grace Elder (a member of Scottish Parliament) also stated in *The Herald* in June 2002, 'put a kilt on it'!

Throughout much of Europe, oxaliplatin or irinotecan are regularly used in combination with 5-FU/FA. In March 2000, the Oncologic Drugs Advisory Committee of the U.S. Food and Drug Administration (FDA) approved the first-line use of combined irinotecan and 5-FU/FA for patients with ACRC. More recently, the FDA has also approved the use of oxaliplatin in combination with 5-FU/FA for patients with ACRC. There is concern, therefore, that the NICE guidelines put UK colorectal oncology practice significantly out of step with its European and North American counterparts.

The NICE guidance is disputed on several issues

Interpretation of survival benefits: cross-over within trial arms

As discussed previously, crossover from the control (5-FU/FA) arms to the 'new agent' treatment arm was seen in all the major clinical trials that randomised patients between 5-FU/FA and irinotecan or oxaliplatin combinations. All trials were analysed on an intention-to-treat basis. While it was morally correct that patients failing on the control arm should be allowed to cross over to receive the new agent, and equally correct that the trial analyses did not formally recognise this, the impact of this crossover effect cannot be ignored. In particular, the randomised study by de Gramont *et al.* (2000) showed a much higher than expected median overall survival in the control 5-FU/FA arm because of the crossover of these patients to the oxaliplatin-containing arm or because they also received irinotecan at some point. If crossover was not allowed, a significant survival benefit may well have been achieved.

Use of single-agent irinotecan rather than in combination

Combinations of irinotecan with 5-FU/FA are well tolerated and a patient's quality of life is no worse than with 5-FU/FA (de Gramont regimen) alone (Douillard *et al.* 2000). However, single-agent irinotecan, as recommended by NICE, is given at approximately twice the dose, and the prevalence of alopecia, and grade III/IV nausea (15% vs 2.1%), diarrhoea (22% vs 13.1%) and vomiting (14% vs 2.8%) is increased compared with the two-weekly irinotecan/de Gramont schedule commonly used in the UK. (Figures quoted are drawn from separate studies by Cunningham *et al.* (1998) and Douillard *et al.* (2000), respectively.)

Delayed use of new agents rather than 'up-front' use

The evidence for the use of Ir.5-FU/FA in the first-line treatment of patients with ACRC is significant. The two published large randomised trials (Douillard *et al.* 2000; Saltz *et al.* 2000) are discussed above, both showing a significant survival benefit when patients receive an Ir.5-FU/FA combination compared with 5-FU/FA alone. Outcomes in the treatment arms, where irinotecan was given 'up-front', were superior to the control arms, where many patients (31% and 56% respectively) received 5-FU/FA followed by Ir.5/FU.FA. Similarly, the FOLFOX/FOLFIRI study (Tournigand *et al.* 2004) showed a first-line response rate to both arms of approximately 55% and a median survival that exceeded that seen in any previous ACRC studies using first-line 5-FU/FA alone.

Use of oxaliplatin to downstage patients with inoperable liver metastases

While the recommendation for the use of oxaliplatin in patients with inoperable liver metastases, which can potentially be made operable with chemotherapy, is welcomed, this applies to a very small number of patients. The characteristics of such patients must be clearly defined at a multidisciplinary level, particularly in conjunction with hepatobiliary surgeons. NICE failed to offer guidance on the type of patients for which this treatment would be appropriate.

No recommendation for raltitrexed

The use of raltitrexed in patients with ACRC was not recommended by NICE outside appropriately designed clinical studies. 5-fluorouracil should be used with care and may even be contraindicated in patients with problematic arrhythmias and ischaemic heart disease. At present the only effective alternative is raltitrexed and some oncologists feel that this drug should be made available and used with caution in this particular situation.

Cost effectiveness

If irinotecan and 5-FU/FA were given 'up-front' to patients with advanced CRC as recommended by the US FDA, they would receive a single period of 'active treatment' until disease progression. Upon disease progression, they may have the opportunity to enter appropriate clinical trials or receive best supportive care (BSC). If the NICE guidance is followed, patients would receive 5-FU/FA until disease progression followed by single agent irinotecan if they are still fit enough. This would lead to two periods of 'active treatment', amounting to 6 to 12 months of chemotherapy, after which they would receive more intensive follow-up than if they received BSC. This is expensive in terms of staff time and, more importantly, patient time, as well as in monetary terms, with additional outpatient visits and increased demand on pharmacy, pathology and radiology services.

Cunningham *et al.* (2002) performed a detailed cost-effectiveness analysis of Douillard *et al.'s* trial (2000), randomising patients to 5-FU/FA with or without irinotecan as first-line treatment of ACRC. This trial showed a significant survival advantage for the irinotecan arm. While drug acquisition costs were higher for the irinotecan arm, drug administration costs and costs associated with complications of disease and treatment were comparable. In the follow-up period, costs associated with further chemotherapy and with disease progression were lower for patients who had received irinotecan first-line and equated to a cost-effectiveness ratio per life year gained (LYG) of £14,794. This compares favourably to a range surmised from a Department of Health review (1999) of available cost-effectiveness studies, which suggests that incremental costs per LYG of £15,000–£20,000 for a cancer treatment can be considered reasonable. Hence, this treatment may be viewed as cost-effective compared with currently accepted best practice (Cunningham *et al.* 2002). While NICE bases its appraisals on clinical- and cost-effectiveness thresholds these measures are not specified.

Implications of NICE guidelines

Evidence is steadily accruing that the use of all three drugs (Ir., Ox., 5-FU) in different combinations and sequencing leads to improved patient survival (Tournigand *et al.* 2004). Restriction of the use of these drugs in line with NICE guidelines has direct implications for individual patients, overall UK CRC survival figures and the future of colorectal cancer research in the UK.

Patient choice

Almost all patients now have direct access to the results of clinical trials and the wealth of additional information that is available on the Internet. Given that informed consent and patient choice are paramount, patients are unlikely to accept they are unable to receive treatment that is standard in much of Europe and North America. This unacceptable situation places oncologists in a difficult predicament on a daily basis.

'Rationing' by treatment deferral

NICE have accepted that only 75% of patients (likely to be an overestimate) will still be fit enough to receive irinotecan after first-line 5-FU/FA (NICE 2002). Therefore, 25% of patients who were initially deemed fit enough to receive a first-line combination of Ir.5-FU/FA or oxaliplatin 5-FU/FA will, in-fact, be denied this therapy because their disease has progressed and their fitness deteriorated. The MRC CR06 trial, which randomised patients between infusional 5-FU (Lokich or de Gramont) and raltitrexed, included a second randomisation (CR06 B) whereby, on completion of the first three months of their randomised treatment, patients with stable or responding disease were randomised again to either continue treatment or to discontinue their chemotherapy until disease progression. Less than half restarted, and although survival was not improved in the arm who continued chemotherapy, these findings emphasise that when treatment is kept in reserve for use on disease progression, most patients will cease to be fit enough to receive it, denying them the chance of an initial response.

A further point of concern is that deferring the use of new agents until 5-FU failure commits patients to at least two periods of 'active treatment' before phase 1 trials of novel agents would be considered. Consequentially, fewer patients are likely to be fit for entry into such evaluating therapies including molecular targeting agents vaccines or gene-therapies, which may ultimately be pivotal in treating colorectal cancer.

The targets of The National Cancer Plan

The five-year survival figures for the UK are already extremely poor compared with Europe and North America (41%, 47% and 63%, respectively) (National Statistics 2000; Office for National Statistics 2000). The government aims to reduce cancer deaths by 10% by 2010 (*Saving Lives: Our Healthier Nation* 1999) and to bring UK cancer survival figures into line with the rest of Europe. Failure to allow the introduction of new agents for ACRC into a first-line setting can only serve to widen the gulf that already exists between cancer treatments in the UK, and the US and Europe. One of the aims of the Government's National Cancer Plan is to 'never fall behind again'. However, in the case of CRC, the baseline from which to fall has yet to be reached.

The future of research in ACRC in the UK

To continue with internationally accepted research, UK trials in advanced colorectal cancer must have a control arm that is acceptable to the rest of the world. If North America and Europe are using irinotecan and oxaliplatin regularly, research using just a 5-FU/FA-control arm may no longer be considered relevant by others outside the UK. Gaining the charitable and pharmaceutical industry funding, on which many trials rely, will become even more difficult since these bodies naturally want to fund research that is up to date with the appropriate control arms.

Review of NICE guidelines: MRC CR08 (FOCUS) study

NICE is due to review its guidance on new drugs for advanced colorectal cancer again this year (2005) when data from the MRC CR08 (FOCUS) study become available. This large multi-centre randomised trial recently just closed in the UK. It aimed to address the questions of first- and second-line use and sequencing of irinotecan and oxaliplatin. Patients with ACRC were randomised into one of 5 treatment arms; all arms included infusional 5-FU and folinic acid administered in a modified de Gramont (MdG) regimen. Patients in the four trial arms received MdG with irinotecan or oxaliplatin given either first-line or on disease progression after MdG alone. Patients in the control arm received MdG, with single-agent irinotecan on disease progression. Approximately halfway through the study, a third line of therapy was added to allow those patients who had not received oxaliplatin or irinotecan in the first two lines of therapy to receive the drug that they had 'missed out'. In this way, all patients had the opportunity to receive all of the drugs at some point, so long as they were fit enough to be given all three lines of chemotherapy. This trial accrued well, and hopes to provide definitive conclusions about the comparable efficacy of these new agents and whether they are best delivered 'up-front' or reserved until disease progression. The final results are eagerly awaited.

Conclusion

Later this year (2005), when NICE plans to review its guidance, the routine use of first-line irinotecan and oxaliplatin combinations will have become even more established in North America and much of Europe. This Atlantic divide between our routine treatment strategies will probably widen even further and the UK may become even more out of step with its management of ACRC. Let us also hope that NICE will allow oncologists in the UK to offer all of the available therapies to their patients, in a similar manner to the rest of the world.

References

Adam, R., Avisar, E., Ariche, A. *et al.* (2001). Five-year survival following hepatic resection after neoadjuvant therapy for nonresectable colorectal cancer. *Annals of Surgical Oncology* **8**, 347–353.

Benjamin, I., Poston, G. & Sherlock, D. (2002). Is the NICE process flawed? *The Lancet* **359**, 2120

Bismuth, H., Adam, R., Levi, F. *et al.* (1996). Resection of nonresectable liver metastases from colorectal cancer after neoadjuvant chemotherapy. *Annals of Surgery* **224**, 509–520, discussion 520–522.

Borner, M., Schoffski, P., de Wit, R. *et al.* (2002). Patient preference and pharmacokinetics of oral modulated UFT versus intravenous fluorouracil and leucovorin: a randomised crossover trial in advanced colorectal cancer. *European Journal of Cancer* **38**, 349–358.

Carmichael, J., Popiela, T., Radstone, D. *et al.* (2002). Randomised comparative study of Tegafur/Uracil and oral leucovorin versus parenteral fluorouracil and leucovorin in patients with previously untreated metastatic colorectal cancer. *Journal of Clinical Oncology* **20**, 3617–3627.

Cassidy, J., Bridgewater, J. *et al.* (2002). Is the NICE process flawed? *The Lancet* **359**, 2120.

Cunningham, D., Pyrhonen, S., James, R D. *et al.* (1998). Randomised trial of irinotecan plus supportive care versus supportive care alone after fluorouracil failure for patients with metastatic colorectal cancer. *The Lancet* **352**, 1413–1418.

Cunningham, D., Falk, S. & Jackson, D. (2002). Clinical and economic benefits of irinotecan in combination with 5-fluorouracil and folinic acid as first line treatment of metastatic colorectal cancer. *British Journal of Cancer* **86**, 1677–1683.

de Gramont, A., Bosset, J. F., Milan, C. *et al.* (1997). Randomised trial comparing monthly low-dose leucovorin and fluorouracil bolus with bimonthly high-dose leucovorin and fluorouracil bolus plus continuous infusion for advanced colorectal cancer: a French intergroup study. *Journal of Clinical Oncology* **15**, 808–815.

de Gramont, A., Figer, A., Seymour, M. *et al.* (2000). Leucovorin and fluorouracil with or without oxaliplatin as first-line treatment in advanced colorectal cancer. *Journal of Clinical Oncology* **18**, 2938–2947.

Department of Health (1999). *Saving Lives: Our Healthier Nation*. London: Stationery Office.

Douillard, J. Y., Cunningham, D., Roth, A. D. *et al.* (2000). Irinotecan combined with fluorouracil compared with fluorouracil alone as first-line treatment for metastatic colorectal cancer: a multicentre randomised trial. *The Lancet* **355**, 1041–1047.

Douillard, J. Y., Hoff, P. M., Skillings, J. R. *et al.* (2002). Multicentre phase III study of uracil/tegafur and oral leucovorin versus fluorouracil and leucovorin in patients with previously untreated metastatic colorectal cancer. *Journal of Clinical Oncology* **20**, 3605–3616.

Giacchetti, S., Itzhaki, M., Gruia, G. *et al.* (1999). Long-term survival of patients with unresectable colorectal cancer liver metastases following infusional chemotherapy with 5-fluorouracil, leucovorin, oxaliplatin and surgery. *Annals of Oncology* **10**, 663–669.

Giacchetti, S., Perpoint, B., Zidani, R. *et al.* (2000). Phase III multicenter randomised trial of oxaliplatin added to chronomodulated fluorouracil-leucovorin as first-line treatment of metastatic colorectal cancer. *Journal of Clinical Oncology* **18**, 136–147.

Goldberg, R. M., Sargent, D. J., Morton, R. F. *et al.* (2004). A randomised controlled trial of fluorouracil plus leucovorin, irinotecan and oxaliplatin combinations in patients with previously untreated metastatic colorectal cancer. *Journal of Clinical Oncology* **22**, 23–30.

Hoff, P. M., Ansari, R., Batist, G. *et al.* (2001). Comparison of oral capecitabine versus intravenous fluorouracil plus leucovorin as first-line treatment in 605 patients with metastatic colorectal cancer: results of a randomised phase III study. *Journal of Clinical Oncology* **19**, 2282–2292.

Maughan, T. S., James, R. D., Kerr, D. J. *et al.* (2002). Comparison of survival, palliation and quality of life with three chemotherapy regimes in metastatic colorectal cancer: a multicentre randomised trial. *The Lancet* **359**, 1555–1563.

Meta-analysis Group in Cancer (1998). Efficacy of intravenous continuous infusion of fluorouracil compared with bolus administration in advanced colorectal cancer. *Journal of Clinical Oncology* **16**, 301–308.

National Institute for Clinical Excellence (NICE) (2002). Guidance on the use of irinotecan, oxaliplatin and raltitrexed for the treatment of advanced colorectal cancer. Technology Appraisal Guidance No. 33.

National Institute for Clinical Excellence (NICE) (2003). Guidance on the use of capecitabine and tegafur with uracil for metastatic colorectal cancer. Technology Appraisal Guidance No. 61.

National Statistics (2000). *The Official UK Statistics Site*. StatStore VI.2.

Nordic Gastrointestinal Tumor Adjuvant Therapy Group (1992). Expectancy or primary chemotherapy in patients with advanced asymptomatic colorectal cancer: a randomised trial. *Journal of Clinical Oncology* **10**, 904–911.

Office for National Statistics. (2000). *Cancer Survival 1991–1998*.

Rougier, P., Van Cutsem E., Bajetta E. *et al.* (1998). Randomised trial of irinotecan versus fluorouracil by continuous infusion after fluorouracil failure in patients with metastatic colorectal cancer. *The Lancet* **352**, 1407–1412.

Saltz, L. B., Cox, J. V., Blanke, C. *et al.* (2000). Irinotecan plus fluorouracil and leucovorin for metastatic colorectal cancer. Irinotecan Study Group. *New England Journal of Medicine* **343**, 905–914.

Saunders, M. P. & Valle, J. W. (2002). Why hasn't the National Institute for Clinical Excellence been 'NICE' to patients with colorectal cancer? *British Journal of Cancer* **86**, 1667–1669.

Tournigand, C., Andre, T., Achille, E. *et al.* (2004). FOLFIRI followed by FOLFOX6 or the reverse sequence in advanced colorectal cancer: A randomised GERCOR study. *Journal of Clinical Oncology* **22**, 229–237.

Van Cutsem, E., Twelves, C., Cassidy, J. *et al.* (2001). Oral capecitabine compared with intravenous fluorouracil plus leucovorin in patients with metastatic colorectal cancer: results of a large phase III study. *Journal of Clinical Oncology* **19**, 4097–4106.

Chapter 16

Risk adjustment in colorectal cancer surgery: the role of hierarchical models in comparative clinical audit

P. P. Tekkis, J. D. Stamatakis, M. R. Thompson and C. G. Marks

Introduction

Surgery is now in the era of objective assessment and professional accountability for clinical outcomes (Spiegelhalter *et al.* 2002). Increasing emphasis is being placed on the clinical effectiveness and quality of healthcare provision, with the individual patient being the focus of quality improvement. Meaningful comparisons of outcomes between or within hospitals may be undertaken by careful adjustment for patient risk factors. However, before making any inference about the effectiveness or quality of care it is essential to make proper adjustments for risk (comparing like with like, i.e., apples with apples).

Clinical audit is primarily concerned with clinical effectiveness and differs from randomised trials whereby investigators attempt to control for patient risk factors by defining eligibility. Randomisation also minimises selection bias, yielding groups that are similar across patient characteristics. Studies of clinical effectiveness are often population based, with no control for risk factors, no randomisation to providers or treatment groups and no defined management protocol (Blumberg 1986).

Historical precedents

Mortality data have been collected for centuries in England primarily to study epidemic illnesses. English hospitals have accumulated statistics on their patients since the 1600s but, as noted by the 1863 Report for the Medical Officer of the Privy Council, '*the public as a rule still look to the death rates of hospitals as the best indication of the relative healthiness*' (Bristowe & Holmes 1864). At the same time, Florence Nightingale (1820–1910) published the third edition of her book, *Notes on Hospitals*, describing the structural defects, principles of construction and proposed hospital plans for reducing deaths from unsanitary conditions. In addition, she made recommendations for '*improving methods of tabulating hospital statistics, together with a proposal for a uniform system for registering statistics of surgical operations, their complications and results*'. Most startling was the 91% mortality among inmates at 24 London hospitals from a total of 106 principal hospitals in England during the year 1861 (see Figure 16.1). Nightingale warned that '*there was undoubtedly some difficulty in arriving at correct statistical comparison to exhibit this. For in the first place, different hospitals receive very different proportions of the same class of diseases. The ages in one hospital may differ considerably from the ages in another. And the state of the cases on admission may differ very much in each hospital. These elements affect considerably the result of treatment altogether apart from the sanitary state of hospitals*' (Nightingale 1863). Nightingale actually highlighted the importance of considering the patients' case-mix and indeed modern methodologies are intended to adjust for this as much as possible so that the remaining variation can be considered as measuring differences in quality of care.

Mortality per Cent. in the principal Hospitals of England. 1861.

	Number of SPECIAL INMATES on the 8th April, 1861.	Average Number of INMATES in each HOSPITAL.	Number of DEATHS registered in the Year 1861.	MORTALITY per Cent. on INMATES.
IN 106 PRINCIPAL HOSPITALS OF ENGLAND	12709	120	7227	56·87
24 London Hospitals	4214	176	3828	90·84
12 Hospitals in Large Towns	1870	156	1555	83·16
25 County and Important Provincial Hospitals	2248	90	886	39·41
30 Other Hospitals	1136	38	457	40·23
13 Naval and Military Hospitals	3000	231	470	15·67
1 Royal Sea Bathing Infirmary (Margate)	133	133	17	12·78
1 Dane Hill Metropolitan Infirmary (Margate)	108	108	14	12·96

Figure 16.1 Extract from Florence Nightingale's *Notes on Hospitals* comparing mortality rates among inmates from a total of 106 principal hospitals in England during the year 1861.

In the field of colorectal cancer, UK regional audits were held in the 1990s in Wessex (1993), Wales and Trent (Mella *et al.* 1997), and in the Scottish health districts of Lothian and Borders (1995). More recently, the Association of Coloproctology of Great Britain and Ireland (ACPGBI) has conducted two national audits:

- A multi-centre malignant bowel obstruction (MBO) study (April 1998 – April 1999) on 1,046 patients from 146 UK hospitals (Stamatakis *et al.* 2000).
- A colorectal cancer (CRC) study to which 73 NHS trusts contributed 8,077 new colorectal cancer cases diagnosed over a 12-month period (April 1999 – 2001) (Tekkis *et al.* 2002).

This chapter illustrates, with representative examples from the MBO and CRC studies, the value of audit of data and the absolute need for risk adjustment in comparing outcomes between or within units. We also describe the principles of hierarchical analysis in deriving risk-adjusted outcomes using audit data from these studies.

Uses of mortality prediction models

Operative mortality is an outcome that can be readily measured and used for monitoring performance within a trust or between trusts. However, for this measure to be truly objective it must be adjusted for patient-related risk factors (case mix). Mortality prediction models are potentially attractive for an increasingly broad range of applications. Many of these applications can be politically sensitive, have potentially significant consequences and can be applied at three levels:

Patient level
- Provision of an estimated numerical probability of survival as part of the process of informed consent.
- Patients may use outcome data, available in the public domain, to compare different hospitals or other institutions.

Clinician level
- Educational use to review quality of local care. Outcomes can be compared with local, regional, national and international results.
- Use of outcome information for individual clinicians' local appraisal.

Institutional level
- Institutional self-monitoring for competitive contractual reasons.
- Formal monitoring by regulatory authorities and agencies.
- To inform local and national resource allocation, for example provision of high-dependency unit (HDU) beds and Confidential Enquiry into Peri-Operative Deaths (CEPOD) list.

Data quality and standardisation

Accurate, reliable data, in which clinicians have confidence, are an absolute prerequisite and demand organised and disciplined methods of collection. Reported data must be precise and detailed enough to withstand robust, and potentially hostile, scrutiny. The quality and scope of audit data will have to be greatly improved before they can be used to compare the performance of clinicians. That this is achieved is of considerable importance because such data will be used for clinical governance and resource allocation and surgeons, together with the multidisciplinary team, should therefore strive to ensure data are recorded as accurately as possible. There is a need for standardisation and uniformity of data collection with a nationwide system, maintained at local hospitals, with direct links for central data analysis and regular feedback. Implementation of such systems within hospitals should lead to an increased awareness in the use of such data, with subsequent improvement in the quality of the data collection. The reliability of the process of data collection should be formally assessed and monitored on a prospective basis. High-quality audit is resource intensive and requires appropriate funding. The initial costs of the Wales, Trent and Wessex colorectal cancer audits were similar, approximating to £40–50 per patient (Stamatakis et al. 2001). This represents less than 1% of the total treatment costs. Successful audit will require dedication from senior clinicians and resources for sophisticated statistical analysis and dissemination of the results.

Defining outcomes

Measuring quality of care is an issue that must be addressed to retain the respect and confidence of those whom we seek to treat (Keogh & Kinsman 2001). The concept of quality should include the entire structure and process of care from the preliminary assessment to the time of discharge and beyond. Individual surgical performance, though significant, constitutes only a small part of this process. Extreme caution should therefore be exercised before attempting to draw conclusions about the quality of surgery, delivered by individual surgeons or units, based simply on in-hospital mortality data. Mortality may be assessed as in-hospital mortality, defined as death during the same hospital admission as the operation, regardless of cause. An alternative outcome is 30-day operative mortality, defined as death from any cause occurring within 30 days of an operative procedure, either in hospital or following discharge from hospital. The latter is more difficult to measure, as patients who are discharged early need to be followed up for a period of 30 days following surgery. A combination of 30-day and in-hospital mortality has also been used in relatively recent risk-adjusted outcome studies (Birkmemeyer et al. 2002). In the MBO and CRC reports, 30-day operative mortality was used as the main outcome measure. From the patients' perspective, other measures such as long-term survival, post-operative complications or quality of life are also important.

Dimensions of risk

Risk adjustment is commonly used to calculate the so-called 'algebra of effectiveness' (Iezzoni 1997) shown in Figure 16.2. The underlying hypothesis is that patients' outcomes are a complex function, not only of the patients' clinical attributes (dimensions of risk) and other factors such as random events, but also of the effectiveness and quality of the services provided. It is imperative to minimise the practical difficulties in data collection and standardisation of data harvesting and to appreciate that no degree of risk adjustment is likely to account for all the patient attributes.

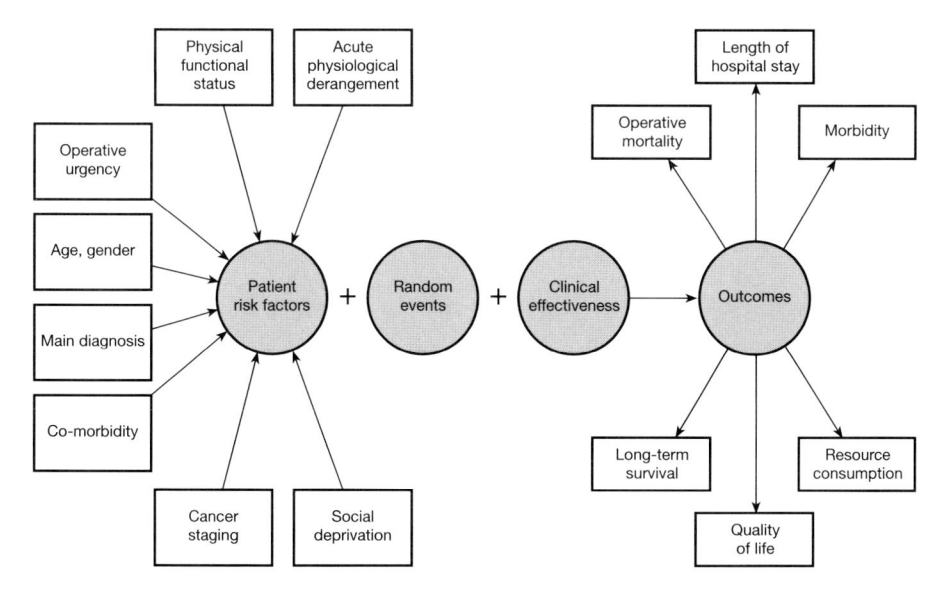

Figure 16.2 The algebra of effectiveness.

Age

Age is one variable that is recorded in most cases and although the physiology of aging is poorly understood, in colorectal surgery older patients are more likely to have worse clinical outcomes than younger patients (see Figure 16.3). The very elderly are a special class of patients. Many believe that these patients are physiologically different from younger patients, possibly due to lack of any physiological reserve, and they need to be addressed as a separate subgroup.

Gender

Although gender is an important factor in epidemiological studies of long-term survival, its statistical value, in predicting short-term outcomes, is often modest, as in the case of the MBO and CRC studies.

Physiological derangement

Identification of physiological derangement involves tests that reflect basic function such as vital signs, haematological and biochemical investigations, level of consciousness, etc. This dimension may be independent of the underlying diagnosis. However, a relatively small number of parameters appear to be sufficient to evaluate physiological derangement and contribute to much of the variation in outcome among patients undergoing surgery (see Figure 16.4). Currently available mortality prediction models take account of physiological derangement in different ways.

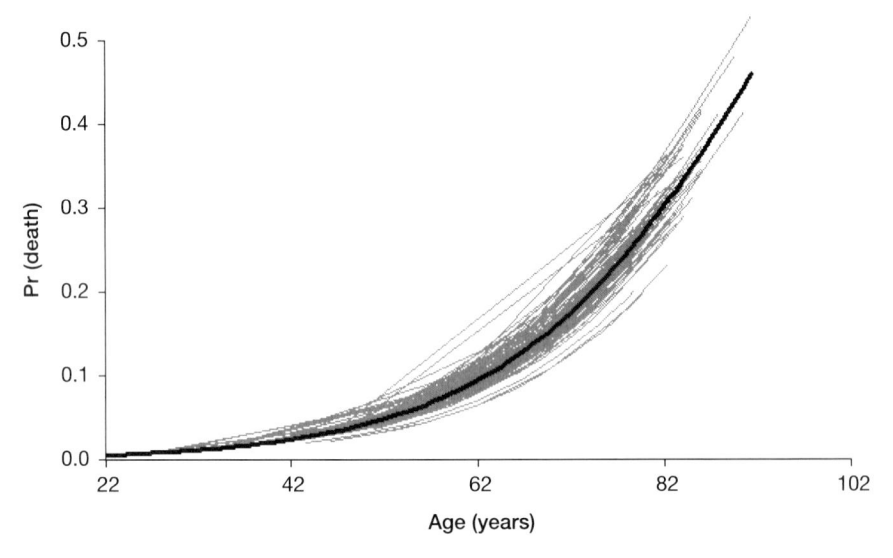

Figure 16.3 Variation of operative mortality with age for patients presenting with malignant large bowel obstruction. Each hospital is represented by individual prediction curves, with the median regression line of the total population superimposed on the curves for individual hospitals.

Jones, H. J. S., de Cossart L. *et al.* (1999) reviewed various scoring systems, including the APACHE and POSSUM grades of the American Society of Anaesthesiologists (ASA), which are currently used to evaluate physiological status (APACHE standing for Acute Physiology and Chronic Health Evaluation and POSSUM for Physiological and Operative Severity Score for the enUmeration of Mortality and morbidity).

The ASA grading is simple and has been widely used since 1963 when it was first proposed (Dripps *et al.* 1963). It is very effective and, when the age is also taken into account, there is an additive, predictive effect (Hall & Hall 1996). The drawback of ASA is that it is subjective and therefore open to manipulation.

The APACHE scoring systems are used exclusively in the intensive therapy setting. The original APACHE (Knaus *et al.* 1981) used 34 physiological variables taking the worst value in the first 24 hours of admission to an intensive therapy unit (ITU). APACHE II (Knaus *et al.* 1985) comprised an acute physiological score from 12 physiological variables added to a score derived for age and chronic health. The APACHE II system has been widely used in the UK and although it is a valid tool in the emergency general surgical population, its applicability to elective surgical admissions to ITU has been questioned. The APACHE III score (Knaus *et al.* 1991) is a development that uses 18 physiological variables and, in the UK, has been mainly used in Scotland and South-West Thames Region. The application of the APACHE system in colorectal surgery is limited to patients requiring ITU admission, which is not representative of patients undergoing surgery for colorectal cancer.

	APACHE II	APACHE III	SAPS	POSSUM	MPM
Temperature	+	+	+		
Blood pressure	+	+	+	+	+
Pulse rate	+	+	+	+	+
Respiratory rate					
Respiratory effort					
PaO$_2$	+	+			
pH	+	+			
Bicarbonate			+		
Haemoglobin				+	
Haematocrit	+	+	+		
White blood cell count	+	+	+	+	
Sodium	+	+	+	+	
Potassium	+		+	+	
Creatinine	+	+			
Albumin		+			
Bilirubin		+			
Glucose		+	+		
Urea	+	+	+		
Urine output		+	+		
Glasgow Coma Scale	+	+	+	+	+
ECG				+	
Capillary refill					
Cardiac signs				+	
Respiratory signs				+	
Chronic health	+	+			+
Age	+		+	+	+

Figure 16.4 Scoring systems and their components utilised in surgery: APACHE (Acute Physiology and Chronic Health Evaluation), SAPS (Simplified Acute Physiological Score), POSSUM (Physiological and Operative Severity Score for the enUmeration of Mortality and morbidity), MPM (Mortality Probability Model).

The POSSUM (Copeland *et al*, 1991) and p-POSSUM (Whiteley *et al*. 1996; Prytherch *et al*. 1998) scoring systems were developed in 1991 and 1998 respectively. Both use 12 physiological variables to give a physiological score and a 6-factor operative severity score, for predicting operative mortality (Figure 16.4). Although the POSSUM scoring systems have been validated in patients undergoing general, colorectal surgery (Sagar *et al*. 1993, 1994; Tekkis *et al*. 2000) and vascular surgery

(Midwinter *et al.* 1999), they were not applicable to emergency vascular surgery, and a recent study has shown that both systems under-predict outcome in the emergency setting and in the elderly colorectal population (Tekkis *et al.* 2001). The question as to whether the weights assigned to acute physiological variables should vary depending on the patient's diagnosis is unresolved. Nevertheless, indices based on physiological parameters are objective and therefore are not generally open to abuse. The fields can be collected automatically by interfacing with hospital IT systems, which may reduce costs.

Emergency admission or operative urgency?

Emergency surgery is an important factor in determining post-operative mortality and long-term survival in colorectal cancer. The precise definition of emergency surgery is critical. In the MBO and CRC audits surgical procedures were defined according to the National Confidential Enquiry into Patient Outcome and Death (NCEPOD) classification (2000) ('elective' and 'scheduled' procedures were grouped together):

- *Elective.* Operation at a time to suit both patient and surgeon.
- *Scheduled.* An early operation but not immediately lifesaving, usually within three weeks.
- *Urgent.* Operation as soon as possible after resuscitation.
- *Emergency.* Immediate life-saving operation, resuscitation simultaneous with surgical treatment.

It is important to note that many patients who have an emergency admission do not have emergency surgery and their risk of dying from surgery approximates to that of an elective case. The post-operative mortality of a true emergency case was twice that of an elective/scheduled operation in the MBO audit (20.0% versus 12.9%) and 3.5 times the elective mortality in the CRC audit (19.3% versus 5.6%). It is therefore important that emergency should refer to surgery rather than the mode of admission.

Disease severity and cancer staging

The severity of disease, for example the extent of cancer spread (staging), is an important determinant of long-term outcome. With regard to short-term outcomes (30-day operative mortality), Dukes' A, B or C did not make a significant contribution to the risk estimate whereas Dukes' D was found to be an independent predictor of outcome in both the MBO and the CRC audits (see Figure 16.5). In the UK, Dukes' staging (Dukes 1932) is still used with most bowel cancers. The original Dukes' classification was based entirely on pathological examination of the level of invasion in the resected specimen. In spite of Dukes' concerns about the accuracy of surgeons' observations, it is now common practice to combine pathological staging with clinical assessment. Turnbull *et al.* (1967), who defined Dukes' stage D as any patient with metastatic or residual local disease, first introduced this clinico-pathological staging in 1967. Other instigators have defined Dukes' stage D as any metastatic disease in the abdomen alone, as in the Wessex audit, or any systemic or residual local disease, as in the Wales and Trent, the MBO, and CRC audits. A further consideration when comparing surgical outcomes based on cancer staging, is the use of increasingly sophisticated pre- and intra-operative liver imaging, which would inevitably mean that Dukes' D stage will no longer be based on clinical assessment alone. A direct consequence of intensive imaging would be the up-staging of cancers and the associated stage migration, known as 'the Will Rogers phenomenon'. (While commenting on the geographic migration of the 1930s, the American humorist Will Rogers is alleged to have said, 'When the Okies left Oklahoma and moved to California, they raised the average intelligence levels of both states' (Feinstein *et al.* 1985).) An analogous phenomenon occurs with stage migration, whereby if a population of patients is more accurately staged, it will improve the survival of all stages because patients with subtle advanced disease are upstaged. Therefore, the staging protocols used by different centres should be clearly defined. In addition, the need for change to the TNM staging systems (1966) may be necessary to overcome the shortcomings of the Dukes' classification.

Cancer site and type of operative procedure

Cancer site was coded in the MBO and CRC audits as in the ICD10 classification. In the CRC audit a total 7,509 entries were collected for tumour site. Rectal cancers constituted 45.5% of all cancers with a ratio of right- to left-sided cancers of 31.1% to 68.9%. Operative mortality for patients presenting with rectal cancers was 6.4% versus 8.3% for colonic cancers (Wald statistic = 6.24, 1 degree of freedom, $p = 0.013$). This difference subsequently disappeared following adjustment for all other risk factors. Using the anterior resection as a reference category (operative mortality (OM) of 4.8%), all palliative procedures (OM ~ 20%) and right-sided colonic resections (OM 7.9%) had a significantly higher operative mortality. The mortality from left hemicolectomy, sigmoid colectomy and abdominoperineal excision of the rectum exceeded the anterior resection group. Non-resection of the tumour, for whatever reason, was associated with the highest post-operative mortality rate, 17.1%. Whether the colonic tumour is excised or not is an independent predictor of outcome in the CRC audit.

The surgeon effect

In both the Trent/Wales and the Wessex regional audits, a subset of patients with Dukes' C colon and rectal carcinomas, having curative, elective resections, had improved overall survival rate after treatment by specialist surgeons. In the Lothian and Borders audit (minimum follow-up 26 months) it has not been possible to show any variation between surgeons or benefit from high-volume or specialist surgeons.

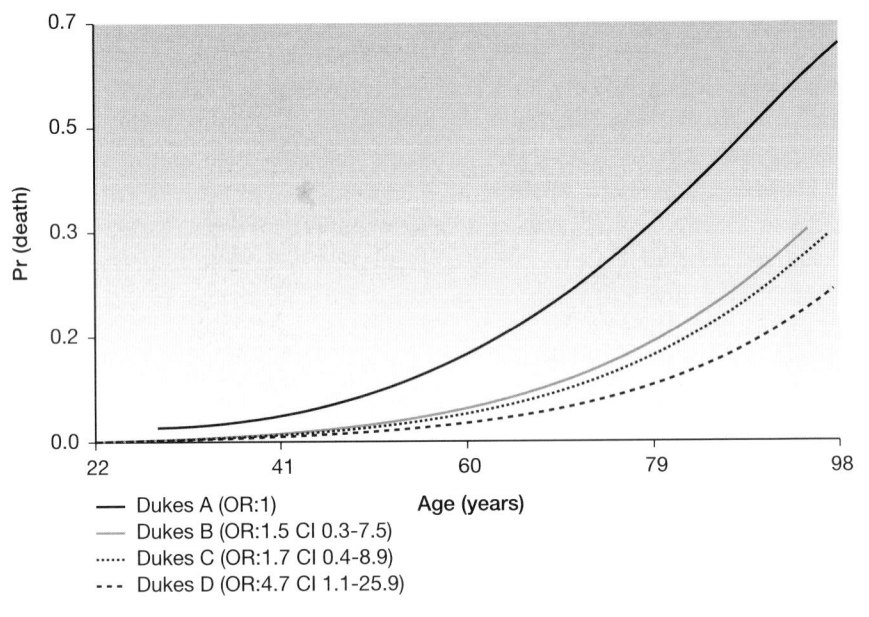

Figure 16.5 Variation of operative mortality by age and Dukes' grading for patients presenting with malignant large bowel obstruction. Odds ratios and their 95% CI are shown in the legend for each of the Dukes' grades.

Legend:
— Dukes A (OR:1)
— Dukes B (OR:1.5 CI 0.3–7.5)
...... Dukes C (OR:1.7 CI 0.4–8.9)
--- Dukes D (OR:4.7 CI 1.1–25.9)

The Wales/Trent audit also failed to show that high-volume surgeons achieve a better outcome. In the acute/emergency situation (MBO audit) there was no difference in outcome between ACPGBI and non-ACPGBI surgeons, using risk-adjusted operative mortality rates. This implies that emergency colorectal surgery may be provided by general surgeons without any apparent short-term disadvantage for patients. As there is no nationally recognised definition on what constitutes a specialist, or high-volume, surgeon, these definitions are arbitrary and we cannot draw definitive conclusions.

Hierarchical models in colorectal surgery

The use of operative mortality to compare quality of care between providers demands comprehensive, accurate and reliable information that is clinically valid. A relatively new statistical methodology was adopted in the MBO and CRC audits called *hierarchical regression* or *multilevel regression analysis*. This method is particularly useful in modelling observations that have a hierarchical or clustered structure. Such data are routinely found in various organisations, such as patients within hospitals or pupils within schools (Goldstein *et al.* 1996). In the past, the hierarchical structure of the data has been ignored, the analysis being based on reducing the data to the lowest level and subsequently applying a standard methodology. The penalty for ignoring the

Hepatic flexure
2.8% (8.0%)

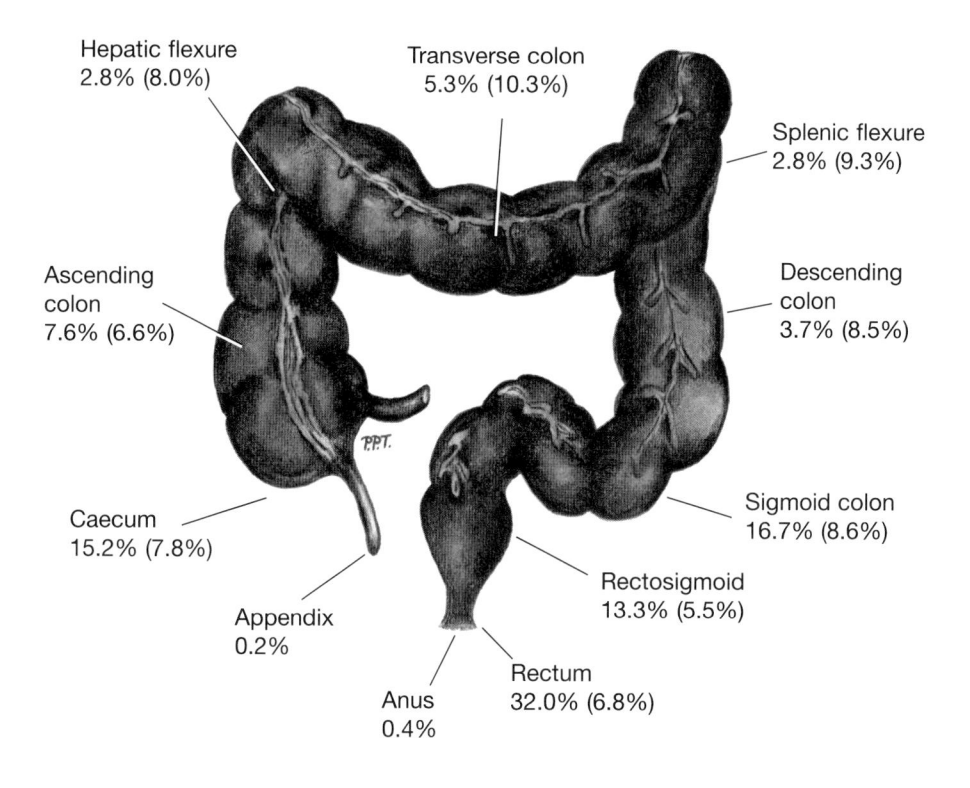

Transverse colon
5.3% (10.3%)

Splenic flexure
2.8% (9.3%)

Ascending colon
7.6% (6.6%)

Descending colon
3.7% (8.5%)

Caecum
15.2% (7.8%)

Sigmoid colon
16.7% (8.6%)

Appendix
0.2%

Rectosigmoid
13.3% (5.5%)

Anus
0.4%

Rectum
32.0% (6.8%)

Figure 16.6 Distribution of colorectal cancers along the large bowel as percentages of all the cancers reported in the ASGBI audit. The 30-day operative mortality is shown in brackets for each site.

clustered nature of patients within hospitals is that the standard error of the regression coefficients, which describes the performance of each hospital, is too low (Greenland 2000). In the traditional non-hierarchical model, more centres are shown to be outliers because they do not take into account the possibility that hospitals with small numbers of operated cases may be divergent or under-performing by chance. This effect may be reversed by larger studies, a concept called *regression to the mean* in which, year by year, the worst centres have the tendency to get better while the better ones tend to get worse! Hierarchical models work on the basic principle that the true performance rates for different centres are drawn from a normal distribution and, as a consequence, the performance rate (unit coefficient) of each hospital is weighted according to the number of cases submitted. The unit coefficients are therefore shrunk towards the population mean, with greater shrinkage for smaller centres. The shrinkage attempts to simulate the regression to the mean, providing a more realistic and accurate estimate of *long-term* performance.

The multilevel regression model for the ACPGBI CRC study used three levels of hierarchy placing the individual patient-related risk factors (subscript i) at the lowest level, named the 'patient level', while hospitals (subscript j) were placed in the second level and regional data (subscript k) were entered at the highest, third level. Conceptually, the model can be viewed as a hierarchical system of regression equations as shown in Figure 16.7. The hierarchical nature of the analysis allows for the possibility that patients from the same hospital will have more similar outcomes than patients chosen at random from different units. Using this approach the variation between regions or centres can be exclusively modelled to produce custom-made regression lines for each unit and region. This is shown in Figure 16.3 where individual prediction curves are produced for each unit, each with a similar shape, while accommodating for the chance effect in low volume units. In addition, the overall median regression line can be superimposed on the individual hospital prediction lines. With increasing age the lines fan out, demonstrating a greater variation in outcome in the elderly patients between centres.

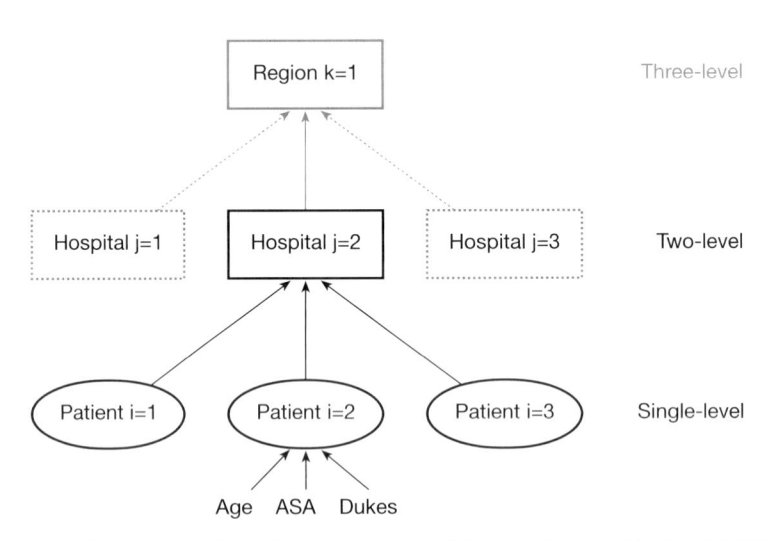

Figure 16.7 Illustration of the three level hierarchical model used in the ACPGBI audit. Patients' related risk factors are placed at the first level while hospitals are placed in the second level. An alternative model could be patient (level 1), surgeon (level 2), hospital (level 3) and so on.

The MBO colorectal cancer model

The MBO colorectal cancer model is intended to provide an estimate of operative mortality for all patients undergoing surgery for malignant large bowel obstruction. Probabilities of outcome (death within 30 days) can be calculated by entering into the model the following risk factors that have been shown to be independent predictors of mortality:

- age;
- American Society of Anesthesiology (ASA) grade;
- operative urgency;
- Dukes' stage.

There were very little specific data relating to other co-morbid conditions, such as ischaemic heart disease, pulmonary disease, diabetes, renal failure, or neurological disease. Risk models often include such factors in their computations as these co-morbidities will affect outcomes. In the MBO study, ASA grade was used as a general measure of fitness for surgery and the predictive model comprised all patients who had had surgery and whose mortality outcome was known.

Adjusted odds ratios and their interpretation

The MBO model provides adjusted odds ratio that can be used to compare the operative risk to a reference category. This is the group of patients with the lowest risk of an adverse outcome and represents patients who are younger than 65 years of age, with an ASA grade I, Dukes' A tumours that are excised on an elective basis (odds ratio of 1 and a probability of death of 0.7%). For example a 72-year-old patient with an ASA grade III having an urgent anterior resection for an obstructing lesion with suspected Dukes' B cancer would have an odds ratio of 3 × 11.7 × 1.6 × 2 = 112.3. In other words the patient is 112 times more likely to die than the 'reference patient'. The patient's odds ratio can be converted into a probability of death by entering the total score from the MBO model into the following equation:

$$\Pr(death) = \frac{MBO\ score \times 0.0018}{1 + (MBO\ score \times 0.0018)}$$

Where MBO score is the product of all the odds ratios as shown in Figure 16.8. The value 0.0018 represents exponent of the estimate of the model constant. For example, a patient with odds of death of 50:1 would have a predicted risk of death of 8.3%.

The performance of any predictive model can be evaluated by three measures of accuracy: (1) model discrimination; (2) model validation; and (3) subgroup analysis.

Model discrimination

Model discrimination measures the accuracy with which the risk-score distinguishes between patients with an adverse outcome (death following surgery) and those patients without an adverse outcome (alive following surgery). Receiver operating characteristic (ROC) curve analysis is an accepted method for determining the accuracy with which a risk score discriminates between positive and negative outcomes. During the ROC curve analysis, two patients are selected at random from the entire data group, one of whom has the post-procedural status of alive and the

		Adjusted Odds Ratios	Score
Age	<65 years	1.0	
	65–74 years	3.0	
	75–84 years	4.3	
	85+ years	5.9	
			X
ASA grade	ASA I	1.0	
	ASA II	3.3	
	ASA III	11.7	
	ASA IV-V	22.3	
			X
Urgency	Elective / Scheduled	1.0	
	Urgent	1.6	
	Emergency	2.3	
			X
Staging	Dukes A	1.0	
	Dukes B	2.0	
	Dukes C	2.0	
	Dukes D	6.0	
	MBO score {Product of the odds ratios} =		

Figure 16.8 The MBO Colorectal Cancer Model. Based on a Bayesian hierarchical regression model using Markov chain Monte Carlo simulation of 50,000 interactions.

other who has the post-procedural status of deceased. The analysis attempts to decide which is the deceased patient, based on the risk score alone. The analysis then records the number of times the choice is correct and the number of times the choice is incorrect. The more accurately the risk score discriminates between alive and dead patients, the fewer errors are made. Perfect discrimination would give a ROC curve area of 1.00 whereas random discrimination, the same power as simply tossing a coin to make the choices, would give a ROC curve area of 0.50. A value between 0.7 and 0.8 represents reasonable discrimination and if the value exceeds 0.8 it is considered to be very good discrimination. In the MBO study the area under the ROC curve for the hierarchical model was 0.816 (standard error = 0.019) and for the empirical Bayesian model 0.779 (standard error = 0.022), a difference which was statistically significant.

Model calibration

Calibration or goodness-of-fit refers to the ability of the model to assign the correct probabilities of outcome to individual patients. The Hosmer-Lemeshow C statistic was used to assess model calibration. In order to obtain this statistic, we computed the estimated probability of death for each patient based on the model, ranked them into 10 equal groups of ascending operative mortality (deciles), and then statistically evaluated the expected and observed number of outcomes in each decile. Smaller values represent better model calibration. Model calibration can also be shown graphically, where the observed and predicted operative mortality rates are plotted side by side, stratified in deciles (see Figure 16.9). The hierarchical MBO model calibrated well, with minimal discrepancies between the observed and expected outcomes as shown by the Hosmer-Lemeshow χ^2 statistic of 13.3 and a p-value of 0.10.

Subgroup analysis

Subgroup analysis is intended to assess the accuracy of the model by internally evaluating the observed and expected mortality rates among relevant strata. For example, the observed 30-operative mortality is shown in Figure 16.10 with its 95% confidence intervals for each of the four ASA groups. The observed mortality, as predicted by the MBO model, is well within the confidence intervals of the observed mortality. We further investigated the accuracy of the model among the age strata. The agreement between observed and expected mortality was adequate, with no significant difference between the observed and predicted group of outcomes.

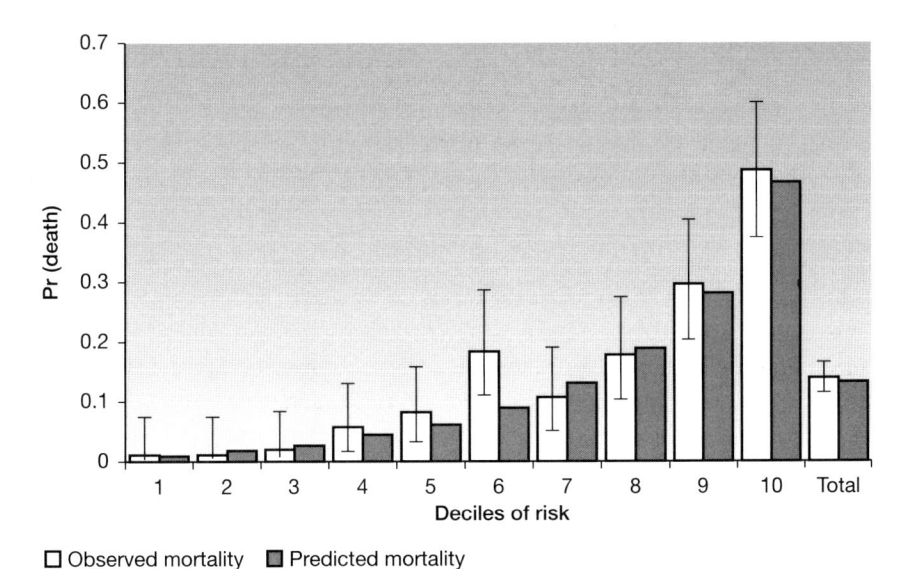

Figure 16.9 Calibration plot for the MBO model comparing the observed and expected operative mortality among deciles of increasing risk.

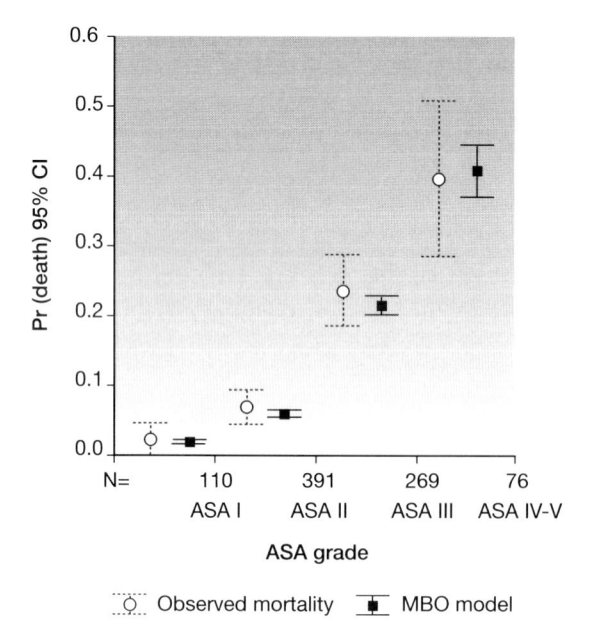

Figure 16.10 Subgroup analysis across different strata of ASA grade comparing the observed and expected operative mortality derived by the MBO model.

Sample size estimation

When relatively few patients are sampled the effects of chance may swamp any true quality effect and a longer period of monitoring may be needed for a meaningful estimate of mortality rates. Using the binomial distribution, the sample size required to detect a doubling of the operative mortality from 7.5% to 15% at 80% power and 5% statistical significance, was approximately 104 cases. Raising the power to 90% and 1% statistical significance, 222 cases would be required to detect such a difference. Operative mortalities higher than 15% require an even smaller sample size to detect a significant difference from the 'norm'. At 40% operative mortality, 18 cases would be sufficient to detect a change at 90% power and 1% statistical significance!

Recommendations

- There is a need for a nationwide system for data collection at all hospitals, with direct links and regular feedback for central data analysis.
- Precise definitions are essential to ensure standardisation and uniformity of data collection.
- In comparative audit, data should be collected from *all* cases including the patients not suitable for surgery and therefore not operated upon.

- At present, data quality may be limited but implementation of prediction systems within hospitals should lead to an increased awareness in the use of such data, with subsequent improvement in the quality of data collection.
- The reliability of the process of data collection should be formally assessed and validated at regular intervals.
- Raw audit data, not corrected for risk factors, is of little value in comparative audit.
- Hierarchical regression analysis provides risk-adjusted outcomes that are appropriately matched for the needs of colorectal practice.

Acknowledgements

The MBO and ACPGBI CRC studies were collaborative projects in which many surgeons, physicians, colorectal cancer coordinators, audit staff and others participated. Without their input neither of these studies would have been possible and we gratefully acknowledge their support.

References

Birkmemeyer, J. D., Siewers, A. E. *et al.* (2002). Hospital volume and surgical mortality in the United States. *New England Journal of Medicine* **346**, 1128–1137.

Blumberg, M. S. (1986). Risk adjusting healthcare outcomes: a methodologic review. *Medical Care Review* **43**, 351–393.

Bristowe, J. S. & Holmes, T. (1864). *Report on the hospitals of the United Kingdom. Sixth Report of the Medical Officer of the Priory Council. 1863.* (ed. G. E. Eyre & W. Spottiswoode) (512 pages). London: Her Majesty's Stationery Office.

Copeland, G. P., Jones, D. *et al.* (1991). POSSUM: a scoring system for surgical audit. *British Journal of Surgery* **78**, 355–360.

Dripps, R. D., Lamont, A. *et al.* (1963). The role of anaesthesia in surgical mortality. *Journal of the American Medical Association* **178**, 261–266.

Dukes, C. E. (1932). The classification of cancer of the rectum. *Journal of Pathology and Bacteriology* **35**, 323–332.

Feinstein, A. R., Sosin, D. M. *et al.* (1985). The Will Rogers phenomenon: stage migration and new diagnostic techniques as a source of misleading statistics for survival of cancer. *New England Journal of Medicine* **312**, 1604–1608.

Goldstein, H. & Thomas, S. (1996). Using examination results as indicators of school and college performance. *Journal of the Royal Statistical Society* **159**, 149–163.

Greenland, S. (2000). Principles of multilevel modelling. *International Journal of Epidemiology* **29**, 158–167.

Hall, J. C. & Hall, J. L. (1996). ASA status and age predict adverse events after abdominal surgery. *Journal of Quality in Clinical Practice* **16**, 103–108.

Iezzoni, L. I. (1997). Dimensions of Risk. In *Risk Adjustment for Measuring Healthcare Outcomes* (ed. L. I. Iezzoni), pp. 43–168. Ann Arbor, Michigan: Health Administration Press.

Jones, H. J. S. & de Cossart, L. (1999). Risk scoring in surgical patients. *British Journal of Surgery* **86**, 149–157.

Keogh, B. E. & Kinsman, R. (2001). *National Adult Cardiac Surgical Database Report 1999–2000*, pp. 10–14. London: The Society of Cardiothoracic Surgeons of Great Britain and Ireland.

Knaus, W. A., Draper, E. et al. (1985). APACHE II. *Critical Care Medicine* **13**, 818–829.

Knaus, W. A., Wagner, D. P. et al. (1991). The APACHE III prognostic system. Risk prediction of hospital mortality for critically ill hospitalised adults. *Chest* **100**, 1619–1636.

Knaus, W. A., Zimmerman, J. E. et al. (1981). APACHE – acute physiology and chronic health evaluation: a physiologically based classification system. *Critical Care Medicine* **1981**, 591–597.

Lothian and Borders Large Bowel Cancer Project (1995). The immediate outcome of surgery. *British Journal of Surgery* **82**, 888–890.

Mella, J., Biffin, A. et al. (1997). Population-based audit of colorectal cancer management in two health regions. *British Journal of Surgery* **84**, 1731–1736.

Midwinter, M. J., Tytherleigh, M. et al. (1999). Estimation of mortality and morbidity risk in vascular surgery using POSSUM and the Portsmouth predictor equation. *British Journal of Surgery* **86**(4), 471–474.

Nightingale, F. (1863). *Notes on Hospitals*. London: Longman, Green, Longman, Roberts and Green.

Prytherch, D. R., Whiteley, M. S et al. (1998). POSSUM and Portsmouth POSSUM for predicting mortality. Physiological and Operative Severity Score for the enUmeration of Mortality and morbidity. *British Journal of Surgery* **85**, 1217–1220.

Sagar, P. M., Hartley, M. N. et al. (1994). Comparative audit of colorectal resection with the POSSUM scoring system. *British Journal of Surgery* **81**, 1492–1494.

Sagar, P. M., Johnston, D. et al. (1993). Significance of circumferential resection margin involvement after oesophagectomy for cancer. *British Journal of Surgery* **80**, 1386–1388.

Spiegelhalter, D. J., Aylin, P. et al. (2002). Commissioned analysis of surgical performance by using routine data: lessons from Bristol inquiry. *Journal of the Royal Statistical Society* **165**, 1–31.

Stamatakis, J. D., Aitken J. et al. (2001). What can we learn from colorectal cancer audits? In *Recent Advances in Surgery*, vol. 24 (ed. I. Taylor & C. Johnson) Edinburgh: Churchill Livingstone.

Stamatakis, J. D., Thompson, M. R. et al. (2000). *National Audit of Bowel Obstruction due to Colorectal Cancer April 1998 – March 1999*. London: Association of Coloproctology of Great Britain and Ireland.

Tekkis, P. P., Kocher, H. M. et al. (2000). Operative mortality rates among surgeons: comparison of POSSUM and p-POSSUM scoring systems in gastrointestinal surgery. *Diseases of the Colon and Rectum* **43**, 1528–1532.

Tekkis, P. P., Kocher, H. M. et al. (2001). How accurate is POSSUM and p-POSSUM in predicting mortality in emergency surgery and in old age? *British Journal of Surgery* **88** (Supplement 1), 42–43.

Tekkis, P. P., Poloniecki, J. et al. (2002). *The ACPGBI Colorectal Database Report 2002 Part A: Unadjusted Outcomes*. London: The Association of Coloproctology of Great Britain and Ireland.

Turnbull, R. B., Kyle, K. et al. (1967). Cancer of the colon: the influence of the no-touch isolation technique on survival rates. *Annals of Surgery* **166**, 420–427.

UICC Committee on TNM Classification(1966). *Malignant tumours of the Oesophagus, Stomach, Colon and Rectum.* Geneva: International Union Against Cancer.

Wessex Colorectal Cancer Audit (1993). First Report. Wessex Cancer Intelligence Unit, Highcroft, Romsey Road, Winchester SO2 5DH.

Whiteley, M. S., Prytherch, D. R. et al. (1996) An evaluation of the POSSUM surgical scoring system. *British Journal of Surgery* **83**(6), 812–815.

Chapter 17

The development of colorectal cancer services through the implementation of the National Cancer Plan and the operation of cancer networks

Roger James

What has happened so far?

The Association of Coloproctology of Great Britain and Ireland (ACPGBI) celebrated its 10th anniversary in 2001, with the publication of *Resources for Coloproctology* (Association of Coloproctology of Great Britain and Ireland 2001), a template for investment, professional development and best practice over the next three years. This coincided with the announcement by the Government of £570 million extra investment in cancer services over three years, linked to a series of ambitious targets (Department of Health 1999, 2000a, 2000b).

Over the past 10 years the ACPGBI has established a series of committees dealing with issues affecting the practice of coloproctology. Locally, members meet in a series of ACPGBI chapters. Policy decisions are taken by Council after discussion between officers and chapter representatives.

The 1995 Calman–Hine report (Department of Health 1995) advised a re-organisation of NHS cancer services (ref). The main recommendations were site-specialisation, multi-disciplinary teamwork, and reorganisation of surgery for rare cancers on a population-base. NHS commissioning Guidance (COG) for colorectal cancer closely matched a previously published joint publication by the ACPGBI and Royal College of Surgeons (1996).

Although implementation of Calman–Hine was patchy and uncoordinated, many colorectal surgical teams in district general hospitals, encouraged by the ACPGBI, began to move towards specialisation and to meet formally on a weekly or fortnightly basis. Multi-disciplinary team (MDT) meetings in colorectal, lung and breast cancer now form the backbone of secondary sector cancer services in the NHS.

In April 2001, based on pioneering work in Scotland, 34 Cancer Networks were established in England and accredited by peer review during the following three months. In April 2002, English health authorities were replaced by strategic health authorities (a net reduction by 60%), and all health commissioning was devolved to the primary sector through primary care trusts (PCTs).

Why networks?

A managed care network has been described as 'A virtual service framework', 'A team of institutions' or 'A Special Health Authority'. Networks are part of the NHS 'modernisation' programme and '*Shifting the Balance of Power*' (October 2001), which includes devolution of health authority (HA) planning to PCTs. External regulation of clinical services is a feature of the Commission for Health Improvement (CHI). Ministers have made it clear that investment will be linked to evidence-based protocols and a reduction in waiting times. Evidence-based guidance is produced by the National Institute for Clinical Excellence (NICE). Networks encourage an approach to care that crosses NHS institutions – the 'patient pathway' – similar to those adopted by American health maintenance organisations (HMOs) and UK health insurance organisations. These exclude cover for high risk conditions and encourage cost control through 'prior authorisation' or protocol-based medicine.

Structure versus functional agenda

Structure

Cancer Networks are based on the catchment area of patients attending oncology centres for radiotherapy. However, their functional agenda is governed by an independent committee structure, and the oncology centre is part of a community which includes cancer units, PCTs and hospices. In Kent, as in most other developed networks, each cancer unit colorectal cancer MDT is represented on a network disease orientated group (DOG). The chairman of the colorectal DOG represents his/her speciality views on a clinical advisory board (CAT) along with chairmen of other site-specialised DOGs. The final arbiter of the network is a chief executive committee, responsible for 'difficult, smoke-filled room' decisions such as hospital closures and mergers.

Function

Cancer networks are intended by ministers to take over many of the duties of HAs, including the co-ordination of cancer service commissioning by PCTs. By the end of 2001, each Network was required to prepare a 3-year 'service delivery plan' (SDP). This is a network strategy to achieve National Cancer Plan targets using the recently announced extra £570 million investment. The SDP covers targets for prevention, screening, primary and community sector services, waiting lists, surgical, oncology and palliative care.

Improving audit and research

Each colorectal network DOG is expected to perform at least one audit per annum. Many clinicians have felt a useful audit is to assess the impact of the '2-week wait' policy on clinical practice. In addition, cancer networks are required to conform with

National Guidance on Research Governance (April 2001) and to register with the National Cancer Research Network (NCRN). The NCRN Colorectal Subcommittee will develop a portfolio of accredited trials. Individual networks are required to demonstrate an intention to improve recruitment through a three-year strategic plan. This identifies a nominated network clinical lead with protected sessions, a full-time infrastructure manager, secretarial staff, data managers and research nurse posts.

Challenges

Politicians have made a commitment to major additional investment in cancer services. Unfortunately, the medical profession is perceived by many as impeding modernisation by restrictive practices. Meanwhile, many clinicians perceive NHS modernisation as politically driven, performance-managed and insensitive to patient or professional needs. Many consultants perform their daily duties with fewer junior staff than five years ago, often with agency nurses and reduced management support. Workforce shortages in radiology and pathology are likely to persist for several years. Furthermore, the combination of NICE with CHI, together with questions over the future of the General Medical Council, raise the spectre of a medical 'Ofsted'.

The challenge to cancer networks is to change institutional thinking in the NHS. Networks are 'horizontal' structures that cut across traditional 'vertical' institutions like hospitals and PCTs. Networking services around one disease like cancer causes tensions unless all diseases are 'networked'. Reducing waiting times for cancer patients may simply increase waiting times for non-cancer patients. Audit departments are in trusts, not networks, so a 'network-wide audit' challenges chief executives to release some of their audit staff. Commissioning is not currently 'ring-fenced' by disease, giving chief executives some flexibility in achieving budgetary control by moving investment around year-on-year. Furthermore, the idea of 'corporate' accountability implied in Networks and MDTs seems at odds with a 'blame-culture' NHS where chief executives are often dismissed for failures of systems outside their direct control.

Finally, networks appear to differ strategically from professional bodies like ACPGBI in that they offer a performance-managed rather than an innovatory, technological approach to patient care. Managers find it easier to measure performance (process) than outcome. However, the goal of many clinicians is to accurately assess the results of their treatment, with an attempt to control for any retrospective bias and to publish in a peer-reviewed journal.

The way forward

How can the ACPGBI and the royal colleges overcome ministerial suspicion over professional aims?

The first task is to convince ministers that professional bodies like the ACPGBI are struggling hard to lead the modernisation programme in coloproctology and to fulfil the recommendations of the Calman–Hine report. Weekly MDT meetings held in cancer units are multi-disciplinary and site-specialised. They are active examples of clinical governance and many collect audit data prospectively. MDTs facilitate access of patients to surgery, radiotherapy or chemotherapy by cutting out delays imposed by referral letters. Many surgeons have agreed protocols for general practitioner follow-up for fully resected Dukes' B colon cancer patients, thereby reducing hospital-based clinics and opening spaces for new referrals. Most cancer units are attempting to implement the '2-week wait' policy by setting up rapid access clinics. Nurses are being encouraged to train to perform endoscopy and to lead assessment clinics. Innovations in practice are generally introduced by doctors, after rigorous clinical trials. Recent examples are stapled anterior resections, total mesorectal excision (TME) surgery and pre-operative radiotherapy. Colorectal audit is widely practiced in the UK, and most members of the ACPGBI audit their own practice.

A second task is to recognise a unique opportunity to drive the cancer modernisation agenda, rather than be driven by it. The committee structure of cancer networks and the chapter structure of the ACPGBI have similar aims and membership. Many ACPGBI members were involved in the National Cancer Network accreditation performed in 2001, and their clinical expertise has helped with difficult decisions in that process.

Most cancer networks cover a population of 1.5–2.0 million and will contain one network colorectal cancer DOG. Most of its members will be in the overlapping ACPGBI chapter, covering populations of 1–4 million, equivalent to between one and four networks. Although the two groups have differing functions, their agendas overlap in many respects and are likely to agree on important issues.

A 'bottom-up' approach from professional organisations could include the ACPGBI, the Royal College of Nursing, the College of Radiographers and other medical colleges. Together, these groups could drive cancer networks by sharing agendas and minutes of local (chapter) meetings, or even by joint meetings. In this way the uniformity of practice required by politicians could be linked with investment to the benefit of patients. There is an exciting opportunity for multidisciplinary professional groups to make a major contribution to the improvement of care for patients with suspected or confirmed colorectal cancer.

References

Association of Coloproctology of Great Britain and Ireland (2001). Resources for Coloproctology. London: Association of Coloproctology of Great Britain and Ireland.

Department of Health (1995). *A Policy Framework for Commissioning Cancer Services*. A Report by the Expert Advisory Group on Cancer to the Chief Medical Officers of England and Wales. London: Department of Health.

Department of Health (1999). *Saving Lives: Our Healthier Nation*. See http://www.archive.officialdocuments.co.uk/documentlcm43/4386/4386.htm.

Department of Health (2000a). *The NHS Cancer Plan*. See http://www.doh.gov.uk/cancer/cancerplan.htm.

Department of Health (2000b). *Manual of Cancer Services Standards*. See http://www.doh.gov uk/cancer/manualcancerservicesstandards.pdf.

National Institute for Clinical Excellence (2002). *Improving Outcomes in Breast Cancer. Guidance on Cancer Services.* See http://www.nice.org.uk/pdf/Improving_outcomes_breastcancer_manual.pdr.

NHS Executive (1997). Improving Outcomes in Colorectal Cancer. Guidance on Commissioning Cancer Services. See http://www.doh.gov.uk/cancer/pdfs/ colorectalmanual.pdf.

Index

abdomino-perineal resection 41, 88
  laparoscopic 78
adenoma carcinoma sequence 3–4, 25
  in HNPCC 29
adenomatous polyps
  inherited susceptibility 14
  see also familial adenomatous
      polyposis (FAP) ; hereditary
      non-polyposis colorectal cancer
      (HNPCC)
adjuvant chemotherapy xii, 121–2, 130
  bevacizumab 128, 129
  capecitabine 126–9
  cetuximab 129
  irinotecan 122–4
  oxaliplatin 122, 123
  value in stage II disease 124–6
  see also chemotherapy
advanced disease xiv
  chemotherapy 133–4
    5FU 134
    capecitabine 135, 140–2
    cost-effectiveness 202–3
    irinotecan 135–6
    optimal combination 139–40
    oxaliplatin 137–9
  COX-2 inhibitors 186
  early intervention, benefits 197
  liver metastases 143–4
  NICE management guidance xvi,
      196–200
  survival rates 195
  targeted therapies 142–3
  see also palliative chemotherapy
adverse effects
  of bevacizumab 183
  of capecitabine 126
  of cetuximab 181
  of irinotecan 135, 136, 201
  of oxaliplatin 122, 138–9
  of palliative chemotherapy 170, 171
  of pre-operative chemoradiation
      160–1

age
  effect on outcome of surgery 213,
      214, 221, 222
  and risk of recurrence 124
algebra of effectiveness 212, 213
altered bowel habit, referral guidelines
    63
American Society of Anaesthesiologists
    (ASA), physiological scoring
    systems 214–16, 222
Amsterdam criteria 10, 11, 30, 51, 52
anaemia, referral guidelines 63
anal cancer, response to chemoradiation
    159
anal preservation 86
anastomotic leaks, incidence after
    pre-operative chemoradiation 93,
    94
angiogenesis 155–6, 182–3
anti-VEGF antibodies
  sensitivity to ix
  see also bevacizumab
APACHE scoring systems 214, 215
APC, and wnt signalling pathway 7
APC gene 4, 5–6, 25
  in attenuated polyposis 50
  FAP genotype-phenotype
      correlations 6, 8
  I1307K variant 15, 17, 50, 53
APOE gene 15
apoptotic index, prognostic significance
    155
Appraisal Committees, NICE 195–6
Ashkenazim 15, 17
aspirin 185
Association of Coloproctology of
    Great Britain and Ireland
    (ACPGBI) 227, 229–30
attenuated FAP (AFAP) 6
  bi-allelic *MYH* mutations 49–50
audit 228, 229, 230
  see also clinical audit
autonomic nerve plexus preservation 86
Avastin see bevacizumab

Bannayan-Rilet-Ruvalcaba (Bannayan-Zonana) syndrome 9, 50
base-excision repair pathway 14
BAT25 12
BAT26 12–13
Bax 13
Bcl2 155
beta-catenin, and wnt signalling pathway 7
beta-catenin (*CTNNB1*) gene 25
Bethesda guidelines 10, 11, 52
bevacizumab (Avastin) xiv, 134, 183–4, 188
  adjuvant use 128, 129
  value in advanced disease 142
biological agents *see* bevacizumab; cetuximab
bladder function preservation 86
'blame culture' 229
BLM[Ash] allele 17, 53
Bloom's syndrome 29, 53
BMPR1A gene mutations 10, 50
BOND (Bowel Oncology with Cetuximab Antibody) study 181–2
bortezomib (Velcade, PS-341) 186–7
brain tumours, risk in HNPCC 27
breast cancer, in Peutz-Jeghers syndrome 8
butyrate 187

CALGB C89803 trial 122–4
Calman-Hine report (DOH, 1995) 227
Cancer Networks 227–30
cancer site, prognostic significance 217, 219
CAO/ARO/AIO-94 protocol 162
capecitabine xiv, 126–9, 130, 134, 195
  in advanced disease 135, 200
    combination therapy 140–2
carcinoembryonic antigen (CEA) measurement, value in follow-up xiii, 105, 106, 107, 108, 110
'caretaker' genes 5
caspase-5 13
CDX2 13

celecoxib, preventive role 185
cervical cancer, in Peutz-Jeghers syndrome 8
cetuximab xiv, 134, 181–2
  adjuvant use 129
  cost of treatment 187–8
  value in advanced disease 143
change in bowel habit, referral guidelines 63
chemoradiation 41–2
  post-operative 153
  pre-operative xii, 89, 152–3, 154
    lymph node response 159–60
    residual cell density 158
    role in sphincter preservation 92, 93–8
    significance of response 159
    toxicity and complications 160–1
  for rectal cancer 151, 153–62
chemotherapy xiii–xv, 41–2, 121–2
  in advanced disease 133–45
  optimal regimens xv
  palliative, MRC CR06B trial 168–76
  pre-operative 88
  role in sphincter preservation 91, 92
  value in stage II disease 124–6
  see also adjuvant chemotherapy; chemoradiation
chemotherapy response ix, 43–4, 45
chromosomal instability 25
chromosome abnormalities 14
  in FAP 5
  in juvenile polyposis syndrome 9–10
  in Peutz-Jeghers syndrome 9
circumferential margin involvement (CMI) 86, 88, 152, 154, 157
CLASSIC trial 82
clinical advisory boards (CATs) 228
clinical audit 209
  data quality and standardisation 211–12
  defining outcomes 212
  hierarchical (multilevel) regression analysis 218–20
  recommendations 224–5

risk adjustment 212–18
clinical governance xvi
clinical trials, cross-over within trial
 arms 198, 201
colonoscopic screening
 value in follow-up 112, 114
 see also surveillance
Colorectal Unit, South Devon NHS
 Trust study x–xi, 63–70
combination chemotherapy 176
 with capecitabine 127–8
Commission for Health Improvement
 (CHI) 228
complications, surgical
 after chemoradiation 93–4
 after laparoscopic surgery 79
computed tomography (CT), value in
 follow-up xiii, 105, 106, 107,
 108, 110
congenital hypertrophy of retinal
 pigment epithelium (CHRPE) 5,
 6, 49
continence after sphincter-sparing
 surgery 95–6
continuous palliative chemotherapy,
 MRC CR06B trial 169–74, 175
conversion rates during laparoscopic
 surgery 80, 82
'corporate' accountability 229
COST (Clinical Outcomes of Surgical
 Therapy), review of laparoscopic
 surgery 0, 77
cost effectiveness
 chemotherapy for advanced disease
 202–3
 of follow-up 114, 116
costs
 of cetuximab treatment 187–8
 of clinical audit 212
 of laparoscopic surgery 81
Cowden syndrome (CS) 9, 50
COX-2 inhibitors xv, 144–5, 184–6, 188
CRAC1 gene 14
cross-over within trial arms 198, 201
CTNNB1 gene 25

cutaneous neoplasms in HNPCC 26, 27
cyclooxygenase-2 inhibitors *see*
 COX-2 inhibitors
CYP1A1 gene 15

data collection 211–12, 224–5
DCC (deleted in colorectal cancer)
 expression, prognostic
 significance 126
delays x, 61, 62
 impact of two week rule 67, 69–70,
 71
 new targets 72
dendritic cells, use in immunotherapy
 144
dental anomalies in FAP 5
desmoid tumours in FAP 5, 8
diagnosis, proteomic pattern analysis
 180
disease orientated groups (DOGs) 228
disease progression, effect of
 continuous palliative chemotherapy
 170, 173
disease severity, prognostic
 significance 216–17
distal cancers ix
 see also left-sided cancers; rectal
 cancer
distal resection margin 92–3
distribution of colorectal cancers 42
 South Devon Healthcare Trust
 Colorectal Cancer Study 67
DNA repair proteins 5
down staging
 of liver metastases 144
 of rectal cancer
 histopathological assessment 158
 significance of response 159
DPC4 gene *see SMAD4* gene
Dukes' stage *see* stage of disease
duodenal carcinoma, risk in FAP 5
duration of palliative chemotherapy
 167–8
Dutch TME study 88–9, 152, 157,
 159, 160, 161

E-cadherin, and wnt signalling pathway 7
E2F-4 13
effectiveness, definition of term 103
efficacy, definition of term 103
efficiency, definition of term 103
elective surgery, definition 216
emergency surgery, as risk factor 216, 222
endometrial cancer, risk in HNPCC 10, 51
endoscopy services, impact of two week rule 72
E3200 142
EORTC, trial of pre-operative chemoradiation 161–2
EORTC-GITCG group, follow-up RCT 113
epidermal growth factor receptor (EGFR) 142–3, 180
   EGFR expression, prognostic significance 156
   as therapeutic target xiv, 129, 144
   see also cetuximab
epidermal growth factor receptor tyrosine kinase (Iressa) 176
epidermoid cysts, in FAP 5
Erbitux *see* cetuximab
erlotinib (Tarceva) 144
evidence-based practice 228
EXO1 gene 14
extra-colonic features
   of FAP 5, 49
   of HNPPC x, 10, 11, 26, 27, 51
   of Peutz-Jeghers syndrome 8, 50
extra-mural detection 104, 105, 110

FACS trial 113
familial adenomatous polyposis (FAP) 5–8, 49
   attenuated 50
   effect of COX-2 inhibitors 185
family history ix, 3, 26
   testing for mutations 51–2
   see also inherited susceptibility

Fanconi's anaemia 29
farnesyl transferase inhibitors 45
   sensitivity to ix
fast-track investigations, impact of two week rule 72
fatigue, post-operative 80
FFCD Group, Follow-up RCT 113
fibroblast growth factor xv
final advisory documents (FADs), NICE 196
fistulae, incidence after pre-operative chemoradiation 93
5-fluorouracil (5FU) 121-2, 130, 167, 195, 197
   in advanced disease 134, 139
   NICE guidelines 196
   combination with gefitinib 182
   combination with irinotecan xiv, 135–6, 198, 201–2
   combination with oxaliplatin 122, 123, 137–8, 198
   down staging of liver metastases 144
   in MRC CR06B trial 168
   post-operative use in rectal cancer 151, 153
   pre-operative use in rectal cancer 154
   sensitivity to ix, 35, 43, 44, 126
   synergy with Cox 2 inhibitors 144
5-fluorouracil and leucovorin therapy xiii–xiv
FOCUS trial 140, 141, 196, 204–5
FOLFIRI regimen (irinotecan, LV/5FU) 139–40
FOLFOX regimens (oxaliplatin, LV/5FU) 122, 123, 125, 138–40
   combination with cetuximab 143
   comparison with XELOX 141, 142
   down staging of liver metastases 144
   OPTIMOX study 138–9
folinic acid 197
   in advanced disease, NICE guidelines 196
follow-up xiii, 101–3, 115
   economic issues 114, 116
   effect on quality of life 114–15

efficacy of surveillance tools 112–14
GILDA trial 108–9
meta-analysis of RCTs 104–7
responses 107–10
ongoing or planned RCTs 113
French Epirubicin Study Group 168
frozen sections xii–xiii
functional results, sphincter-sparing surgery 95–6

gastric cancer, risk in HNPCC 10, 11, 27
'gatekeeper' genes 4–5
gefitinib (ZD 1839) xv, 176, 182
gender, effect on outcome of surgery 213
gene chips 145
genetic counselling 51–3
germline mutations in HNPCC 11, 27
testing for 51–2
GILDA trial 108–9, 110, 113
G° (8-oxoguanine) mutations, repair 16
Gorlin syndrome 9
grade of tumour, prognostic significance 154
GSTM1 gene 15
GSTT1 gene 15

H-ras-VNTR gene 15
hamartomatous polyps
associated syndromes 8–10, 50
'landscaper' effect 5
hepato-biliary tumours in HNPCC 27
hepatoblastoma, risk in FAP 5
HER-1 *see* epidermal growth factor receptor (EGFR)
hereditary non-polyposis colorectal cancer (HNPCC) x, 10–13, 26–7, 50–1
COX-2 expression 185
diagnosis 30–1
MMR dysfunction 28, 29
pathological features 29–30
testing for mutations 51–2
tumour analysis 31–5

hierarchical (multilevel) regression analysis 218–20, 225
histone deacetylase inhibitors (HDACs) xvi, 187
histopathological examination
lymph nodes, effect of chemoradiation 160
residual cell density 158
role in quality control 158–9
histopathological features, of HNPCC 10
HRAS-1 gene VNTR polymorphism 17
hyperpigmentation, in Peutz-Jeghers syndrome 8
hypoxic tumours 159

ibuprofen 185
ICER (incremental cost-effectiveness ratio), follow-up 114, 116
IFL (irinotecan/5-FU/leucovorin), combination with bevacizumab 183
IGFIIR gene 13
IMC-C225 *see* cetuximab
immunohistochemistry, detection of MMR abnormalities 31, 32, 35, 52
incidence ix, 41, 133
incremental cost effectiveness ration (ICER), follow-up xiii
indomethacin 185
inflammatory response, post-operative 79
INFORM study 182
infusional 5FU regimens 134
inherited susceptibility ix, 3, 13–15, 18
familial adenomatous polyposis (FAP) 5–8
hamartomatous polyp syndromes 8–10
hereditary non-polyposis colorectal cancer (HNPCC) 10–13
low-penetrance genes 15, 17
mechanisms 4–5
surveillance 49, 53
testing for mutations 51–2

integrins xv
intensive follow-up 101–3, 115
  economic issues 114, 116
  effect on quality of life 114–15
  meta-analysis of RCTs 104–7
    responses 107–10
  ongoing or planned RCTs 113
Intergroup 0144 study 153, 160
intermittent palliative chemotherapy
  advantages 174–5
  MRC CR06B trial 168–74
International Collaborative Group
  (ICG), definition of HNPCC 30
intra-mural detection 104, 105, 110
intussusception 8
Iressa *see* gefitinib
irinotecan 122–4, 128, 134, 167
  combination with 5-FU xiv, 201–2
  combination with capecitabine 141–2
  combination with celecoxib 186
  combination with cetuximab 181, 187
  combination with oxaliplatin
    199–200
  in MRC CR06B trial 169
  'rationing' by treatment deferral
    203–4
  sensitivity to ix
  use in advanced disease 135–6,
    197–8
    NICE guidelines xvi, 196, 201
    value in left-sided colorectal cancers
      44
  see also FOCUS trial; FOLFIRI
    regimen; IROX regimen
iron deficiency anaemia, referral
  guidelines 63
IROX regimen (irinotecan and
  oxaliplatin) 139, 199–200

J-pouch reconstruction 95, 96
juvenile polyposis syndrome (JPS)
  9–10, 50
  'landscaper' effect 5

K-ras oncogene ix, 25, 45

Ki67, prognostic significance 155
'landscaper' genes 5, 9
laparoscopic surgery xi, 77, 82–3
  clearance and survival 77–8
  disadvantages 80–1
  port site metastases 77, 78–9
  quality of life studies 80
  short-term outcome 79
  Yeovil District Hospital practice
    81–2
left-sided cancers ix, 42
  characteristics 41, 45
  p53 gene mutations 44
  thymidylate synthase expression 44
leucovorin 121–2
levamisole 121
LIFE study 138
liver metastases 143–4
  downstaging with oxaliplatin 199,
    202
LKB1 gene mutations 9, 50
local recurrence, after pre-operative
  chemoradiation 93
local recurrence rates, after TME
  86–7, 88
lomustine 121
low-penetrance genes 15, 17
lymph node yields, from laparoscopic
  surgery 77
lymph nodes, effect of pre-operative
  chemoradiation 159–60
lymphocytic infiltration, and
  microvessel density 156
Lynch syndromes 26
  see also hereditary non-polyposis
    colorectal cancer (HNPCC)

magnetic resonance imaging, prior to
  TME xii, 86, 88
malignant bowel obstruction (MBO)
  MBO colorectal cancer model 220–4
  national audit 210
managed care networks 228
management of colorectal cancer 41–2
markers, prognostic 154–5

matrix metalloproteinases 184
MBO colorectal cancer model 220–4
melanin pigmentation, in Peutz-Jeghers syndrome 8
metastases
  at laparoscopic port sites 77, 78–9
  hepatic 143–4
    downstaging with oxaliplatin 199, 202
  risk in rectal cancer 152
metastatic disease *see* advanced disease; palliative chemotherapy
MFTR^{val/val} mutation 17
MGMT (06-methylguanine DNA methyl transferase) ix, 44–5
MHS3 13
microarrays 179
microsatellite instability (MSI) ix–x, 12–13, 25–6, 43–4, 51
  incidence 29–30
  as prognostic marker 126
  testing for 31, 33–4, 35, 52
  see also MSI-H; MSI-L
microsatellites 25, 42–3
microvessel density, prognostic significance 155–6
mismatch repair (MMR) deficiency ix–x, 25–6, 43
  from conception, phenotype 29
  immunohistochemical detection 31, 32, 35
  mutations in HNPCC 11–13
  promotion of tumour progression 2–8
mismatch repair(MMR) system, function 27–8
mitomycin C
  in MRC CR06B trial 169
  use in pre-operative chemoradiation 154
MLH1 gene mutations 11, 13, 25, 51
  in HNPCC 27
  MLH1 promoter hypermethylation 33, 35
MLH1 protein 43

immunohistochemical analysis 31, 32
monoclonal antibodies *see* bevacizumab (Avastin); cetuximab; pantumumab
morbidity, after conversion from laparoscopic surgery 80–1
mortality ix, 42
  assessment in clinical audit 212
  operative 217
  see also prognostic factors; survival rates
mortality data collection 209–11
mortality prediction models 211
MOSAIC 2 trial 129
MOSAIC trial xiv, 42, 122, 124, 125
MPM (Mortality Probability Model) 215
MRC 2 rectal cancer study 159
MRC CR06B trial 167, 168–75, 203–4
MRC CR08 (FOCUS) trial 140, 141, 196, 204–5
MRCCR07 study 152
MS-275 187
MSH2 gene mutations 11, 13, 51
  in HNPCC 27
MSH2 protein 43
  immunohistochemical analysis 31, 32
MSH3 gene mutations 27
MSH6 gene 13, 27, 51
MSH6 protein, immunohistochemical analysis 31
MSI-H 28, 33
  prognostic significance 43–4
MSI-L 45
MTHFR gene 15
Muir-Torre syndrome 26
multi-disciplinary teams 227, 230
multilevel (hierarchical) regression analysis 218–20, 225
multimodal rehabilitation 83
mutations, adenoma carcinoma sequence 3–4
MYH gene 14–15
  and attenuated polyposis 49–50
MYH protein, functions 16

NASBP C-06 trial 126
NAT2 gene 15
national audits 210
National Cancer Plan 204
National Cancer Research Network (NCRN) 229
National Institute for Clinical Excellence (NICE) xvi, 195–6, 228
  guidelines for management of advanced disease 196–200
  controversial issues 201–2
  cost-effectiveness 202–3
  implications 203–4
  review 204–5
  recommendations for laparoscopic surgery 77
NCCTG N0147trial 129
neoadjuvant therapy *see* pre-operative chemoradiation; pre-operative radiotherapy
networks 229
  see also cancer networks
NHS Cancer Plan 61
NHS Cancer Survey, delays 62
NICE *see* National Institute for Clinical Excellence
Nightingale, Florence 209–10
nitrosoureas 45
NO16968 trial 127–8
non-steroidal anti-inflammatory drugs (NSAIDs) 184, 185
Nordic GI Tumour Adjuvant Therapy Group 197
Norweigian rectal cancer project 152
NSABP C-08 trial 129
nurse specialists 230

OGG1, functions 16
operability rates, South Devon Healthcare Trust Colorectal Cancer Study 64
OPTIMOX study 138–9
oral fluoropyrimidines 126–9, 134, 195
  in advanced disease 134–5, 200

osteomas, in FAP 5
ovarian cancer
  in Peutz-Jeghers syndrome 8
  risk in HNPCC 10, 11, 27
oxaliplatin xiv, 134, 136, 167
  adverse effects 138–9
  combination with capecitabine 127–8
  combination with irinotecan 199–200
  down staging of liver metastases 144, 199, 202
  in MRC CR06B trial 169
  NICE guidance xvi, 203
  OPTIMOX study 138–9
  sensitivity to ix
  use in advanced disease 137–8, 198–9
    NICE guidelines 196
  use in early stage disease 122, 123, 127–8, 130
  use in left-sided colorectal cancers 44
  XELOX trial 140–2
  see also FOCUS trial; FOLFOX regimens; IROX regimen
8-oxoguanine (G°) mutations, repair 16

P27^{kip1} 155
p53 mutations ix, 25, 44
  prognostic significance 154–5
pain, post-operative 80
palliative chemotherapy 167–8
  MRC CR06B trial 168–76
  optimal regimens xv
  see also advanced disease
palliative procedures, South Devon Healthcare Trust Colorectal Cancer Study 66
pancreatic tumours in HNPCC 27
pantumumab (ABX-EGF) 144
papillary thyroid cancer, risk in FAP 5
patient choice, implication of NICE guidelines for management of advanced disease 203–4
patient pathway 228
PCR, MSI testing 33, 34

pelvic abscess, incidence after pre-operative chemoradiation 93
pelvic radiotherapy, adverse effects 161
PETACC3 trial 124, 129
Peutz-Jeghers syndrome (PJS) 8–9, 50
physiological derangement, effect on outcome of surgery 213–16, 222
piroxicam 185
PLA2G2A gene 15
PMS1 gene 27, 51
PMS2 gene mutations 27, 51
PMS2 protein, immunohistochemical analysis 31
port site metastases 77, 78–9, 82
POSSUM scoring systems 214, 215–16
post-operative chemoradiation 153
post-operative morbidity, after laparoscopic surgery 79
power calculations in RCTs 111
pre-operative chemoradiation xii, 152–3, 154
  lymph node response 159–60
  residual cell density 158
  role in sphincter-sparing surgery 92, 93–8
  significance of response 159
  toxicity and complications 160–1
pre-operative radiotherapy, in rectal cancer 151
presentation 41
  of Peutz-Jeghers syndrome 8
prognosis, in HNPCC 10
prognostic factors 212–18
  EGFR 180
  MSI-H 43
  p53 gene mutations 44
  in rectal cancer xv, 154–60
  for recurrence 124, 126
  VEGFR 142
progression of disease, effect of continuous palliative chemotherapy 170, 173
prospective randomised controlled trial (PRCT)

of pre-operative chemoradiation 94–5
and TME 85, 89
proteasome inhibitors 186–7
protein truncation test (PTT) 6
proteomics 145, 179–80
proteosome inhibitors xv–xvi
provisional advisory documents (PADs), NICE 196
PS-341 (Velcade, bortezomib) 186–7
PTEN gene mutations 50

quality of care, measurement 212
quality control, role of histopathological examination 158–9
quality of life
  after laparoscopic surgery 80
  during palliative chemotherapy 170, 171–2
  effect of follow-up 114–15
  in metastatic disease 133
Quasar (Quick and simple and reliable) 1 trial 42, 121, 124, 125
Quasar II trial 128

R0 resection 151, 157
radiotherapy 41
  combination with TME 89
  pre-operative, in rectal cancer 151
  role in sphincter preservation 91–2
  see also chemoradiation; pre-operative chemoradiation
raltitrexed
  in MRC CR06B trial 168, 169
  NICE guidelines xvi, 196, 200, 202
randomised controlled trials
  evaluation of follow-up 102, 104–7, 115
    general principles 111
    ongoing or planned trials 113
  of pre-operative chemoradiation 94–5
  and TME 85, 89
rapid referral clinics, impact on services 72

'rationing' by treatment deferral 203–4
receiver operating characteristic (ROC) curve analysis 221–2
rectal bleeding 41
  in Peutz-Jeghers syndrome 8
  referral guidelines 63
rectal cancer xv
  distal resection margin 92–3
  incidence 41
  K-*ras* mutations 45
  lymph nodes, effect of chemoradiation 159–60
  management 51–3
    chemotherapy 41–2
    laparoscopic surgery 78
    post-operative chemoradiation 153
    pre-operative chemoradiation 154–62
  microsatellite instability 25, 33
  operative mortality 217
  prognostic factors 154–7
  residual cell density 158
  see also sphincter-saving surgery; total mesorectal excision (TME)
recurrence
  after laparoscopic surgery 77–8, 82
  local recurrence rates after TME 86–7, 88
  port site metastases 78–9
  risk factors for 87
referral, delays 62
referral guidelines 62–3, 72
referral routes, South Devon Healthcare Trust Colorectal Cancer Study 64
regression to the mean 219
rehabilitation, multimodal 83
research, implications of NICE guidance for management of advance disease 204
resection *see* surgery
residual cell density, after pre-operative chemoradiation 158
right-sided colon cancer ix, 42
  characteristics 41, 45

K-*ras* mutations 45
MSI-H 43
risk adjustment 212–18
risk factors
  family history ix, 53
  for recurrence 87
  see also inherited susceptibility
rofecoxib 185
  combination with 5FU 144–5
  VICTOR study 185–6
  withdrawal 188
'Russian Doll' phenomenon 101–2

SAHA (suberoylanilide hydroxamic acid) 187
SAPS scoring system 215
scheduled surgery, definition 216
scoring systems 72
screening *see* surveillance
SEER (Surveillance Epidemiology and End Results) data 112
segregation analyses 13–14
Sertoli cell tumours, in Peutz-Jeghers syndrome 8
service delivery plans (SDPs) 228
service provision xvi
services, impact of two week rule 72
sexual function, preservation of xii, 86
short course palliative chemotherapy 167–8
  MRC CR06B trial 168–76
short course radiotherapy 89
site of cancer, prognostic significance 217, 219
skin neoplasms in HNPCC 26, 27
SMAD4 (*DPC4*) gene 9–10, 25, 50
small bowel tumours, risk in HNPCC 27
SN38 135
South Devon Healthcare Trust Colorectal Cancer Study 63–70
sphincter-saving surgery xii–xiii, 91–2
  distal resection margin 92–3
  late functional results 95–6
  pre-operative chemoradiation 93–8

sporadic CRC, microsatellite instability 12, 33
staff shortages 229
stage of disease
   impact of two week rule 68, 69, 71
   prognostic significance 154, 216–17, 218, 222
stage II disease, value of chemotherapy 124–6, 130
stage migration 217
staging xii, xv
standardisation of treatment, in RCTs 111
Stockholm TME workshops, impact 87
stomach cancer, risk in HNPCC 10, 11, 27
stratification, in RCTs 111
stress response to surgery 79
stroma, 'landscaper effect' 5
suberoylanilide hydroxamic acid (SAHA) 187
sulindac 185
surgeons, experience and specialist status 217–18
surgery
   clinical audit 209
      data collection 211–12
      defining outcomes 212
      hierarchical regression analysis 218–20
      risk adjustment 212–18
   distal resection margin 92–3
   for liver metastases 144
   MBO colorectal cancer model 220–4
   R0 resection 151
   resection of metastases 195
   South Devon Healthcare Trust Colorectal Cancer Study 65–6
   stress response 79
   see also laparoscopic surgery; pre-operative chemoradiation; sphincter-saving surgery; total mesorectal excision (TME)
surveillance 53
   in FAP 49
   in HNPCC 29, 51
   in Peutz-Jeghers syndrome 50
   see also follow-up
survival rates x, 195, 204
   after laparoscopic surgery 78
   effect of intensive follow-up 101, 104, 106–7, 110
   effect of palliative chemotherapy 170, 173–4
Swedish Rectal Cancer Trial 151, 154

Tarceva (erlotinib) 144
targeting therapy 145
TCF-4 13
Technology Appraisal Guidance, NICE 196
TGFBR2 gene 13
thymidylate synthase expression ix, 44
   prognostic significance 126
thyroid cancer, risk in FAP 5
TNM stage xv
   impact of two week rule 68, 69, 71
total mesorectal excision (TME) xi–xii, 41, 85–6, 88–9, 151–2
   follow-up data 86–7
   impact of teaching programme 87
   laparoscopic 78
   quality control, role of pathologist 158–9
TREE2 142
trichostatin A 187
tumour analysis 31–5, 52
tumour necrosis, assessment 158
tumour regression grade (TRG) 158
tumour suppressor genes 4–5
twin studies, inherited susceptibility 13
'two hit' hypothesis 4
two week referral system, uptake 70–1
two week rule x–xi, 61, 72–3, 230
   impact on waiting times 67, 69–70, 71
tyrosine kinase inhibitors xv, 182
   sensitivity to ix

ubiquitin-proteasome pathway 186

UFT *see* uracil tegafur
UKCCCR Colorectal Cancer Group, follow-up RCT 113
uracil tegafur 126, 135, 200
urgent surgery, definition 216
uroepithelial tumours risk in HNPCC 10, 11, 25

value in follow-up 112, 114
vascular endothelial growth factor (VEGF) xv, 156, 183
　as therapeutic target xiv, 129
　see also bevacizumab
vascular endothelial growth factor (VEGF) expression ix, 45, 142
vascular invasion, prognostic significance 154
Velcade (PS-341, bortezomib) 186–7
VICTOR study 185–6
　termination 188

vincristine 121
waiting times 62, 229
　impact of two week rule 67, 69–70, 71
　targets 61–2, 72
'Will Rogers phenomenon' 217
wnt signalling pathway 7

X-act trial xiii–xiv, 126–7
Xeloda *see* capecitabine
XELOX regimen (capecitabine and oxaliplatin) 140–1, 142
xeroderma pigmentosum 29

ZD 1839 (gefitinib) xv, 182